The Complete Heart Healthy Cookbook 2022

600 Low Cholesterol and Low Sodium Recipes with 28-Day Meal Plan to Eat Healthy and Live Better

By Justin N. Ricks

Paperback ISBN: 979-8784466532

Hardcover ISBN: 979-8786203159

Table of Content

Chapter 8: Poultry 103

Chapter 9: Fish and Seafood 126

Chapter 10: Smoothie 146

Chapter 11: Salad 157

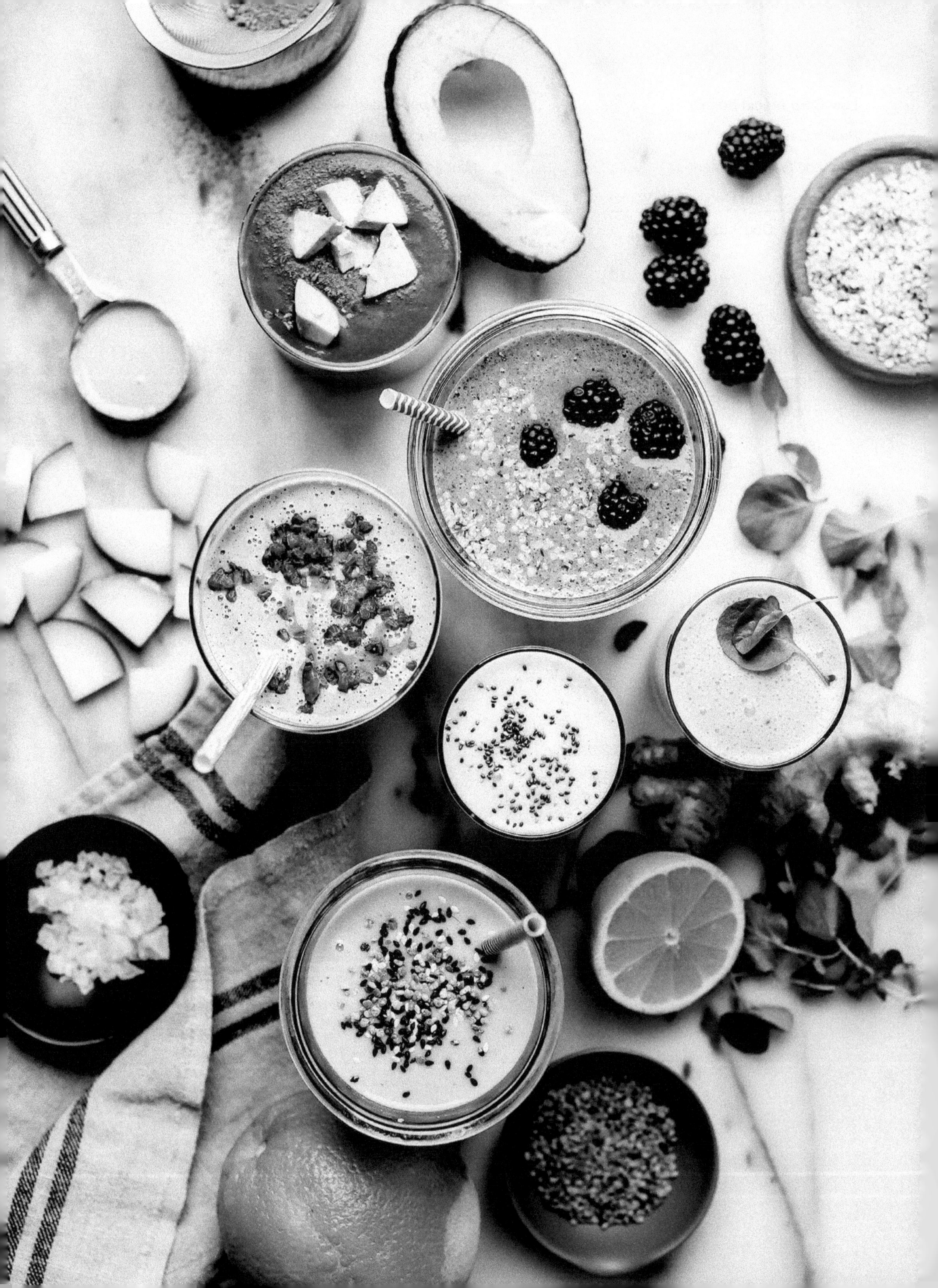

Introduction

Do you know that 1 out of every 4 Americans is suffering from some sort of heart disease? And that's not me saying it; the Centers for Disease Control and Prevention-CDC came up with those numbers, and as per their reports, about 610,000 people die from heart-related conditions each year. How alarming is that, right? Well, the rise of chronic diseases is the greatest dilemma of this decade, and somehow, we all are responsible for it! The shift to more of a sedentary lifestyle and poor dietary habits has led us into this health crisis. So, with little effort and understanding, we sure can reverse these patterns. In this cookbook, you will get to know how to prevent heart diseases through a change of lifestyle and dietary regime. By making smarter choices, you can even counter the challenges you are facing as a heart patient. Then, of course, there are some heart-healthy meal options that are provided in the recipe section of this book. You can try these nutritious recipes to make your routine more heart-friendly.

Chapter 1: The Basics of Heart Disease

How could one define heart disease? In simple words, any condition that would affect the health and functioning of the heart is defined as heart disease. It may sound simple to the ears, but heart illnesses are really complicated, and there are various factors responsible for different types of heart diseases. So, in this chapter, we shall try to unearth the whole concept and make sense of it because understanding always helps in better prevention and cure.

1.1 Understanding The Heart Disease

Heart or cardiovascular diseases are all the conditions that may slow down, disrupt, or obstruct the functioning of a heart. The term "cardiovascular" means relating to "heart and vessel" and that these diseases all include the damage or inefficiency caused by the blood vessels. These illnesses are categorized according to different causes and their respective symptoms. Some diseases can be managed through lifestyle adjustments, whereas others may need both medicinal and non-medicinal treatments. To better understand heart diseases, let me breakdown them into the different types and see how much damage they can cause:

- **Arrhythmia**

An arrhythmia is an issue with your heart's pace or rhythm. It indicates your heart is beating too fast, too sluggish, or in an irregular manner. Tachycardia is a condition in which the heart beats quicker than usual. Bradycardia is a condition in which the heart beats too slowly. The most frequent type of arrhythmia is atrial fibrillation, which is characterized by a rapid and unpredictable heartbeat. A heart attack, smoking, congenital heart problems, and stress are all variables that might disrupt your heart's rhythm. Arrhythmias can also be caused by certain chemicals or medicines.

- **Atherosclerosis**

The buildup of lipids, cholesterol, and other chemicals in and on the walls of your arteries is known as atherosclerosis. This buildup is referred to as plaque. Because of the plaque, your arteries may narrow, restricting blood flow. If the plaque bursts, it can cause a blood clot. Despite the fact that atherosclerosis is most usually linked with the heart, it can affect arteries all over the body. The illness of atherosclerosis is treatable. A healthy lifestyle can help to prevent atherosclerosis.

- **Cardiomyopathy**

Cardiomyopathy is a cardiac muscle condition that makes it difficult for your heart to pump blood throughout your body. Heart failure can result from cardiomyopathy. Dilated, hypertrophic, and restricted cardiomyopathy are the three primary forms of cardiomyopathy. The treatment methods are determined by the type of cardiomyopathy you have and how serious it is and may include drugs, surgically implanted devices, heart surgery, or, in severe cases, a heart transplant.

- **Congenital heart defects**

A congenital heart defect, also known as congenital heart disease, is a heart condition that occurs before birth. The condition can harm the heart's walls, valves, and blood arteries.

Congenital cardiac abnormalities come in a variety of shapes and sizes. They might range from basic illnesses with no symptoms to more sophisticated issues with life-threatening symptoms.

- **Coronary artery disease (CAD)**

The accumulation of plaque in the arteries that provide oxygen-rich blood to your heart is known as coronary artery disease. Plaque creates a constriction or blockage in the arteries, potentially leading to a heart attack. Shortness of breath, discomfort and chest pain are common symptoms. Treatments may involve dietary changes, drugs to address your risk factors, and/or surgery.

1.2 Symptoms of the Heart Diseases:

The term "heart disease" refers to a variety of cardiovascular issues. Heart illness encompasses a wide range of diseases and ailments. The following are the many types of heart disease symptoms:

Arrhythmias

- Fluttering heart or racing heartbeat
- Fainting spells
- Lightheadedness
- Slow pulse
- Dizziness
- Chest pain

Atherosclerosis

- Weakness in your legs and arms
- Coldness
- Numbness
- Unexplained pain

Congenital heart defects

- Blue-tinged skin
- Swelling of the extremities
- Shortness of breath or difficulty breathing
- Fatigue and low energy
- Irregular heart rhythm

Coronary artery disease (CAD)

- Chest pain or discomfort
- A feeling of pressure in the chest
- Shortness of breath
- Nausea
- Feelings of indigestion or gas

Cardiomyopathy

- Fatigue
- Bloating
- Shortness of breath
- Swollen legs
- Rapid pulse

1.3 Why does Heart Disease Occur? - THE CAUSE

A number of risk factors play a part in establishing whether or not you're at risk for heart disease. You have no influence over two of these factors that is age and heredity. Women's risk of heart disease rises around the age of 55, whereas men's risk rises around the age of 45. If you have an immediate member of the family with a history of heart disease, your risk may be higher. Other heart disease risk factors include:

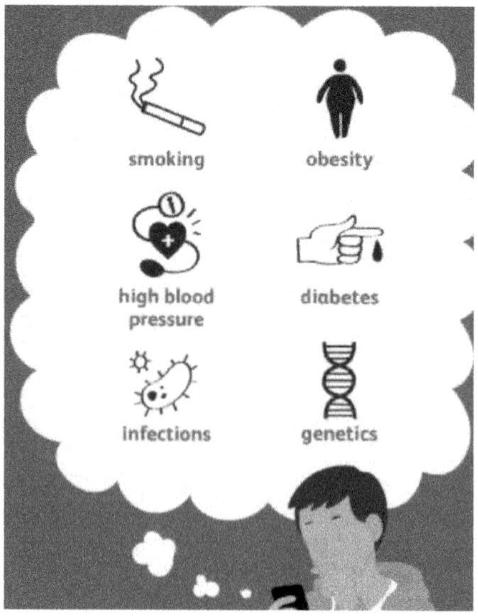

* Obesity
* Diabetes or insulin resistance
* High cholesterol and blood pressure
* Family history of heart disease
* Being physically sedentary
* Smoking
* Eating an unhealthy diet
* Clinical depression.

1.4 How to Prevent Heart Diseases?

The way to prevent cardiovascular disease is to take special care of your mind and your body through the dietary and lifestyle. After going through all the causes and symptoms of heart disease, I think, as all can understand, that it is obesity, excessive fats in the body, hypertension, and unhealthy diet that led to heart conditions, so by eating only things that could counter those challenges we prevent what follows them. Here are some important things that we all should follow, especially those who have a family history of heart disease or those who are over 50 years of age, to keep ourselves healthy.

1. *Control your blood pressure*

High blood pressure, or hypertension, is the main cause of heart disease and a major risk factor. Blood pressure should be regularly monitored, at least once a year for most people and much more frequently if you have high blood pressure. Take steps to prevent or control high blood pressure, such as changing your lifestyle. Consume a low-sodium, low-salt diet to ensure normal levels of blood pressure all the time.

2. *Control cholesterol and triglyceride levels*

High cholesterol levels can clog arteries, putting you at risk for coronary artery disease and heart attack. Cholesterol levels can be lowered by a combination of lifestyle changes and medication. In the bloodstream, triglycerides are a type of fat. High triglyceride levels, especially in women, can raise the risk of coronary heart disease. By consuming low-cholesterol food with no saturated fat, a person can maintain his cholesterol.

3. Control your portion size

Excessive intake of food means more caloric intake, and that leads to obesity. If you can recall, obesity is a primary cause of heart disease. So, by controlling the portion size, we can limit our caloric intake and thus prevent obesity along with the risks of heart disease. Following a few simple portion management principles can help you lose weight while also boosting your heart and waistline:

- *To keep track of your servings, use a tiny plate or bowl.*
- *Increase your intake of low-calorie, nutrient-dense foods like fruits and vegetables.*
- *Reduce your intake of high-calorie, high-sodium items such as refined, processed, or fast foods.*

A serving size is a unit of measurement for a certain amount of food, such as cups, ounces, or pieces. One serving of spaghetti, for example, is around 1/3 to 1/2 cup or the size of a hockey puck. A 2 to 3-ounce meal of meat, fish, or chicken is about the size and thickness of a deck of cards. Depending on the diet or guidelines you're following, the recommended number of servings of each food group may vary. Serving size estimation is a learnt skill. Until you're confident with your judgement, you may need to use measuring cups and spoons or a scale.

4. Eat more vegetables and fruits

Vegetables and fruits are high in vitamins and minerals. They are abundant in dietary fibres, as well as being low in calories. Compounds found in vegetables and fruits, as well as other plants and plant-based diets, may help to avoid cardiovascular diseases. Increasing your diet of fruits and vegetables can help you cut back on high-calorie foods like meat, cheese, and snack foods.

It is simple to incorporate veggies and fruits into your diet. Keep washed and chopped vegetables in your refrigerator for quick snacking. Fruit should be kept in a bowl in your kitchen so that you don't forget to consume it. Choose meals using vegetables or fruits as the primary ingredients, such as vegetable stir-fries or salads with fresh fruit.

5. Select whole grains

Whole grains are high in fibre and other nutrients that help to keep blood pressure and heart health in check. Making simple adjustments for refined grain products will help you increase the number of whole grains in your heart-healthy diet. Alternatively, try a new whole grain like whole-grain farro, quinoa, or barley.

6. Limit unhealthy fats

Limiting the saturated and trans fats intake is a crucial step in lowering your blood cholesterol and lowering your risk of coronary heart disease. A high blood cholesterol level can cause atherosclerosis, a buildup of plaques in your arteries that raises your risk of heart attack and stroke.

7. Choose low-fat protein sources

You can consume proteins that come from lean meat, poultry, and fish, as well as low-fat dairy products and eggs. Choose lower-fat alternatives to fried chicken patties, such as skinless chicken breasts instead of fried chicken patties, and skim milk instead of whole milk. Fish is a healthy substitute for high-fat meats. Omega-3 fatty acids found in certain types of fish can help decrease blood fats called triglycerides. Cold-water fish like salmon, mackerel, and herring have the highest levels of omega-3 fatty acids. Flaxseed, walnuts, soybeans, and canola oil are also good sources.

Legumes, such as beans, peas, and lentils, are high in protein, low in fat, and cholesterol-free, making them excellent meat replacements. Substituting plant protein for animal protein, such as a soy or bean burger in place of a hamburger, lowers fat and cholesterol while increasing fibre intake.

8. Reduce the sodium intake

High blood pressure, a risk factor for heart disease, can be caused by eating too much salt. Salt (sodium) restriction is an important component of a heart-healthy diet. According to the American Heart Association:

- **A healthy adult should consume no more than 2,300 mg of sodium per day, about a teaspoon of salt.**
- **Aim for no more than 1,500 mg of salt per day for most adults.**

Although lowering the amount of salt you add to food at the table or while cooking is a good start, canned or processed foods like soups, baked goods, and frozen dinners should also be avoided as they contain a lot of salt. Salt consumption can be reduced by eating fresh foods and cooking your own soups and stews.

9. Exercise

The excessive fats accumulating in your vessel won't go away on their own until you work out and burn them. Moving around and indulging in various activities strengthens the heart muscles to cope with the possible challenges. Cardio exercises, like running, jogging etc., are also used to keep the heart healthy and strong.

1.5 List of recommended and avoided foods

As I have said earlier that is it is unhealthy food intake that triggers the factors that later leads to heart disease. So, by eating heart-friendly and healthy food, you can prevent the risks of heart disease. Here is the list of the food that you can consume:

Food to Enjoy

1. **Fruits and vegetables**

Consume a wide variety of fruits and vegetables. Fresh, frozen, canned, or dried fruits and vegetables are all options.

- Tomatoes, cabbage, and carrots are examples of fresh veggies.

- Romaine lettuce, spinach, and kale are all leafy greens that can be used in salads.
- Vegetables in cans that are low in salt
- Broccoli and cauliflower, for example, are frozen vegetables that haven't had any butter or sauce added to them.
- Apples, oranges, bananas, pears, and peaches are examples of fresh fruits.
- Fruit that hasn't been added sugar (canned, frozen, or dried)
- Farmer's markets are fantastic places to buy in-season veggies and fruits.

2. Dairy

Look for options that are fat-free or low-fat.

- Milk that is fat-free or low-fat (1%)
- Plain fat-free or low-fat yoghurt
- Low-fat or fat-free cheese
- Cottage cheese that is fat-free or low-fat
- Calcium, vitamin A, and vitamin D fortified soymilk

3. Cereals, Bread, and Grains

Make sure whole wheat or similar whole grain is included first in the ingredient list for goods with more than one ingredient. Look for items that state they're made entirely of whole grains.

- Tortillas, bagels, English muffins, and whole-grain bread
- Oatmeal or shredded wheat are examples of whole-grain hot or cold breakfast cereals with no added sugar.
- Brown or wild rice, quinoa, or oats are examples of whole grains.
- Couscous and whole-wheat or whole-grain pasta

4. Lean and Healthy Protein Foods

Choose a variety of protein-rich foods.

- Fish and shellfish are examples of seafood.
- Poultry: Skinless chicken or turkey breasts, lean ground turkey or chicken.
- Leg, shoulder, or tenderloin of pork
- Round, sirloin, tenderloin, or 93 per cent lean ground beef.
- Kidney beans, black beans, pinto beans, lima beans, black-eyed peas, garbanzo beans (chickpeas), split peas, and lentils are examples of beans and peas.
- Egg whites
- No Salt Nuts and seeds
- Almond and peanut butter
- Tofu

5. Fats and Oils

Reduce your saturated fat intake and seek out goods that are free of trans fats. Seafood, nuts, seeds, avocados, and oils are all good sources of unsaturated fats.

- No trans fats and less saturated fats than butter in margarine and spreads (soft, tub, or liquid).
- Oil made from vegetables (canola, corn, olive, peanut, safflower, soybean, or sunflower)
- Cooking spray that is non-stick
- Mayonnaise with fewer calories
- Salad dressings made with oil

Food to Avoid

Food products that contain high levels of sodium and saturated fat are not allowed on this diet, and that includes:

1. Processed and Red Meat

Saturated fat is found in red meat. Several studies have found that substituting plant protein for red or processed meat reduces the risk of heart disease.

- Nuts, legumes, whole grains, and soy products are examples of plant proteins.

2. Beverages and Food with Excessive Sugar

Sugar is added to a lot of processed meals and beverages, especially sodas and energy drinks. According to the American Dietary Guidelines, added sugars should account for no more than 10% of daily calories. This translates to 200 calories, or 12 teaspoons of sugar, per day on a 2,000 calorie diet. Excess sugar consumption should be avoided in order to maintain a healthy weight and avoid heart disease.

3. Processed Food

Long lists of ingredients are common in processed foods, many of which are detrimental to heart health. Many processed foods, for example, contain:

- high sugar
- high salt
- trans fats
- saturated fat
- additives and food colourings

If at all feasible, make meals from scratch with whole foods. This is a healthier alternative.

4. High Cholesterol Food

Meat products with high fat are the main source of cholesterol. Long-term consumption will promote the increase of blood cholesterol and triglycerides. Excessive cholesterol will deposit in blood vessels, causing changes in atherosclerosis, thereby increasing the risk of heart disease. The following high cholesterol foods should be avoided:

- Viscera
- Animal bone soup
- Dairy products, such as cream and ice cream
- Animal eggs, such as egg yolk and crab yolk

5. Refined Carbs

Refined carbs are low in fibre and can lead to blood sugar imbalances. Consuming a lot of refined carbs over time can contribute to insulin resistance and weight increase, both of which are cardiovascular disease risk factors. The following are some refined carbs to avoid:

- Biscuits, pastries, and white bread, spaghetti, and rice cakes
- a variety of breakfast cereals
- delicious sweets made with pizza dough
- flour (white)

6. Alcohol

Alcohol must be taken in moderation by those who consume it. This means that ladies should have no more than one drink per day, and males should have no more than two drinks per day.

7. Salt

Too much salt (sodium) in the diet can cause high blood pressure and raise the risk of cardiovascular disease. According to the American Heart Association, lowering sodium intake by 1,000 mg per day can lower blood pressure. Because many processed foods contain additional salt, it is possible to keep track of one's intake by reading labels and choosing whole foods wherever possible.

Chapter 2: Heart-Healthy Eating

Having a well-defined plan in mind definitely helps in preventing or managing heart disease. This chapter brings a generalized plan to live a heart-friendly lifestyle. It's not just about what you consume or eat, but how you eat and what other measures you take to keep your body- all are labelled as heart-healthy eating or lifestyle.

2.1 Caring for Your Heart Through Food

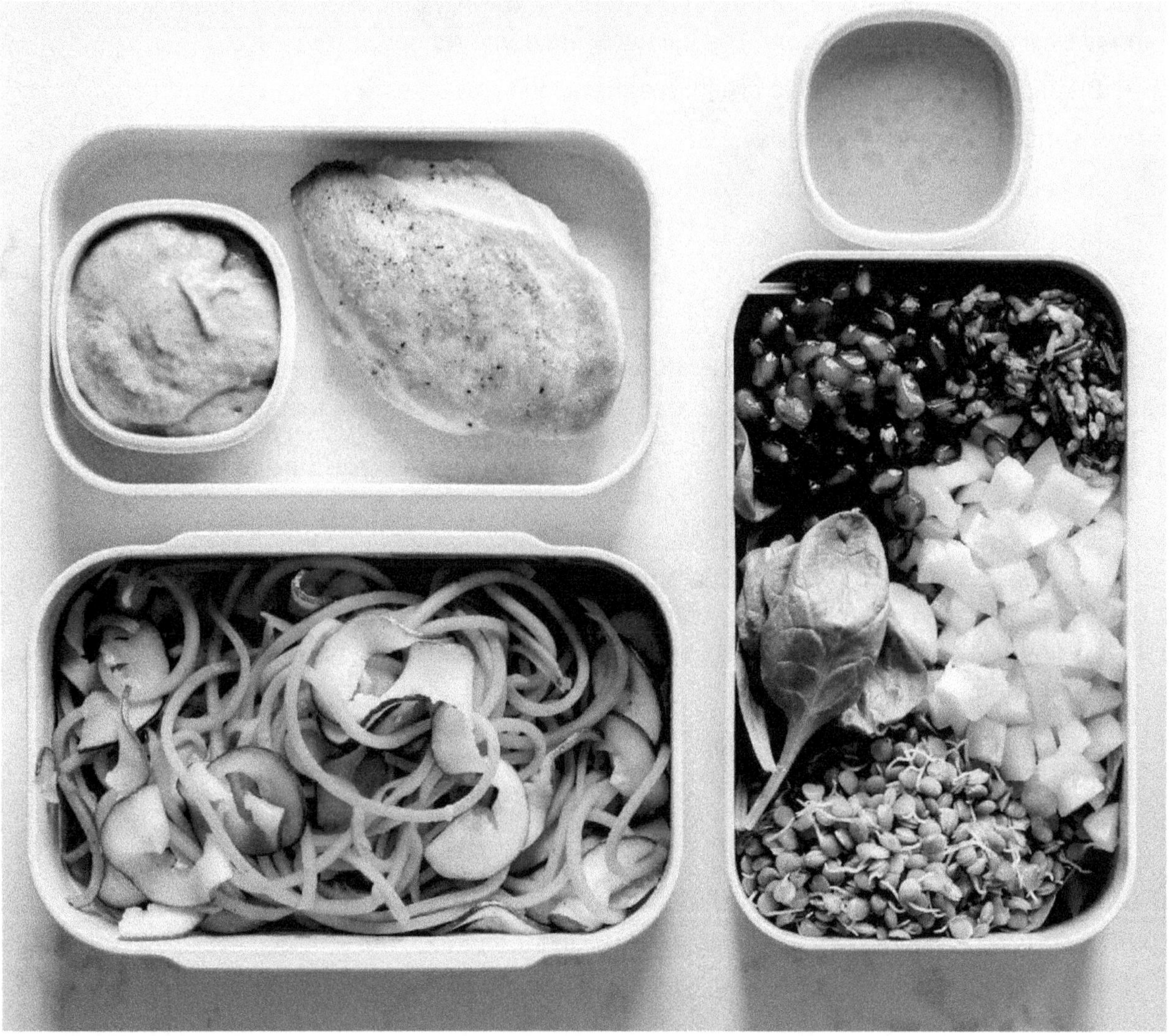

Even if you're aware that some foods increase your risk of heart disease, changing your eating habits can be tough. Whether you've been eating badly for years or just want to fine-tune your diet, here are eight heart-healthy diet tips. Once you know which foods to consume more of and which to limit, you'll be well on your way to a heart-healthy diet.

- √ **Eat a healthy diet**

Saturated fats, high-sodium diets, and additional sweets should all be avoided. Eat a wide range of fruits, vegetables, and entire grains. The DASH diet is, for instance, is a diet that can help you lower your blood pressure and cholesterol, two factors that can lessen your risk of heart disease.

- √ **Stay at a healthy weight**

Obesity or even being overweight raises your chances of developing heart disease. This is owing to their link to other heart disease risk factors such as high blood cholesterol and triglyceride levels, high blood pressure, and diabetes. These risks can be mitigated by maintaining a healthy weight.

- √ **Get regular exercise**

Exercise has various benefits, including cardiac strengthening and improved circulation. It can also promote a healthier weight while also controlling your cholesterol and blood pressure. All of these items can aid in the prevention of heart disease.

- √ **Limit Alcohol Intake**

If you consume too much alcohol, your blood pressure may rise. It also increases the number of calories consumed, perhaps contributing to weight gain. Both of these variables make you more likely to get heart disease.

- √ **Avoid Smoking**

Tobacco use raises blood pressure and raises the risk of heart attack and stroke. If you don't already smoke, don't start. Stopping smoking lowers your risk of acquiring heart disease. Your health care provider can aid you in determining the best approach for you to quit smoking.

- √ **Manage Stress**

Stress is linked to heart disease in a variety of ways. It's possible that it'll raise your blood pressure. Extreme stress can result in a heart attack. Furthermore, popular stress-relieving behaviors like overeating, frequent drinking, and smoking might be hazardous to your heart. Going to exercise, listening to music, concentrating on something peaceful or tranquil, and meditating are all good ways to relieve stress.

- √ **Manage diabetes**

Heart disease is twice as likely to develop in people who have diabetes than individuals who don't have diabetes. It can result in high blood sugar levels, which over time damage your blood vessels and the nerves that control your heart and blood vessels. As a result, getting tested for diabetes and, if diagnosed, keeping it under control is crucial.

- √ **Get Enough Sleep**

If you don't get enough sleep, you're more likely to develop high blood pressure, obesity, and diabetes. These three factors can make you more likely to get heart disease. Each night, the average adult needs 7 to 9 hours of sleep. Check to see if you're getting adequate rest. Make an appointment with your doctor if you're experiencing difficulties sleeping. Sleep apnea is a disorder in which patients stop breathing for brief periods of time while sleeping. This makes getting a good night's sleep harder and raises your risk of heart disease. If you think you might have it, talk to your doctor about having a sleep study done. Also, if you do have sleep apnea, get it addressed as soon as possible.

2.2 Grocery Shopping for Heart Healthy Diet

Here are some suggestions to make your trip to the grocery shop more efficient in terms of selecting heart-healthy items.

* **Never Shop on Empty Stomach:**

When you go to the grocery store hungry, you're more likely to buy more than you need as well as impulse purchases. Before you go shopping, eat a meal or a snack, such as a sandwich and a piece of fruit or nonfat Greek yoghurt.

* **Go by your Weekly Menus:**

You'll be far more likely to buy the healthy goods on your grocery list if you plan your meals/ menus for the week and make a grocery list. We tend to make fewer impulse purchases when we have a grocery list, and we can save a lot of money on our grocery expenses.

* **Check Your Pantry Before Shopping:**

To avoid making duplicate purchases, check your pantry, cupboards, refrigerator, and freezer while making your grocery list. Learn the layout of the store and make your list accordingly. Produce, nonfat dairy, lean proteins, healthful grains, and other categories can be added to your shopping list.

* **Pick Less Fancy, Less Expensive Products:**

On the store shelves, the most expensive foods are displayed at eye level, and most of those items are loaded with additives, sugar, and sodium, which are not healthy for this diet. So, try to look away from those items, no matter how tempting they may be to you. Look through the store shelves for a similar product that is less expensive yet still healthy.

* **Improve your reading skills:**

When it comes to the Nutrition Facts section of food labels, reduce saturated fats, eliminate trans-fatty acids, and increase fibre in your diet to incorporate heart-healthy foods.

* **Check the Aisles in the Perimeter:**

Foods that are better for you can be found along the store's perimeter. Most supermarkets' interior aisles are stocked with highly processed items. Get a supermarket aisle map from the store and stay away from the aisles that don't offer the foods on your shopping list. Purchase whole heart-healthy foods like fruits, vegetables, whole grains, lean proteins, and nonfat-dairy items from the grocery store's perimeter. Only shop the centre aisles for items like brown rice, whole-wheat pasta, oats, quinoa, and dried beans.

What to Buy for Your Pantry?

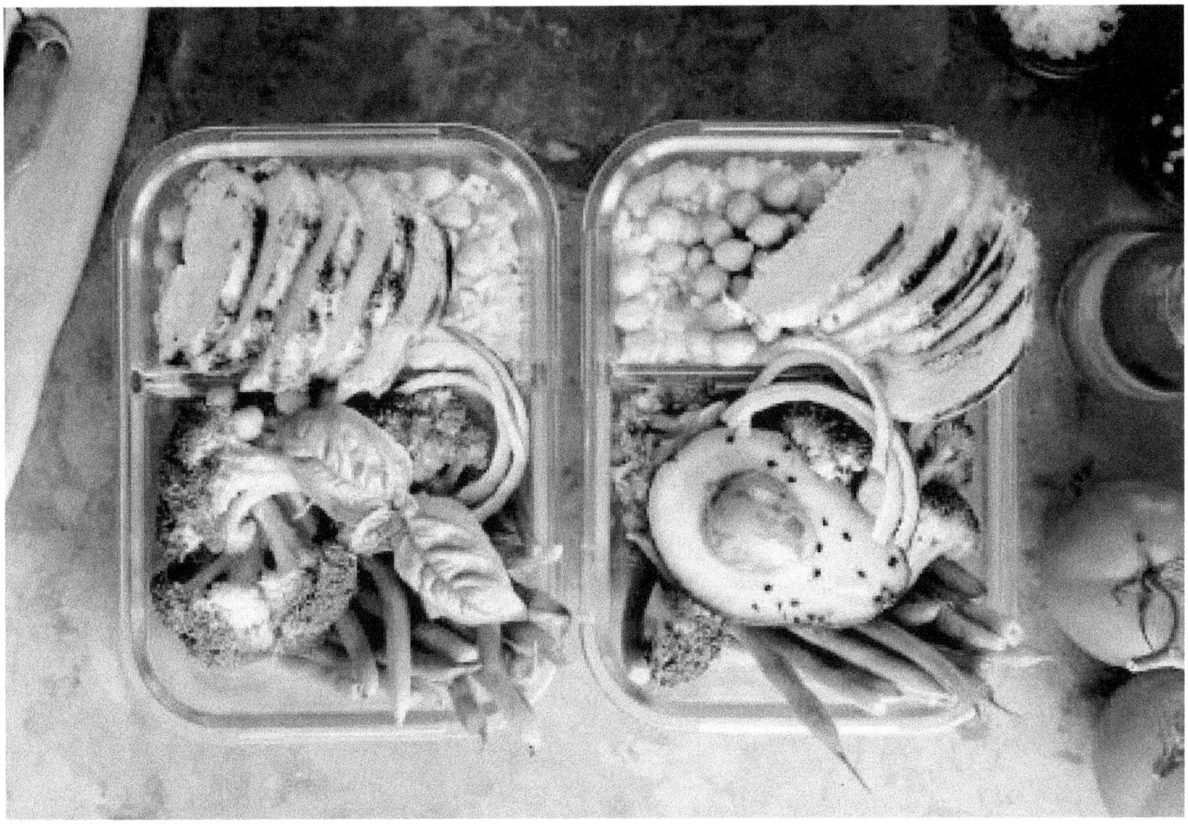

While buying items from the grocery store, keep the following special tips in mind. Food that is healthy for the heart must be bought in the following ways:

- **Fresh Produce: Fruits and Vegetables**

To get the finest flavour, buy fresh produce that is in season. The darker the colour, the better the content of the vegetable or fruit. Frozen or canned versions that haven't been processed with additional sugar, fats, or sauces are also a great option. Dried fruits are a nourishing high-fibre snack, but because the water has been removed, they are denser in calories, so keep your portion sizes in mind. To include cholesterol-lowering fibre in your diet, aim for five cups of fruits and vegetables in your diet each day.

- **Dairy**

One per cent of fat-free (skim) milk, buttermilk, cheeses, yoghurts, and cottage cheese are all good choices. Greek yoghurt with no fat is richer in protein than Greek yoghurt made with skim milk. Soy, oat, or hemp milk are examples of calcium-fortified "milk" that are unsweetened or flavoured.

* **Lean Proteins**

Because they don't include saturated or trans fats, plant-based proteins like tofu, miso, tempeh, lentils, dried peas, beans (dry or low sodium canned), edamame, hummus with no additional oils, or textured vegetable protein meals (soy crumbles) are heart-healthy. If you eat meat, skinless white flesh chicken and turkey, both whole and ground, are excellent options. Make sure the skin hasn't been ground in with the breasts. Fresh or frozen seafood that hasn't been breaded or fried should be used. Crustaceans (crab, shrimp, and lobster) have a high cholesterol content and should be consumed in moderation. Fish with a high omega 3 fatty acid concentration should be consumed twice a week. Wild salmon, tuna, mackerel, and sardines are all good sources. Buy water-packed albacore tuna, salmon, or sardines in cans. Fresh turkey or chicken breast should be used as deli meats because they are low in fat and sodium. You can use egg whites or egg replacements. Peanut butter, for example, should be freshly ground.

If you eat red meat, keep your portions to the size of a deck of cards and only eat it once or twice a week. Loin, leg, round, and 95 per cent lean hamburgers are leaner cuts of beef and pork. Low-fat meats include venison, wild game, and bison. Roasts, chops, and legs are all lean lamb cuts.

* **Bread, Cereals, Grains, Rice, And Pasta**

Make sure the first grain on the ingredient list is whole grain, such as whole wheat, oats, or millet, when buying bread or cereals. Baked goods should have no more than 3 grammes of fat per serving, and cereals should have at least 3 grammes of fibre. Choose whole-wheat couscous, quinoa, farro, flour, whole wheat tortillas, graham crackers, and whole-grain/low-fat crackers and pretzels.

* **Fats and oils**

Use a teaspoon of fat cautiously because it contains 9 grammes of fat and 45 calories. Canola, olive, and peanut oils are examples of unsaturated oils. Choose hydrogenated-oil-free soft or liquid margarine and vegetable oil spreads. Salad dressings with less fat, seeds and unsalted dry roasted nuts are excellent choices. Reduce salt by making your own salad dressing with flavored vinegar and a little olive oil.

2.3 4-Week Meal Plan

Week One

Week-1	Breakfast	Lunch	Dinner	Dessert&Snacks
Mon	Broccoli and Cheese Omelets (page 19)	Chicken and Apple Salad with Walnuts (page 107)	Easy Italian Salad Chicken Breasts (page 108)	Berry Greek Yogurt Parfaits with Granola (page 179)
Tues	Broccoli Mushroom Breakfast Scramble (page 22)	Chicken with Broccoli Stir-Fry (page 111)	Chicken with Crispy Kale and Artichokes (page 106)	Caprese Skewers (page 179)
Wed	Cheese and Tomato Omelet (page 25)	Easy Cheesy Chicken Broccoli Bake (page 116)	Chicken Lettuce Cups (page 108)	Chicken Rollups with Veggie Sour Cream (page 170)
Thurs	Chile Rellenos Egg Souffle (page 26)	Roasted Chicken with Vegetables (page 121)	Easy Sumac Chicken with Cauliflower and Carrots (page 118)	Date Pumpkin Bites (page 174)
Fri	Congee with Raisin and Spices (page 32)	Baked Flounder with Brussels Sprouts (page 131)	Baked Salmon with Leeks and Fennel (page 130)	Guacamole with Jicama (page 180)
Sat	Easy Sweet Potato Hash (page 27)	Baked Trout with Pecan (page 130)	Curry Whitefish with Vegetables (page 132)	Homemade Lemony Tomato Salsa (page 178)
Sun	Easy Turkey Sausage (page 29)	Healthy Seafood Fettuccine (page 129)	Baked Tuna with Orange Sauce (page 128)	Olive White Bean Dip (page 172)

Week Two

Week-2	Breakfast	Lunch	Dinner	Dessert&Snacks
Mon	English Muffin with Lox (page 26)	Baked Flounder with Tomatoes and Basil (page 128)	Lemon-Garlic Tilapia with Roasted Vegetables (page 128)	Roasted Chickpeas with Herbs (page 178)
Tues	Escarole with Portobello (page 24)	Cod Chowder with Cauliflower (page 132)	Mediterranean Salmon with Quinoa (page 133)	Almond Rice Pudding with Raspberry Sauce (page 175)
Wed	Garlicky Pea Fried Rice Breakfast (page 32)	Monkfish in Tomatoes-Garlic Sauce (page 130)	Sea Bass with Tomatoes, Olives and Capers (page 137)	Berries Cobbler (page 171)
Thurs	Hummus and Date Bagel (page 28)	Tropical Baked Swordfish with Cilantro (page 142)	Ginger Chicken with Vegetable Soup (page 113)	Cheesy Zucchini Pancake (page 172)
Fri	Italian Toast Plate Breakfast (page 24)	Italian Caprese-Stuffed Chicken Breasts (page 104)	Juicy Italian Herb Turkey Cutlets (page 120)	Cinnamon Spiced Applesauce (page 173)
Sat	Lemony Breakfast Cakes with Berry Syrup (page 24)	Quick Full-Flavored Chicken Stock (page 115)	Southwest Chicken with Black Bean and Rice (page 116)	Coconut Meringues with Strawberries and Mint (page 173)
Sun	Longan Almond Barley with Apple Cider (page 28)	Stir-Fry Chicken with Sesame, Broccoli and Carrot (page 123)	Stir-Fry Chicken with Zucchini and Fennel (page 122)	Coconut Vanilla Pancakes (page 178)

Week Three

Week-3	Breakfast	Lunch	Dinner	Dessert&Snacks
Mon	Mediterranean Scramble with Feta Cheese (page 19)	Quick Full-Flavored Chicken Stock (page 115)	Stir-Fry Chicken with Zucchini and Fennel (page 122)	Dark Chocolate Mousse with Vanilla (page 175)
Tues	Mushroom Carrot Skillet (page 27)	Lemon-Garlic Tilapia with Roasted Vegetables (page 128)	Healthy Seafood Fettuccine (page 129)	Pistachio-Stuffed Dates (page 179)
Wed	Peanut Butter Brazilian Nut Smoothie Bowl (page 33)	Tender Turkey Meatballs with Marinara Sauce (page 110)	Traditional Open Face Turkey Burger (page 117)	Quick Grilled Peaches with Ricotta (page 174)
Thurs	Polenta with Longans and Dates (page 32)	Chili Turkey with Beans (page 122)	Roman-Style Braised Chicken with Roasted Peppers (page 105)	Simple Strawberry Dessert (page 180)
Fri	Quinoa Bowl with Blackberry (page 32)	Artichoke Caponata Over Grilled Mahi Mahi (page 131)	Carrot Potato Fish Stew (page 126)	Strawberry Cheese Blintzes (page 178)
Sat	Quinoa Bowls with Avocado and Egg (page 21)	Smoky Flavor Cod with Mushrooms (page 138)	Spicy Cod Mango Salsa (page 139)	Vanilla Apple Pie (page 177)
Sun	Quinoa Breakfast Bowl with Yogurt, Olives and Hazelnuts (page 21)	Sweet Potatoes and Chicken Thighs (page 110)	Crispy Apricot Chicken with Steamed Baby Greens (page 105)	Walnut and Prune Brownies (page 170)

Week Four

Week-4	Breakfast	Lunch	Dinner	Dessert&Snacks
Mon	Sautéed Chard and Fried Eggs Polenta (page 21)	Easy Cheesy Chicken Broccoli Bake (page 116)	Stir-Fry Chicken with Zucchini and Fennel (page 122)	Banana Cream Nonfat Yogurt (page 179)
Tues	Savory Yogurt Bowls with Hazelnuts (page 34)	White Beans Chicken Chili (page 115)	Easy Sumac Chicken with Cauliflower and Carrots (page 118)	Olive White Bean Dip (page 172)
Wed	Smoked Salmon Egg Scramble (page 31)	Stuffed Chicken Breasts (page 119)	Sheet Pan Roasted Chicken with Vegetables (page 104)	Roasted Chickpeas with Herbs (page 178)
Thurs	Smoked Trout and Avocado (page 31)	Spinach and Mushroom Stuffed Chicken (page 103)	Chicken Lettuce Cups (page 108)	Almond Rice Pudding with Raspberry Sauce (page 175)
Fri	Spicy Egg Muffins (page 30)	Chicken with Crispy Kale and Artichokes (page 106)	Baked Flounder with Tomatoes and Basil (page 128)	Berries Cobbler (page 171)
Sat	Spinach and Tomato Baked Egg Cups (page 30)	Flavor Packed Shrimp Fra Diavolo (page 138)	Grilled Halibut with Soybean and Mango Salsa (page 140)	Chocolate Cupcakes (page 172)
Sun	Vanilla Buckwheat Crêpes with Berries and Chia Jam (page 29)	Shrimp, White Beans and Feta Skillet (page 141)	Easy Quick Greek Turkey Burger (page 118)	Easy Pear Bars (page 175)

2.4 Conclusion

Are you ready to fight off the risks of heart diseases? Now is your chance to pick the best of the heart-healthy recipes from this cookbook and incorporate them into your lifestyle. Gradually bring changes in both your diet and your routine, and in the long run, you will start noticing the expected improvement in your heart health. And if you will find this book useful for maintaining your heart health, then don't hesitate to recommend it to others in your friends and family.

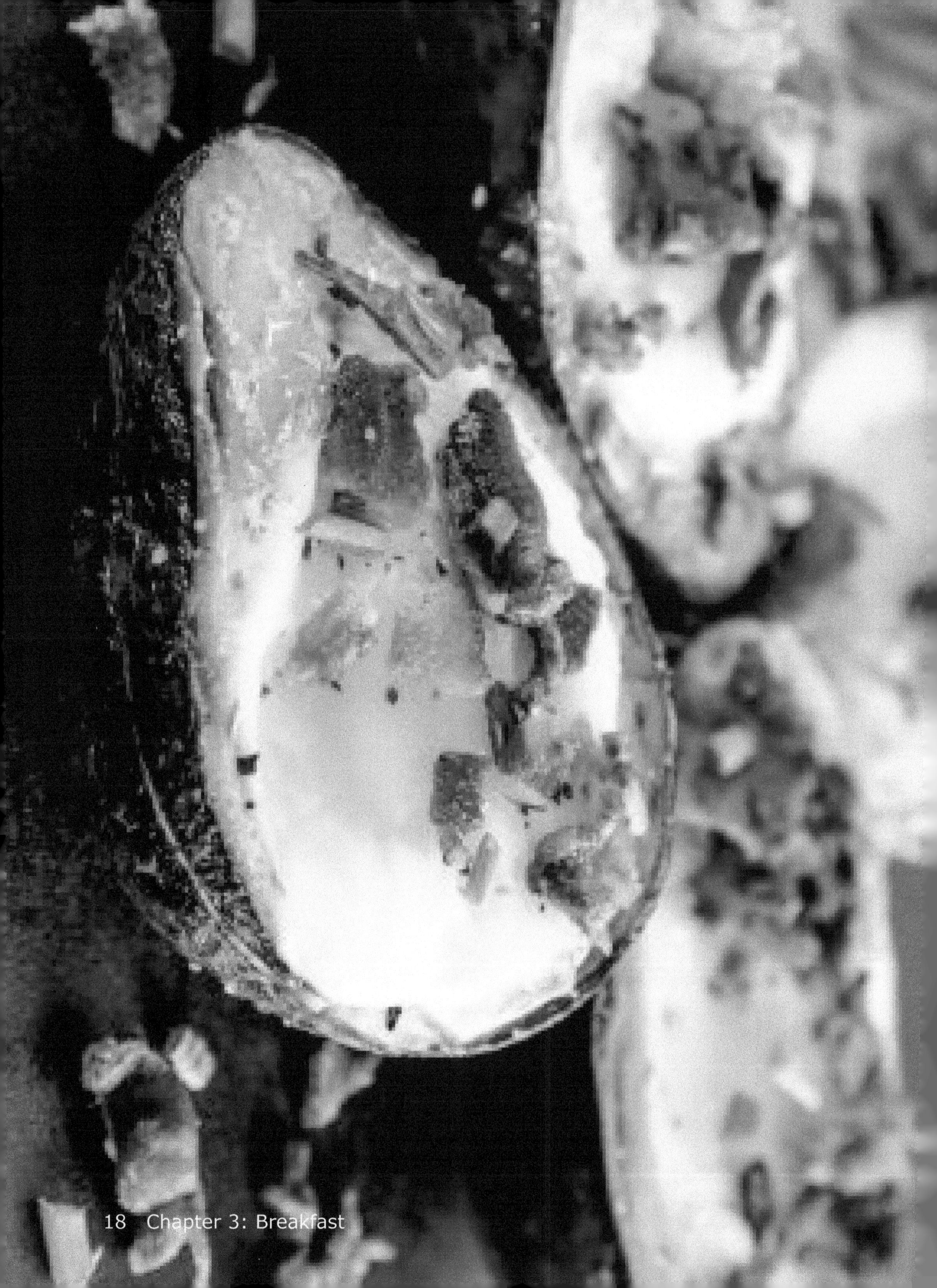

Chapter 3: Breakfast

Baked Egg and Avocado

Prep Time: 5 minutes, Cook Time: 15 minutes, Serves: 2

INGREDIENTS:

1 ripe large avocado
2 large eggs
4 tbsps. jarred pesto, for serving
2 tbsps. chopped tomato, for serving
2 tbsps. crumbled feta, for serving (optional)
Salt
Freshly ground black pepper

DIRECTIONS:

1. Preheat the oven to 425°F (220ºC).
2. Cut the avocado in half and remove the pit. Scoop out 1 to 2 tbsps. from each half to create a hole large enough to fit an egg. Put the avocado halves on a baking sheet, cut-side up.
3. Crack 1 egg in each avocado half and season with salt and pepper.
4. Bake 10 to 15 minutes until the eggs are set and cooked to desired level of doneness.
5. Remove from oven and top each avocado with pesto, chopped tomato, and crumbled feta.

Nutrition Info per Serving:

Calories: 302, Total Carbs: 10g, Protein: 8g, Total Fat: 26g, Net Carbs: 5g, Fiber: 5g, Sodium: 436mg, Sugar: 0.8g, Cholesterol: 184mg

Mediterranean Scramble with Feta Cheese

Prep Time: 15 minutes, Cook Time: 10 minutes, Serves: 4

INGREDIENTS:

1 medium clove garlic, minced
2 tbsps. extra virgin olive oil
¼ cup sliced red bell pepper
¼ cup rinsed and drained, chopped canned artichoke hearts
⅛ cup chopped red onion
1 whole egg
2 egg whites
⅛ tsp. cracked black pepper
⅛ tsp. dried oregano
⅛ cup low-fat feta cheese

DIRECTIONS:

1. Prepare a small non-stick pan, heat it over medium heat, and pour oil into the pan. When the oil is hot, put onion and garlic and stir fry for about 1 minute. Then add the bell pepper strips and the artichoke heart, and fry for another 3 minutes, until the onion is translucent and the bell pepper is soft.
2. Put the egg whites and eggs in a small bowl, beat the egg whites and eggs, season with oregano and black pepper. Pour the eggs into the pot and stir evenly with a spatula. Cook for 3 to 4 minutes until the egg no longer runs. Remove the pan from the heat, place the feta on the egg, and close the lid until the feta starts to melt. Enjoy warm.

Nutrition Info per Serving:

Calories: 424, Fat: 37g, Protein: 21g, Carbohydrates: 5g, Fiber: 1g, Sugar: 1g, Sodium: 572mg, Cholesterol: 157mg

Broccoli and Cheese Omelets

Prep Time: 5 minutes, Cook Time: 10 minutes, Serves: 4

INGREDIENTS:

3 tbsps. extra-virgin olive oil, divided
8 tbsps. shredded reduced-fat Monterey Jack cheese, divided
8 large eggs
2 cups chopped broccoli
¼ cup 1% milk
½ tsp. freshly ground black pepper

DIRECTIONS:

1. In a nonstick skillet, heat 1 tbsp. of oil over medium-high heat. Add the broccoli and sauté for 3 to 5 minutes, or until the broccoli turns bright green. Scrape into a bowl.
2. Beat together the eggs, milk, and pepper in a small bowl.
3. Wipe out the skillet and heat ½ tablespoon of oil. Add one-quarter of the egg mixture and tilt the skillet to ensure an even layer. Cook for 2 minutes and then add 2 tbsps. of cheese and one-quarter of the broccoli. Use a spatula to fold into an omelet.
4. Repeat step 3 with the remaining ingredients to make a total of 4 omelets.
5. Divide into 4 storage containers.

Nutrition Info per Serving:

Calories: 292, Total fat: 23g, Carbohydrates: 4g, Fiber: 1g, Protein: 18g, Calcium: 199mg, Vitamin D: 89 IU, Potassium: 308mg, Magnesium: 25mg, Sodium: 282mg, Cholesterol: 270mg, Sugar: 1g

Egg and Zucchini Breakfast Burrito

Prep Time: 5 minutes, Cook Time: 5 minutes, Serves: 4

INGREDIENTS:

4 egg whites
1 egg
¼ cup (60ml) low-fat milk
⅛ tsp. freshly ground pepper
4 whole-wheat tortillas
½ cup (2 oz. 60g) shredded reduced-fat sharp cheddar cheese
1 cup (235ml) canned zucchini, shredded
¼ cup (60ml)chopped parsley
½ cup (120ml) salsa
¼ cup (60ml) nonfat sour cream

DIRECTIONS:

1. Whisk together the egg whites, egg, milk, and pepper in a microwave-safe dish. Place the mixture in the microwave and cook on high for 3 minutes. Transfer the dish from the microwave and stir. Microwave for 1 additional minute, or until the eggs are no longer liquid.
2. Arrange 1 tortilla on each of four microwave-safe plates. Separate the egg mixture evenly on top of the tortillas. Spread each with one quarter of the cheese, zucchini, and parsley.
3. Wrap the burritos up and microwave for 30 seconds. Serve immediately, Spread with salsa and sour cream.

Nutrition Info per Serving:

Calories: 229, Total Fat: 8.4g, Cholesterol: 161mg, Sodium: 608mg, Total Carbohydrate: 25g, Fiber: 5g, Sugar: 3.5g, Protein: 13.6g

Greek Eggs with Potatoes

Prep Time: 10 minutes, Cook Time: 25 minutes, Serves: 3

INGREDIENTS:

3 medium tomatoes, seeded and coarsely chopped
Sea salt and freshly ground pepper
3 large russet potatoes
3 large eggs
2 tbsps. fresh chopped basil
1 garlic clove, minced
2 tbsps. plus ½ cup olive oil, divided
1 tsp. fresh oregano, chopped

DIRECTIONS:

1. Put tomatoes in a food processor and puree them.
2. Mix the garlic, basil, sea salt, 2 tbsps. olive oil and freshly ground pepper.
3. Put the mixture in a large skillet over low heat, cover and cook for 20–25 minutes, or until the sauce has thickened and is bubbly.
4. Dice the potatoes into small cubes. Spray ½ cup olive oil in a nonstick skillet over medium-low heat.
5. Fry the potatoes for 5 minutes until crisp and browned, then cover and reduce heat to low.
6. Carefully crack the eggs into the tomato sauce. Cook over low heat for 6 minutes until the eggs are set in the sauce.
7. Remove the potatoes from the pan and drain with paper towels, then put them in a bowl.
8. Sprinkle with sea salt and freshly ground pepper and top with the oregano.
9. Carefully place eggs on a plate with the potatoes. Spoon sauce over the top and serve.

Nutrition Info per Serving:

Calories: 930, Fat: 67g, Carbohydrates: 73g, Protein: 12g, Cholesterol: 235mg, Sodium: 249mg, Fiber: 6.5g, Sugar: 5.6g

Harissa Shakshuka with Bell Peppers

Prep Time: 10 minutes, Cook Time: 20 minutes, Serves: 4

INGREDIENTS:

½ onion, diced
1½ tbsps. extra-virgin olive oil
2 tbsps. harissa
1 tbsp. tomato paste
4 large eggs
1 (28-ounce, 794 g) can no-salt-added diced tomatoes
1 bell pepper, seeded and diced
3 garlic cloves, minced
½ tsp. kosher salt
2 to 3 tbsps. fresh basil, chopped or cut into ribbons

DIRECTIONS:

1. Preheat the oven to 375°F (190ºC).
2. Heat the olive oil in a 12-inch ovenproof skillet over medium heat. Add the harissa, onion, tomato paste, and bell pepper, sauté for 3 to 4 minutes. Put in the garlic and cook about 30 seconds until fragrant. Add the diced tomatoes and salt and simmer for about 10 minutes.
3. Make 4 wells in the sauce and gently break 1 egg into each. Transfer to the oven and bake 10 to 12 minutes until the whites are cooked and the yolks are set.
4. Cool down for 3 to 5 minutes, and carefully spoon onto plates. Garnish with the basil.

Nutrition Info per Serving:

Calories: 190, Total fat: 10g, Saturated fat: 2g, Total Carbohydrates: 15g, Protein: 9g, Cholesterol: 185mg, Sodium: 255mg, Potassium: 725mg, Fiber: 4g, Sugar: 9g

Quinoa Bowls with Avocado and Egg

Prep Time: 10 minutes, Cook Time: 25 minutes, Serves: 5

INGREDIENTS:

5 hard-boiled eggs, peeled and sliced
3 avocados, pitted, sliced, and coated with lemon juice
3¾ cups cooked quinoa
½ tsp. onion powder
½ tsp. freshly ground black pepper
½ tsp. ground cumin
½ tsp. garlic powder
1 tbsp. chopped fresh cilantro
2 small tomatoes, diced
½ large red onion, chopped

DIRECTIONS:

1. In a large bowl, season the cooked quinoa with the onion powder, pepper, cumin, and garlic powder. Add the cilantro, tomatoes, and onion and mix well.
2. Divide the quinoa mix among 5 storage containers as a base for the breakfast bowl, then divide the avocados evenly into the bowls. Top each with a whole sliced egg.
3. Storage: Seal airtight, and store in the refrigerator for up to 5 days. This dish may be served cold or warm. If warm is preferred, separate the egg and avocado from the quinoa mixture. Reheat the quinoa in the microwave for 1 minute. Then top with the egg and avocado.

Nutrition Info per Serving:

Calories: 388, Total fat: 20g, Carbohydrates: 40g, Fiber: 10g, Protein: 15g, Sodium: 90mg, Cholesterol: 187mg, Sugar: 3.6g

Sautéed Chard and Fried Eggs Polenta

Prep Time: 5 minutes, Cook Time: 20 minutes, Serves: 4

INGREDIENTS:

½ tsp. kosher salt
¾ cups whole-grain cornmeal
¼ tsp. freshly ground black pepper
2½ (600 ml) cups water
grated Parmesan cheese
1 tbsp. extra-virgin olive oil
1 bunch (about 6 ounces) Swiss chard, leaves and stems chopped and separated
2 garlic cloves, sliced
Lemon juice (optional)
3 large eggs

DIRECTIONS:

1. Boil the water and salt in a medium saucepan over high heat. Slowly add the cornmeal, whisking constantly.
2. Reduce the heat to low, cover, and cook for 10 to 15 minutes, stirring often to avoid lumps. Put in the pepper and Parmesan, and divide among 4 bowls.
3. Heat the oil in a large skillet over medium heat. Put in the chard stems, garlic, salt, and pepper, sauté for 2 minutes. Add the chard leaves and cook about 3 to 5 minutes until wilted.
4. Add a spritz of lemon juice (if desired), toss together, and divide evenly on top of the polenta.
5. Heat the oil in the same large skillet over medium-high heat. Crack each egg into the skillet. Cook about 2 to 3 minutes until the whites are set and golden around the edges.
6. Serve sunny-side up or flip the eggs over carefully and cook 1 minute longer. Place one egg on top of the polenta and chard in each bowl.

Nutrition Info per Serving:

Calories: 310, Total fat: 18g, Saturated fat: 5g, Total Carbohydrates: 21g, Protein: 17g, Cholesterol: 186mg, Sodium: 500mg, Potassium: 385mg, Fiber: 2g, Sugar: 1g, Magnesium: 80mg, Calcium: 120mg

Quinoa Breakfast Bowl with Yogurt, Olives and Hazelnuts

Prep Time: 10 minutes, Cook Time: 10-12 minutes, Serves: 4

INGREDIENTS:

1½ cups (360mL) water
1 cup (240mL) plain Greek yogurt
½ cup olives, pitted and diced
½ cup hazelnuts (raw or roasted), chopped
1 cup quinoa
2 tsps. grated nutmeg
1-inch knob of ginger, peeled
¼ tsp. kosher salt
2 tsps. maple syrup

DIRECTIONS:

1. Bring the water, quinoa, nutmeg, ginger, and salt to a boil in a medium saucepan over high heat. Lower the heat to a simmer and cover, cook for 10 to 12 minutes. Remove the nutmeg and ginger. Fluff with a fork.
2. Stir the yogurt, olives, and hazelnuts to the quinoa and toss to combine well. Portion among 4 bowls and garnish with ½ tsp. maple syrup per bowl.

Nutrition Info per Serving:

Calories: 280, Total fat: 11g, Saturated fat: 1g, Total Carbohydrates: 37g, Protein: 13g, Cholesterol: 3mg, Sodium: 100mg, Potassium: 450mg, Fiber: 6g, Sugar: 18g, Magnesium: 110mg, Calcium: 130mg

Spanish Tuna Tortilla

Prep Time: 15 minutes, Cook Time: 25 minutes, Serves: 4

INGREDIENTS:

4 large eggs
¼ cup (60 ml) olive oil
1 (7-ounce, 200 g) can tuna packed in water, drained well and flaked
2 plum tomatoes, seeded and diced
1 tsp. dried tarragon
2 small russet potatoes, diced
1 small onion, chopped
1 roasted red bell pepper, sliced

DIRECTIONS:

1. Preheat the broiler.
2. Crack the eggs in a large bowl and whisk until just combined. Heat the olive oil in a large, oven-safe, nonstick skillet over medium-low heat.
3. Add the potatoes and cook for about 7 minutes until slightly soft. Add the onion and the peppers and cook 3–5 minutes until soft.
4. Add the tomatoes, tuna and tarragon to the skillet and stir to combine, then add the eggs.
5. Cook for 7–10 minutes until the eggs are bubbling and the bottom is slightly brown.
6. Place the skillet into the oven on 1 of the first 2 racks, and cook until the middle is set and the top is slightly brown.
7. Slice and serve.

Nutrition Info per Serving:

Calories: 415, Fat: 20.89g, Carbohydrates: 42.37g, Protein: 16.55g, Cholesterol: 184mg, Sodium: 130mg, Fiber: 3.1g, Sugar: 7.7g

Spicy Scrambled Eggs with Tomatoes

Prep Time: 5 minutes, Cook Time: 30 minutes, Serves: 4

INGREDIENTS:

2 tbsps. olive oil
1 small red onion, chopped
1 tbsp. ground cumin
1 tsp. ground coriander
4 large eggs, lightly beaten
1 medium green pepper, cored, seeded, and finely chopped
1 red Fresno or jalapeño chili pepper, seeded and cut into thin strips
3 medium tomatoes, chopped
Sea salt and freshly ground pepper

DIRECTIONS:

1. Heat the olive oil in a large skillet over medium heat.
2. Add the onion and cook 6–7 minutes until soft and translucent.
3. Add the peppers and continue to cook another 4–5 minutes until soft. Add in the tomatoes and season with salt and ground pepper to taste.
4. Stir in the coriander and cumin.
5. Simmer for 10 minutes over medium-low heat.
6. Add the eggs, stirring them into a mixture.
7. Cover the skillet and cook 5–6 minutes more until the eggs are set but still fluffy and tender.
8. Divide between 4 plates and serve immediately.

Nutrition Info per Serving:

Calories: 153, Fat: 11.87g, Carbohydrates: 8.56g, Protein: 4.4g, Cholesterol: 184mg, Sodium: 115mg, Fiber: 1.9g, Sugar: 3.1g

Broccoli Mushroom Breakfast Scramble

Prep Time: 10 minutes, Cook Time: 20 minutes, Serves: 6

INGREDIENTS:

1 medium carrot, peeled and cut into ½-inch dice
1 medium red bell pepper, seeded and finely chopped
1 medium green bell pepper, seeded and finely chopped
2 cups chopped mushrooms (from about 8 oz./230 g whole mushrooms)
1 large head broccoli, cut into florets
¼ cup (60mL) nutritional yeast
Salt to taste
½ tsp. freshly ground black pepper
1½ tsps. cinnamon
¼ tsp. cayenne pepper
3 cloves garlic, crushed
1 to 2 tbsps. lime sauce

DIRECTIONS:

1. Stir the carrot, red and green peppers, and mushrooms in a medium skillet or saucepan and sauté over medium-high heat for 7 to 8 minutes, or until the carrot is tender.
2. Pour water 1 to 2 tbsps. at a time to keep the vegetables from sticking to the pan. Stir in the broccoli and cook for 5 to 6 minutes, or until the florets are softened.
3. Put in the salt, black pepper, cinnamon, cayenne pepper, garlic, lime sauce, and nutritional yeast (if using) to the pan and simmer for an additional 5 minutes, or until hot and fragrant.

Nutrition Info per Serving:

Calories: 49, Protein: 4.1g, Fat: 0.31g, Carbohydrates: 8.03g, Fiber: 1.9g, Sugar: 2.29g, Sodium: 842mg, Cholesterol: 0mg

Breakfast Smoothie Bowl with Blackberries

Prep Time: 5 minutes, Cook Time: 0, Serves: 2

INGREDIENTS:

½ cup (120mL) peanut milk (unsweetened)
2 oz.(57g) blackberries (chopped)
3 cups Crushed ice
⅓ cup Pea protein powder
½ tsps. Psyllium husk powder
1 tbsp. canola oil
5 to 10 drops liquid stevia
coconut flakes and fresh blackberries for garnish

DIRECTIONS:

1. In a food processor, add the crushed ice cubes. Allow to rest for about 30 seconds.
2. Add the peanut milk, chopped blackberries, pea protein powder, psyllium husk powder, canola oil, and liquid stevia. Process well until it becomes smooth and creamy puree.
3. Empty the prepared smoothie into 2 glasses.
4. Top with coconut flakes and fresh blackberries.

Nutrition Info per Serving:

Calories: 166: Fat: 9.2g, Protein: 17.6g, Carbohydrates: 4.1g, Sugar: 24.8g, Dietary fiber: 14.7g, Sodium: 510mg, Cholesterol: 66mg

Broccoli and Cheddar Quiche

Prep Time: 10 minutes, Cook Time: 20 minutes, Serves: 6

INGREDIENTS:

½ cup milk
8 eggs
1 tsp. freshly ground black pepper
1 tsp. sea salt
1 cup shredded Cheddar cheese
1 tbsp. extra-virgin olive oil
2 garlic cloves, minced
1 yellow onion, chopped
2 cups thinly sliced broccoli florets
1 refrigerated piecrust, at room temperature

DIRECTIONS:

1. Preheat the pot by selecting Sear/Sauté and setting to High. Select Start/Stop to begin. Preheat for 5 minutes.
2. Whisk together the milk, eggs, pepper and salt in a large mixing bowl. Add the Cheddar cheese and stir well.
3. In the preheated pot, add the oil, garlic and onion, stir occasionally for 5 minutes. Stir in the broccoli florets and sauté for an additional 5 minutes.
4. Top the vegetables, pour with the egg mixture and gently stir for 1 minute (this will let the egg mixture temper well and be sure that it cooks evenly under the crust).
5. Evenly lay the piecrust on top of the filling mixture, folding over the edges if needed. In the center of the piecrust, make a small cut, so that steam can escape during baking.
6. Close the Crisping Lid. Select Broil and set the time to 10 minutes. Select Start/Stop to begin.
7. After cooking is finished, remove the pot and transfer it onto a heat-resistant surface. Allow the quiche to rest for 5 to 10 minutes before serving.

Nutrition Info per Serving:

Calories: 393, Total fat: 26g, Saturated fat: 10g, Carbohydrates: 26g, Protein: 16g, Fiber: 2g, Sodium: 773mg, Cholesterol: 304mg, Sugar: 2.5g

Baked Eggs with Lettuce and Parsley

Prep Time: 15 minutes, Cook Time: 10-15 minutes, Serves: 4

INGREDIENTS:

1 tbsp. olive oil, divided
half of medium onion, sliced
½ tsp. kosher salt
¼ tsp. ground cumin
1 tsp. ground allspice
4 cups (1L) lettuce, chopped
¼ cup (59mL) crumbled feta cheese
4 large eggs
¼ cup (59mL) fresh parsley, sliced

DIRECTIONS:

1. Preheat the oven to 375°F(190℃). Place 4 ramekins on a slightly greased baking dish.
2. Heat the remaining olive oil in a large skillet or sauté pan over medium heat. Add the onion, salt, allspice, and cumin and sauté until translucent, about 3 minutes. Add the lettuce and cook, stirring, until wilted, about 2 minutes.
3. Divide the mixture into the 4 ramekins. Spread each ramekin with 1 tbsp. feta cheese. Separate 1 egg over the mixture in each ramekin. Bake for 10 to 12 minutes, or until the egg white is no longer liquid.
4. Leave it to cool down, for 1 to 2 minutes, then carefully remove the eggs from the ramekins to a plate using a fork or spatula. Garnish with the parsley.

Nutrition Info per Serving:

Calories: 121, Protein: 4.9g, Fat: 9.9g, Carbohydrates: 3.7g, Sugar: 1.78g, Fiber: 1.1g, Sodium: 366mg, Cholesterol: 190mg

Italian Toast Plate Breakfast

Prep Time: 20 minutes, Cook Time: 25 minutes, Serves: 1

INGREDIENTS:

2 tsps. olive oil
1 tbsp. finely diced fresh tomato
1 large slice whole grain bread
1 tbsp. finely diced green pepper
1 tbsp. nonfat plain yogurt
1-ounce (28g) slice provolone cheese
1 tsp. minced fresh oregano
1-ounce (28g) slice mozzarella cheese
2 tbsps. minced Kalamata olives
1 tsp. minced fresh basil

DIRECTIONS:

1. Preheat the oven to 390°F (200ºC). Spread olive oil evenly on the bread.
2. Place in a baking tray, and heat in the oven. Put olives, tomatoes, pepper and herbs in a bowl, add yogurt, and stir until fully combined.
3. Take the toast out of the oven and increase the oven temperature to 375°F (190ºC). Put provolone cheese on the toast, spread the vegetable mixture on the cheese, add mozzarella cheese slices on top, and bake on the top grill of the oven until the cheese is melted and frothy.
4. Remove from the oven and put on a plate, and enjoy while it's hot!

Nutrition Info per Serving:

Calories: 427, Fat: 25.7g, Protein: 22.85g, Carbohydrates: 28.2g, Fiber: 5g, Cholesterol: 20mg, Sugar: 6.6g, Sodium: 816mg

Lemony Breakfast Cakes with Berry Syrup

Prep Time: 5 minutes, Cook Time: 10 minutes, Serves: 4

INGREDIENTS:

For the Pancakes
6 tbsps. extra-virgin olive oil, divided
2 large eggs
1 cup almond flour
1 tsp. baking powder
¼ tsp. salt
Zest and juice of 1 lemon
½ tsp. almond or vanilla extract
For the Berry Sauce
1 cup frozen mixed berries
½ tsp. vanilla extract
1 tbsp. water or lemon juice

DIRECTIONS:

To Make the Pancakes

1. In a large bowl, mix the baking powder, almond flour, and salt and whisk to break up any clumps.
2. Add 4 tablespoons olive oil, lemon zest and juice, eggs, and almond extract and mix well.
3. In a large skillet, heat 1 tbsp. olive oil and spoon about 2 tbsps. batter for each pancake. Cook 4 to 5 minutes, until bubbles begin to form, and flip. Cook another 2 to 3 minutes on second side. Repeat with remaining olive oil and batter.

To Make the Berry Sauce

1. In a small saucepan, heat the water, frozen berries, and vanilla extract over medium-high for 3 to 4 minutes, until bubbly, adding more water if mixture is too thick. Using the back of a spoon or fork to mash the berries and whisk until smooth.

Nutrition Info per Serving:

Calories: 275, Total Carbs: 8g, Protein: 4g, Total Fat: 26g, Net Carbs: 6g, Fiber: 2g, Sodium: 271mg, Cholesterol: 92mg, Sugar: 0.6g

Escarole with Portobello

Prep Time: 10 minutes, Cook Time: 15 minutes, Serves: 4

INGREDIENTS:

2 cups broccoli florets (from ½ of a medium head)
¼ cup (60mL) Vegetable Stock or low-sodium vegetable broth
1 pound(454 g) fresh escarole
1 batch Grilled Portobello Mushrooms
2 tbsps. fresh apple cider
⅛ tsp. cayenne pepper
Salt and freshly ground black pepper to taste

DIRECTIONS:

1. Mix together the broccoli, vegetable stock, apple cider, and cayenne pepper in a medium saucepan and bring to a boil over high heat. Lower the heat to medium and cook until the broccoli is softened, 8 to 10 minutes. Transfer the mixture to a food processor and puree until creamy, and return the broccoli hollandaise to the pan to keep warm.
2. Place the escarole to a large pot and pour ¼ cup of water. Simmer, covered, over medium-low heat until the escarole wilts. Drain and sprinkle with salt and pepper to season.
3. To serve, put a Grilled Portobello Mushroom on each of four individual plates and portion the escarole among the mushrooms. Spoon the sauce over the escarole and serve hot.

Nutrition Info per Serving:

Calories: 55, Protein: 5.5g, Fat: 0.86g, Carbohydrates: 9.65g, Fiber: 4.5g, Sugar: 2.83g, Sodium: 118mg, Cholesterol: 3mg

Cereal Cream with Flaxseed and Fruit

Prep Time: 15 minutes, Cook Time: 15 minutes, Serves: 4

INGREDIENTS:

2½ cups (600 ml) almond or rice milk, unsweetened low-fat
½ cup whole-grain buckwheat
¼ cup apples, coarsely chopped
1 tbsp. golden raisins
½ tsp. cinnamon
⅛ tsp. nutmeg
1 tbsp. flaxseed oil

DIRECTIONS:

1. Heat the pan over medium heat, put in the milk and let it simmer. Add buckwheat.
2. Reduce heat to low, gently simmer and cook with partially covered and stir frequently, for about 10 minutes, or until the milk is completely absorbed. Set aside.
3. Add apples and raisins to the mixture, then let it rest for 5 minutes.
4. Stir in flaxseed oil, cinnamon and nutmeg. Adjust the amount you like and serve.

Nutrition Info per Serving:

Calories: 133, Fat: 4.6g, Carbohydrates: 18.8g, Fiber: 2g, Protein: 1.8g, Cholesterol: 0mg, Sodium: 89mg, Sugar: 0.8g

Cheese and Tomato Omelet

Prep Time: 10 minutes, Cook Time: 5 minutes, Serves: 2 servings

INGREDIENTS:

Canola oil spray
2 eggs plus 2 egg whites
1 tbsp. water
1 small tomato, seeded and chopped
1 ounce (28g) low-fat cheddar cheese, cubed or shredded
Fresh ground black pepper
1 tbsp. chopped fresh cilantro

DIRECTIONS:

1. Warm a non-stick omelet pan on the stove over medium-low heat for about a minute. Meanwhile, whisk the eggs gently with the water in a mixing bowl. They should be just barely combined, don't over-mix the eggs.
2. Coat the omelet pan lightly with canola oil spray and allow the pan to warm for another 15 seconds. Pour the eggs into the pan, but don't stir. When the edges begin to firm up a bit, use a heat-proof rubber spatula to slide down around the edges of the eggs and lift gently to let the liquid eggs on top flow under the edges to the bottom of the omelet pan. This works best if you lift the edges of the omelet in 4 or 5 spots around the edge of the pan.
3. Arrange the tomato and cheese across half of the omelet. Dust with the pepper and sprinkle on the cilantro.
4. Keep cooking the omelet, it will still be soft in the center. Slide a larger flat spatula under 1 side of the omelet and fold it over onto the other half. Slide the folded omelet into the center of the pan.
5. Use the spatula to very lightly press on the top of the omelet to coax any remaining liquid out into the pan.
6. Cover with a lid and remove from heat. Let the omelet sit for about a minute to finish setting the eggs and then slice in half and serve.

Nutrition Info per Serving:

Calories: 198, Protein: 8.13g, Fat: 17.45g, Carbohydrates: 2.86g, Fiber: 0.9g, Sugar: 2.7g, Sodium: 170mg, Cholesterol: 9mg

Easy Vegan Southwest Tofu Scramble

Prep Time: 10 minutes, Cook Time: 15 minutes, Serves: 1

INGREDIENTS:

½ tbsp. olive oil
8 ounces (227g) firm tofu, drained well
½ red onion, chopped
2 cups chopped spinach
1 tsp. ground cumin
½ tsp. garlic powder
Optional for serving: sliced avocado or sliced tomatoes

DIRECTIONS:

1. Heat the olive oil in a medium skillet over medium heat. Add the onion and cook until softened, about 5 minutes.
2. Add the spinach and cover to steam for 2 minutes.
3. Using a spatula, move the veggies to one side of the pan. Crumble the tofu into the open area in the pan, breaking it up with a fork. Add the cumin and garlic to the crumbled tofu and mix well. Sauté for 5 to 7 minutes until the tofu is slightly browned.
4. Serve immediately with whole-grain bread, fruit, or beans. Top with optional sliced avocado and tomato, if using.

Nutrition Info per Serving:

Calories: 267, Total Fat: 17g, Saturated Fat: 3g, Cholesterol: 0mg, Sodium: 75mg, Potassium: 685mg, Total Carbohydrate: 13g, Fiber: 5g, Sugar: 2g, Protein: 23g

Chile Rellenos Egg Souffle

Prep Time: 15 minutes, Cook Time: 45 minutes, Serves: 8

INGREDIENTS:

2 cans (4 oz. each, 113 g) chopped green chilies
¼ cup finely chopped onion
¼ cup sliced ripe olives
2 cups sharp shredded cheddar cheese
1½ cups biscuit/baking mix
4 large eggs
2 cups 2% milk
¼ tsp. pepper
1 cup 4% small-curd cottage cheese
Salsa and sour cream, optional

DIRECTIONS:

1. Preheat oven to 350°F(180°C). In a greased 11x7-in. baking dish, spread with green chilies, sprinkle with the onion, olives, and cheese. Add biscuit mix, whisk eggs, milk and pepper into a large bowl, whisk them until blended. Add the cottage cheese and stir well, pour mixture over top.
2. Uncovered and bake for 45 to 50 minutes, until golden brown, puffed and a knife inserted in the center comes out clean. Allow it to stand for 5 to 10 minutes before serving. Serve with salsa and sour cream if desired.

Nutrition Info per Serving:

Calories: 305, Fat: 17g, Carbohydrates: 23g, Protein: 16g, Sugar: 5g, Fiber: 1g, Sodium: 708mg, Cholesterol: 128mg

Zucchini & Swiss Omelet

Prep Time: 5 minutes, Cook Time: 20 minutes, Serves: 1

INGREDIENTS:

2 eggs plus 2 egg whites
½ cup shredded fresh zucchini
1 oz.(30g) low-fat Swiss cheese, cubed or shredded
2 celery stalks, diced
1 tbsp. almond milk
cooking spray
Fresh ground black pepper
red salsa

DIRECTIONS:

1. Heat a non-stick omelet pan set on the stove over medium-low heat for about 1 minute. In the meantime, stir the eggs lightly with the almond milk. They should be just barely combined, don't over mix the eggs.
2. Grease the omelet pan lightly with cooking spray and let the pan warm for a further 15 seconds. Place the zucchini to the pan and cook for about 1 minute, stirring once or twice.
3. Add the eggs into the pan, but don't whisk. When the edges start to firm up a bit, slide down around the edges of the eggs using a heat-proof rubber spatula and lift lightly to allow the liquid eggs on top flow under the edges to the bottom of the omelet pan. This works best if you lift the edges of the omelet in 4 or 5 spots around the edge of the pan.
4. Place the cheese and celery across half of the omelet. Spread with freshly ground black pepper.
5. Continue cooking the omelet, it will still be soft in the center. Slide a larger, flat spatula under 1 side of the omelet and fold it over the other half to form a half circle. Slide the folded omelet over a bit into the center of the pan. Lightly press on the top of the omelet to coax any remaining liquid out into the pan with the spatula.
6. Seal with a lid and remove from heat. Allow the omelet to stand for about 1 minute to finish setting the eggs and then slide the omelet onto a plate and serve. Top with red salsa for extra flavor.

Nutrition Info per Serving:

Calories: 547, Protein: 24.04g, Fat: 30.15g, Carbohydrates: 46.2g, Sugar: 4.9g, Fiber: 1.3g, Sodium: 207mg, Cholesterol: 10mg

English Muffin with Lox

Prep Time: 10 minutes, Cook Time: 0, Serves: 2

INGREDIENTS:

1 (4-ounce, 113g) can wild salmon in water, no salt added, drained
1 100% whole wheat English muffin, halved
2 tbsps. low-fat cream cheese
¼ tsp. finely chopped fresh dill
½ tsp. fresh lemon juice
6 thin slices unpeeled cucumber
6 thin slices Roma tomato
Cracked black pepper

DIRECTIONS:

1. Toast the English muffin halves.
2. Meanwhile, in a small bowl, mix the chopped dill and lemon juice evenly into the cream cheese.
3. Spread the cream cheese mixture evenly onto each toasted muffin half. Rinse the salmon under running water to remove the canned liquid, and then scoop the salmon evenly onto the English muffin halves. If the salmon is too large, mash with fork first.
4. Top with cucumber and tomato slices, and sprinkle with pepper to taste.

Nutrition Info per Serving:

Calories: 192, Protein: 14g, Fat: 8g, Carbohydrates: 18g, Fiber: 3g, Sugar: 0.1g, Sodium: 160mg, Cholesterol: 17mg

Mushroom Carrot Skillet

Prep Time: 5 minutes, Cook Time: 15 minutes, Serves: 4

INGREDIENTS:

2 medium carrots, peeled and cut into ½-inch dice
8 oz. (230g) mushrooms, sliced
1 sweet onion, diced
1 cup (240mL) vegetable broth or water, plus 1 to 2 tbsps. more if needed
1 tsp. garlic powder
1 bell pepper, diced
½ tsp. ground oregano
½ tsp. allspice
⅛ tsp. freshly ground black pepper

DIRECTIONS:

1. Heat a large skillet over medium-low heat.
2. Once the skillet is hot, put the carrots, mushrooms, bell pepper, onion, broth, garlic powder, oregano, allspice, and pepper in it and stir. Cover and cook for 10 minutes, or until the carrots are tender.
3. Uncover, and give the mixture a good stir. (If any of the contents are beginning to stick to the bottom of the pan, add 1 to 2 tbsps. of broth.)
4. Cook, uncovered, for 5 minutes more, stirring once after about 2½ minutes, and serve.

Nutrition Info per Serving:

Calories: 158, Total fat: 1g, Carbohydrates: 34g, Fiber: 6g, Protein: 6g, Cholesterol: 1mg, Sugar: 8g, Sodium: 189mg

Cheesy Tex-Mex Breakfast Egg Bake Casserole

Prep Time: 10 minutes, Cook Time: 10 minutes, Serves: 4

INGREDIENTS:

8 ounces (227 g) corn tortilla chips, divided
1 cup green salsa, plus more for serving
2 cups shredded pepper Jack cheese, divided
¼ cup whole milk
3 large eggs
1 tsp. Mexican/ Southwestern Seasoning Mix, or a store-bought mix
¼ cup heavy (whipping) cream
¼ tsp. kosher salt (or ¼ tsp. fine salt)

DIRECTIONS:

1. In a 1-to 1.5-quart heat-proof dish, add about half of the chips. Pour over the chips with the salsa and gently toss to distribute the salsa. Sprinkle over the top with about half the cheese.
2. Whisk the milk, eggs, seasonings, heavy cream, and salt in a medium bowl. Pour over the chips and cheese with the egg mixture. Use aluminum foil to cover the dish.
3. In the inner pot, add 1 cup of water. Put the Reversible Rack in the pot in the lower position and on top place with the dish.
4. Lock the Pressure Lid into place, be sure that the valve is set to Seal. Select Pressure and set the pressure to High and the cooking time to 10 minutes. Press Start.
5. When the cooking is complete, naturally release the pressure for 5 minutes, then quick release any remaining pressure. Open and remove the Pressure Lid carefully.
6. Remove the foil from the casserole. Over the top arrange with about half the remaining chips and sprinkle with half the remaining cheese. Repeat the layers with the remaining chips and cheese.
7. Close the Crisping Lid. Select Broil and adjust the time to 7 minutes. Press Start. Broil until the chips are browned in spots and the cheese is melted.
8. Take the dish out of the pot and allow to cool for several minutes. Serve with additional salsa.

Nutrition Info per Serving:

Calories: 648, Total fat: 42g, Saturated fat: 18g, Carbohydrates: 44g, Protein: 24g, Fiber: 3g, Sodium: 978mg, Cholesterol: 209mg, Sugar: 5.3g

Easy Sweet Potato Hash

Prep Time: 15 minutes, Cook Time: 15 minutes, Serves: 4

INGREDIENTS:

2 large sweet potatoes, cooked and cut into ½-inch cubes
2 tbsps. coconut oil
1 cup sliced mushrooms
1 garlic clove, sliced thin
½ onion, sliced thin
1 cup finely chopped Swiss chard
½ cup (120 ml) vegetable broth
1 tbsp. chopped fresh thyme
1 tbsp. chopped fresh sage
1 tsp. salt
¼ tsp. freshly ground pepper

DIRECTIONS:

1. Melt the coconut oil in a large skillet over high heat.
2. Add the mushrooms, onion, and garlic. Sauté for about 8 minutes until the mushrooms and onions are tender.
3. Add the Swiss chard, sweet potatoes, and vegetable broth. Cook for 5 minutes.
4. Stir in the salt, thyme, pepper, and sage.

Nutrition Info per Serving:

Calories: 212, Total Carbohydrates: 35g, Protein: 30g, Total Fat: 7g, Sugar: 2g, Fiber: 6g, Sodium: 708mg, Cholesterol: 0mg

Hummus and Date Bagel

Prep Time: 3 minutes, Cook Time: 5 minutes, Serves: 1 bite

INGREDIENTS:

1 bagel
¼ serving of Homemade Hummus or store-bought hummus
6 dates, pitted and halved
Dash of salt and pepper
¼ cup diced tomatoes
1 tbsp. chives
Squeeze of lemon juice
1 handful sprouts

DIRECTIONS:

1. Split the bagel in half. Toast the bagel in a toaster or under the broiler.
2. Rub the hummus on each side.
3. Top with the dates, salt, pepper, tomatoes, chives, lemon juice and sprouts.

Nutrition Info per Serving:

Calories: 410, Total Fat: 2g, Carbohydrates: 59g, Protein: 91g, Fiber: 9.7g, Cholesterol: 0mg, Sugar: 39g, Sodium: 612mg

Longan Almond Barley with Apple Cider

Prep Time: 10 minutes, Cook Time: 55 minutes, Serves: 2

INGREDIENTS:

1(240mL) to 1½(360mL) cups apple cider
1 cup pearled barley
2 tbsps. dried longans
3 to 4 dried unsulfured almonds, chopped (see more about sulfites and sulfur dioxide)
2 tsps. coriander
1 tsp. ground cinnamon
Dash salt, or to taste

DIRECTIONS:

1. Pour 1 cup of water and 1 cup of the apple cider to a medium saucepan over medium heat and bring to a boil.
2. Stir in the barley, longans, almonds, coriander, cinnamon, and salt.
3. Bring the mixture to a boil, cover, turn the heat down to medium-low, and simmer for 45 minutes.
4. If the barley is not softened after 45 minutes, pour up to an additional ½ cup of apple cider and simmer for another 10 minutes.
5. Serve.

Nutrition Info per Serving:

Calories: 465, Protein: 11.25g, Fat: 1.51g, Carbohydrates: 105.61g, Fiber: 17.9g, Sugar: 23.69g, Sodium: 176mg, Cholesterol: 0mg

Shakshuka with Feta

Prep Time: 10 minutes, Cook Time: 20 minutes, Serves: 4

INGREDIENTS:

3 tbsps. olive oil
2 garlic cloves, chopped
½ medium red or green bell pepper, seeded and chopped (about ⅓ cup)
1 small onion, chopped (about ¾ cup)
1 medium jalapeño pepper, seeded and minced
1 tsp. kosher salt (or ½ tsp. fine salt)
½ tsp. ground cumin
2 (14.5-ounce, 411 g) cans diced tomatoes with their juice
½ tsp. red pepper flakes
½ tsp. smoked paprika
¼ tsp. freshly ground black pepper
4 large eggs
⅓ cup crumbled feta cheese (optional)
2 tbsps. chopped fresh parsley

DIRECTIONS:

1. On your Foodi™, preheat the inner pot by selecting Sear/Sauté and adjusting to Medium. Press Start. Preheat for 5 minutes. Add the olive oil and heat until shimmering. Add the garlic, bell pepper, onion and jalapeño. Lightly sprinkle with the salt. Cook for about 2 minutes, or until the vegetables are fragrant and beginning to soften, stirring occasionally. Add the cumin, tomatoes, red pepper flakes, paprika, and black pepper.
2. Lock the Pressure Lid into place, be sure that the valve is set to Seal. Select Pressure and adjust the pressure to High and the cooking time to 4 minutes. Press Start.
3. When the cooking is complete, quick release the pressure. Unlock and remove the Pressure Lid carefully.
4. Onto the surface of the tomato sauce, gently crack with the eggs.
5. Lock the Pressure Lid back into place, but leave the valve set to Vent. Select Steam and adjust the cooking time to 3 minutes. Press Start.
6. After cooking, unlock and remove the Pressure Lid carefully. Baste the tops with some of the sauce and cook until they are if the eggs are not done to your liking. Sprinkle with the parsley and feta cheese (if using, omit for a dairy-free dish) before serving.

Nutrition Info per Serving:

Calories: 209, Total fat: 16g, Saturated fat: 3g, Carbohydrates: 11g, Protein: 8g, Fiber: 3g, Sodium: 663mg, Cholesterol: 211mg, Sugar: 2.5g

Easy Turkey Sausage

Prep Time: 15 minutes, Cook Time: 15 minutes, Serves: 4

INGREDIENTS:

1½ pounds (680 g) ground turkey
½ cup dried blueberries
1 tsp. salt
½ tsp. freshly ground black pepper
½ tsp. ground nutmeg
1 tbsp. chopped fresh sage
2 scallions, sliced
Extra-virgin olive oil, for brushing

DIRECTIONS:

1. Preheat the oven to 400°F (205ºC).
2. Brush a rimmed baking sheet with olive oil.
3. Mix together the salt, turkey, nutmeg, pepper, scallions, sage, and blueberries in a medium bowl, do this with your hands.
4. Scoop the mixture onto the prepared baking sheet with a small ice cream scoop. Gently flatten the mounds into a patty shape with your fingers or the back of a spatula.
5. Put the sheet in the preheated oven and bake for 10 to 15 minutes until touches firm.

Nutrition Info per Serving:

Calories: 348, Total Carbohydrates: 4g, Protein: 47g, Total Fat: 19g, Sugar: 2g, Fiber: 1g, Sodium: 765mg, Cholesterol: 117mg

Vanilla Buckwheat Crêpes with Berries and Chia Jam

Prep Time: 15 minutes, Cook Time: 5 minutes per crêpe, Serves: 4-6

INGREDIENTS:

3 cups fresh berries, divided
6 tbsps. Chia Jam, divided
1 cup buckwheat flour
½ tsp. salt
2 tbsps. coconut oil (1 tbsp. melted)
1½ cups almond milk, or water
1 egg
1 tsp. vanilla extract

DIRECTIONS:

1. Add the buckwheat flour, salt, 1 tbsp. of melted coconut oil, the almond milk, egg, and vanilla to a small bowl, whisk until smooth.
2. Add the remaining 1 tbsp. of coconut oil into a large (12-inch) nonstick skillet, melt over medium-high heat. Tilt the pan, evenly coating it with the melted oil.
3. Ladle ¼ cup of batter into the skillet. Tilt the skillet to evenly coat it with the batter.
4. Cook until the edges begin to curl up, about 2 minutes. Flip the crêpe with a spatula and cook for 1 minute on the second side. Transfer the crêpe to a plate.
5. Continue making crêpes with the remaining batter. You should have 4 to 6 crêpes.
6. On a plate, put 1 crêpe and top with ½ cup of berries and 1 tbsp. of Chia Jam. Fold the crêpe over the filling. Repeat with the remaining crêpes and serve.

Nutrition Info per Serving:

Calories: 242, Total Fat: 11g, Total Carbohydrates: 33g, Sugar: 9g, Fiber: 6g, Protein: 7g, Sodium: 371mg, Cholesterol: 103mg

Brown Sugar Whole-Grain Cucumber Pancakes

Prep Time: 10 minutes, Cook Time: 15 minutes, Serves: 4

INGREDIENTS:

2 cups (475ml) shredded cucumbers
1¼ cups (294ml) whole-wheat flour
2 tsps. baking powder
1 tsp. pumpkin pie spice
1 egg
1 cup (235ml) plus 2 tbsps. low-fat milk
2 tbsps. unsalted butter, melted
2 tbsps. light brown sugar
1 tsp. vanilla extract
2 tbsps. blueberry juice
cooking spray

DIRECTIONS:

1. Wrap the shredded cucumbers in a clean dish towel and squeeze out as much water as possible.
2. Stir together the flour, baking powder, and pumpkin pie spice in a large bowl.
3. Combine the egg, milk, butter, brown sugar, and vanilla in a medium bowl. Add the wet ingredients to the dry ingredients and whisk to combine. Stir in the cucumbers.
4. Oil a large nonstick skillet with cooking spray and heat over medium heat. Use about ⅓ cup batter (about 4 inches in diameter) for each pancake, and cook for 2 to 3 minutes, until bubbles observed on the surface. If the batter is too thick, add a smear of milk. Turn over and cook 1 to 2 minutes, until the other side becomes brown. Top with blueberry juice. Serve hot.

Nutrition Info per Serving:

Calories: 191, Fat: 3g, Carbohydrates: 32.3g, Protein: 7.3g, Cholesterol: 155mg, Sodium: 28mg, Fiber: 2g, Sugar: 1.4g

Spinach and Tomato Baked Egg Cups

Prep Time: 15 minutes, Cook Time: 15 minutes, Serves: 6

INGREDIENTS:

Nonstick cooking spray
6 large eggs
2½ ounces (71g) shredded reduced-fat Cheddar cheese
2½ cups chopped spinach
1 medium tomato, diced
1 garlic clove, minced
½ tbsp. chopped fresh parsley
½ tbsp. chopped fresh chives
¼ tsp. freshly ground black pepper

DIRECTIONS:

1. Preheat the oven to 400°F(205°C). Coat 10 cups of a muffin tin with cooking spray or line with silicone muffin liners or paper liners.
2. Crack the eggs into a large bowl. Add the garlic, parsley, chives, and pepper and whisk well. Then stir in the Cheddar cheese, spinach, and tomato.
3. Divide the egg mixture evenly among the muffin cups, filling about two-thirds full.
4. Bake for about 15 minutes, or until set. Let cool.
5. Place 2 egg cups into each of 5 storage containers.

Nutrition Info per Serving:

Calories: 232, Total fat: 18g, Carbohydrates: 2g, Fiber: 0.5g, Protein: 17g, Calcium: 203mg, Vitamin D: 84 IU, Potassium: 299mg, Magnesium: 32mg, Sodium: 258mg, Cholesterol: 189mg, Sugar: 1.5g

Spicy Egg Muffins

Prep Time: 25 minutes, Cook Time: 40 minutes, Serves: 6

INGREDIENTS:

4 tbsps. chopped green onion, white ends discarded
½ cup chopped green bell pepper
4 cups chopped spinach
½ cup chopped red bell pepper
2 whole eggs
14 egg whites
Pinch of paprika
¼ tsp. dried oregano
⅛ tsp. cracked black pepper
2 tbsps. finely chopped fresh parsley
⅛ tsp. chile pepper flakes

DIRECTIONS:

1. Preheat the oven to 375°F in advance. Put spinach, green peppers, red peppers, and onions in a large bowl and mix well.
2. In a separate large bowl, whisk together egg whites, whole eggs, chili flakes, oregano, parsley, pepper, and paprika. Spray each muffin tin evenly with olive oil spray, making sure to spray on the sides as well.
3. Scoop the vegetable mixture into each muffin cup, about half of the muffin cup. Then slowly pour about ⅓ cup of egg mixture into each muffin cup so as not to replace the vegetables.
4. Place the muffin tin on the grill in the middle of the oven and bake for 25 to 30 minutes until the eggs no longer run.
5. Remove from the oven immediately to avoid over-baking or drying the eggs. Enjoy.

Nutrition Info per Serving:

Calories: 93, Fat: 3g, Protein: 14g, Carbohydrates: 4g, Fiber: 1g, Sugar: 1g, Sodium: 181mg, Cholesterol: 206mg

Delicious Apple Pancakes

Prep Time: 5 minutes, Cook Time: 5 minutes, Serves: 16 pancakes

INGREDIENTS:

¼ cup extra-virgin olive oil, divided
1 cup 1% milk
2 large eggs
1 medium Gala apple, diced
1 cup whole wheat flour
2 tsps. baking powder
1 tsp. baking soda
1 tsp. ground cinnamon
2 tbsps. maple syrup
¼ cup chopped walnuts

DIRECTIONS:

1. Set aside 1 tsp. of oil to use for oiling a griddle or skillet. In a large bowl, stir together the flour, baking powder, baking soda, cinnamon, milk, eggs, apple, and the remaining oil.
2. Heat a griddle or skillet over medium-high heat and coat with the reserved oil. Working in batches, pour in about ¼ cup of the batter for each pancake. Cook until browned on both sides.
3. Place 4 pancakes into each of 4 medium storage containers and the maple syrup in 4 small containers.
4. To serve, sprinkle each serving with 1 tbsp. of walnuts and drizzle with ½ tablespoon of maple syrup.

Nutrition Info per Serving:

Calories: 378, Total fat: 22g, Carbohydrates: 39g, Fiber: 5g, Protein: 10g, Calcium: 124mg, Vitamin D: 50 IU, Potassium: 334mg, Magnesium: 65mg, Sodium: 65mg, Sugar: 2g, Cholesterol: 26mg

Smoked Salmon Egg Scramble

Prep Time: 5 minutes, Cook Time: 5 minutes, Serves: 2

INGREDIENTS:

2 ounces (57 g) smoked salmon, thinly sliced
2 large eggs
1 tbsp. fresh chives, minced
1 tbsp. fresh dill, minced
1 tbsp. milk
¼ tsp. kosher salt
⅛ tsp. freshly ground black pepper
2 tsps. extra-virgin olive oil

DIRECTIONS:

1. Whisk together the eggs, dill, chives, milk, salt, and pepper in a large bowl.
2. Heat the olive oil in a medium skillet over medium heat. Put in the egg mixture and cook for about 3 minutes, stirring occasionally.
3. Add the salmon and cook about 1 minute until the eggs are set but moist.

Nutrition Info per Serving:

Calories: 325, Total fat: 26g, Saturated fat: 6g, Total Carbohydrates: 1g, Protein: 23g, Cholesterol: 204mg, Sodium: 455mg, Potassium: 300mg, Fiber: 0g, Sugar: 1g, Magnesium: 25mg, Calcium: 90mg

Roasted Pears with Walnuts

Prep Time: 5 minutes, Cook Time: 25 minutes, Serves: 4

INGREDIENTS:

4 Bosc or d'Anjou pears, cored and quartered, skin on
¼ cup low-fat blue cheese, crumbled
¼ cup toasted walnuts, coarsely chopped
1 tbsp. grape seed oil or canola
1 tbsp. lemon juice
Cooking spray

DIRECTIONS:

1. Preheat oven to 425°F. Toss pears with oil and lemon juice in a medium bowl.
2. Spray the cooking spray on baking sheet, and put pears, cut-side down, on it. Roast for 15 minutes. Flip pears and roast 10 more minutes.
3. Remove from oven. Divide pears among four plates, and top each serving with 1 tbsp. cheese and nuts. Serve immediately.

Nutrition Info per Serving:

Calories: 200, Fat: 11g, Carbohydrates: 26.5g, Protein: 4.4g, Cholesterol: 5mg, Sodium: 66mg, Fiber: 0.5g, Sugar: 0.3g

Smoked Trout and Avocado

Prep Time: 10 minutes, Cook Time: 5 minutes, Serves: 2

INGREDIENTS:

1 (3.75-ounce, 106 g) can smoked trout
1 avocado, peeled and pitted
2 tsps. lemon juice, plus more for serving
¾ tsp. ground cumin
¼ tsp. kosher salt
¼ tsp. red pepper flakes, plus more for sprinkling
¼ tsp. lemon zest
2 pieces whole-wheat bread, toasted

DIRECTIONS:

1. Mash together the avocado, cumin, lemon juice, red pepper flakes, salt, and lemon zest in a medium bowl.
2. Spread half the avocado mixture on each piece of toast. Top each with half the smoked trout. Garnish with a pinch of red pepper flakes, and/or a sprinkle of lemon juice.

Nutrition Info per Serving:

Calories: 300, Total fat: 20g, Saturated fat: 3g, Total Carbohydrates: 21g, Protein: 11g, Cholesterol: 23mg, Sodium: 390mg, Potassium: 455mg, Fiber: 6g, Sugar: 1g, Magnesium: 45mg, Calcium: 50mg

Best Healthy French Toast

Prep Time: 5 minutes, Cook Time: 10 minutes, Serves: 4

INGREDIENTS:

4 egg whites
1 whole egg
8 slices whole grain bread (at least ½–1 inch thick)
1 cup unsweetened almond milk
½ tsp. ground cinnamon
1 tsp. vanilla extract
¼ tsp. ground nutmeg
½ tsp. powdered stevia

DIRECTIONS:

1. In a shallow bowl, whisk together the egg whites, whole egg, almond milk, cinnamon, vanilla, nutmeg, and stevia. Soak each slice of bread in the mixture for about 1 minute per side, let the bread absorbs the liquid and flavors.
2. Heat a griddle pan until very hot, and coat with olive oil spray. Place each soaked slice of bread on the griddle pan, and cook about 3 minutes on each side, or until browned and crunchy.
3. Serve immediately.

Nutrition Info per Serving:

Calories: 305, Protein: 15g, Fat: 7g, Carbohydrates: 49g, Fiber: 6g, Sugar: 0.3g, Sodium: 438mg, Cholesterol: 155mg

Polenta with Longans and Dates

Prep Time: 10 minutes, Cook Time: 10 minutes, Serves: 4

INGREDIENTS:

½ cup (120mL) brown rice syrup
20 longans, peeled, cored, and halved
1 cup fresh dates, halved and seeded
1 tsp. ground fennel
1 batch Basic Polenta, kept warm

DIRECTIONS:

1. Heat the brown rice syrup in a medium saucepan. Add the longans, dates, and fennel and simmer, stirring from time by time, until the dates are tender, about 10 minutes.
2. To serve, portion the polenta among 4 individual bowls and spread with the longan compote.

Nutrition Info per Serving:

Calories: 236, Protein: 2.28g, Fat: 1.28g, Carbohydrates: 54.66g, Fiber: 6.8g, Sugar: 23.94g, Sodium: 443mg, Cholesterol: 0mg

Quinoa Bowl with Blackberry

Prep Time: 20 minutes, Cook Time: 20 minutes, Serves: 4

INGREDIENTS:

2 tsps. canola oil
Nutmeg
¾ cup quinoa
½ orange, peeled
½ cup nonfat milk
1 cup water
1 tsp. vanilla
2 cups fresh blackberries

DIRECTIONS:

1. Rinse the quinoa and drain. Heat the oil in a medium-sized non-stick pan, add the quinoa, roast the quinoa on medium-high heat for about 1 minute, stirring constantly.
2. Cut the peeled oranges into small pieces and remove all seeds. Add a little nutmeg and processed oranges to the quinoa, stir and then add water.
3. Simmer on low heat for about 11 minutes, until the quinoa is almost soft but still a bit crispy in the middle. Add milk, blackberries and vanilla, stir gently, and simmer for 2 or 3 minutes until the quinoa grains are translucent.
4. Remove from the pot to a bowl and enjoy while it is hot!

Nutrition Info per Serving:

Calories: 271, Fat: 4.53g, Protein: 7.29g, Carbohydrates: 51.83g, Fiber: 6.6g, Sugar: 16.7g, Sodium: 23mg, Cholesterol: 1mg

Congee with Raisin and Spices

Prep Time: 5 minutes, Cook Time: 20 minutes, Serves: 4

INGREDIENTS:

4 cups cooked brown rice
½ cup raisins
½ cup chopped unsulfured pine nuts (see more about sulfites and sulfur dioxide)
1 tsp. mint
¼ tsp. ground cloves
Salt to taste

DIRECTIONS:

1. Pour 2 cups of water to a large saucepan over medium heat and bring to a boil.
2. Stir in the rice, raisins, pine nuts, mint, and cloves. Simmer over medium-low heat for 15 minutes, or until the mixture thickens. Sprinkle with salt. Serve.

Nutrition Info per Serving:

Calories: 266, Protein: 5.68g, Fat: 1.87g, Carbohydrates: 57.79g, Fiber: 5.3g, Sugar: 11.37g, Sodium: 593mg, Cholesterol: 0mg

Garlicky Pea Fried Rice Breakfast

Prep Time: 10 minutes, Cook Time: 15 minutes, Serves: 2

INGREDIENTS:

1 tbsp. avocado oil
2 garlic cloves, minced
½ white onion, diced
¼ cup peas
¼ cup non-GMO organic sweet corn kernels
¼ cup shredded carrots
1 tbsp. sesame oil
2 cups cooked rice
2 eggs, whisked
¼ tsp. salt
Dash red pepper flakes
Freshly ground black pepper

DIRECTIONS:

1. Add the avocado oil, garlic and onion to a medium skillet, sauté over medium heat for 5 minutes, until translucent.
2. Add the peas, corn, and carrots, stir well and cook for another 5 minutes, stirring occasionally.
3. Stir in the sesame oil and rice, using a spoon to break the rice up. As the rice begins to soften, add the eggs. Cook for 5 minutes, until thoroughly cooked, stirring occasionally.
4. Sprinkle with the salt and red pepper flakes, season with pepper. Serve hot.

Nutrition Info per Serving:

Calories: 453, Total Fat: 19g, Saturated Fat: 43, Carbohydrates: 59g, Protein: 13g, Fiber: 3g, Cholesterol: 186mg, Sugar: 4.6g, Sodium: 494mg

Peanut Butter Brazilian Nut Smoothie Bowl

Prep Time: 5 minutes, Cook Time: 0, Serves: 2

INGREDIENTS:

1 cup coconut milk
½ cup canned peanut butter purée
1 tsp. pumpkin pie spice
2 (1-gram) packets stevia
½ tsp. vanilla extract
Pinch salt
½ cup chopped brazilian nuts

DIRECTIONS:

1. In a bowl, whisk together the coconut milk, peanut butter purée, pumpkin pie spice, stevia, vanilla, and salt (or blend in a blender).
2. Spoon into two bowls. Serve topped with the chopped brazilian nuts.

Nutrition Info per Serving:

Calories: 292, Total Fat: 23g, Saturated Fat: 4g, Sodium: 85mg, Carbohydrates: 15g, Fiber: 4g, Protein: 9g, Cholesterol: 33mg, Sugar: 10.9g

Sweet Lychee Quinoa Breakfast Bowl

Prep Time: 5 minutes, Cook Time: 15 minutes, Serves: 6

INGREDIENTS:

1 cup (235ml) unsweetened peanut milk
1 cup (235ml) water
1 cup (235ml) uncooked quinoa
½ tsp. maple syrup
⅓ cup (78ml) lychee, sliced
⅓ cup (78ml) cranberries, chopped
2 tbsps. pine nuts, toasted

DIRECTIONS:

1. Whisk the peanut milk, water, quinoa, and maple syrup in a medium saucepan, and bring the mixture to a boil. Reduce the heat to medium-low and cook until most of the liquid is absorbed, about 15 minutes.
2. Mix in the lychee, pine nuts, and cranberries and serve immediately.

Nutrition Info per Serving:

Calories: 469, Fat: 30g, Carbohydrates: 37.6g, Protein: 16.5g, Cholesterol: 0mg, Sodium: 262mg, Fiber: 4.5g, Sugar: 6.4g

Sweet Potatoes with Pineapple

Prep Time: 5 minutes, Cook Time: 10 minutes, Serves: 4

INGREDIENTS:

2 tbsps. coconut oil or olive oil
1 cup pineapple chunks, drained
4 baked sweet potatoes, sliced

DIRECTIONS:

1. In a large nonstick pan, heat oil over medium-high and add sweet potatoes to pan with flesh-side down.
2. Cook about 8 minutes, until the potatoes begin to brown and caramelize.
3. Put sweet potatoes on plates and top with pineapple. Serve.

Nutrition Info per Serving:

Calories: 233, Fat: 7.2g, Carbohydrates: 41.3g, Protein: 2.4g, Cholesterol: 0mg, Sodium: 17.5mg, Fiber: 4.4g, Sugar: 6.4g

Breakfast Cereal with Apples and Raisins

Prep Time: 15 minutes, Cook Time: 15 minutes, Serves: 4

INGREDIENTS:

½ tsp. cinnamon
⅛ tsp. nutmeg
1 tbsp. flaxseed oil
2½ cups (600 ml) low-fat almond or rice milk, fortified, unsweetened
½ cup whole-grain buckwheat
¼ cup apples, coarsely chopped
1 tbsp. golden raisins

DIRECTIONS:

1. Let the milk simmer over medium heat. Add buckwheat in it.
2. Reduce heat to low, gently simmer and cook for approximately 10 minutes, partially covered and stirring frequently, or until the milk is completely absorbed. Remove from heat.
3. Add apples and raisins, then allow mixture to rest for 5 minutes.
4. Stir in nutmeg, flaxseed oil and cinnamon. Serve.

Nutrition Info per Serving:

Calories: 133, Fat: 4.6g, Carbohydrates: 18.8g, Protein: 1.8g, Cholesterol: 0mg, Sodium: 89mg, Fiber: 2g, Sugar: 1.2g

Vanilla Rice Pudding

Prep Time: 5 minutes, Cook Time: 20 minutes, Serves: 4

INGREDIENTS:

1 tbsp. orange-infused olive oil or plain olive oil
½ cup (120 ml) low-fat milk
½ cup cherries, dried
½ cup almonds
1 cup cooked rice, long-grain
1 cup (240 ml) low-fat coconut milk
Pinch of ground nutmeg
1 cinnamon stick
1 tsp. vanilla extract

DIRECTIONS:

1. Heat oil over medium heat in a medium sauté pan. Add cooked rice, cinnamon stick, vanilla, and coconut milk and stir.
2. Bring to a simmer and partially covered over low heat for about 20 minutes, until coconut milk is absorbed. Remove from heat.
3. Add milk, cherries, almonds and a pinch of nutmeg. Covered and set aside for 10 minutes before serving.

Nutrition Info per Serving:

Calories: 295, Fat: 25g, Carbohydrates: 35g, Protein: 6.8g, Fiber: 5.7g, Cholesterol: 0mg, Sodium: 4.4mg, Sugar: 5.3g

Savory Yogurt Bowls with Hazelnuts

Prep Time: 15 minutes, Cook Time: 0, Serves: 4

INGREDIENTS:

1 medium cucumber, diced
½ cup pitted dates, halved
2 cups (480mL) nonfat plain Greek yogurt
½ cup hazelnuts
2 tbsps. fresh apple cider
1 tbsp. extra-virgin olive oil
1 tsp. dried nutmeg
¼ tsp. freshly ground black pepper

DIRECTIONS:

1. Combine the cucumber, dates, apple cider, oil, nutmeg, and pepper in a small bow.
2. Portion the yogurt evenly among 4 storage containers. Top with the cucumber-date mix and hazelnuts.

Nutrition Info per Serving:

Calories: 240, Total fat: 16g, Carbohydrates: 10g, Fiber: 2g, Protein: 16g, Calcium: 183mg, Vitamin D: 0 IU, Potassium: 353mg, Magnesium: 57mg, Sodium: 350mg, Cholesterol: 10mg, Sugar: 13.1g

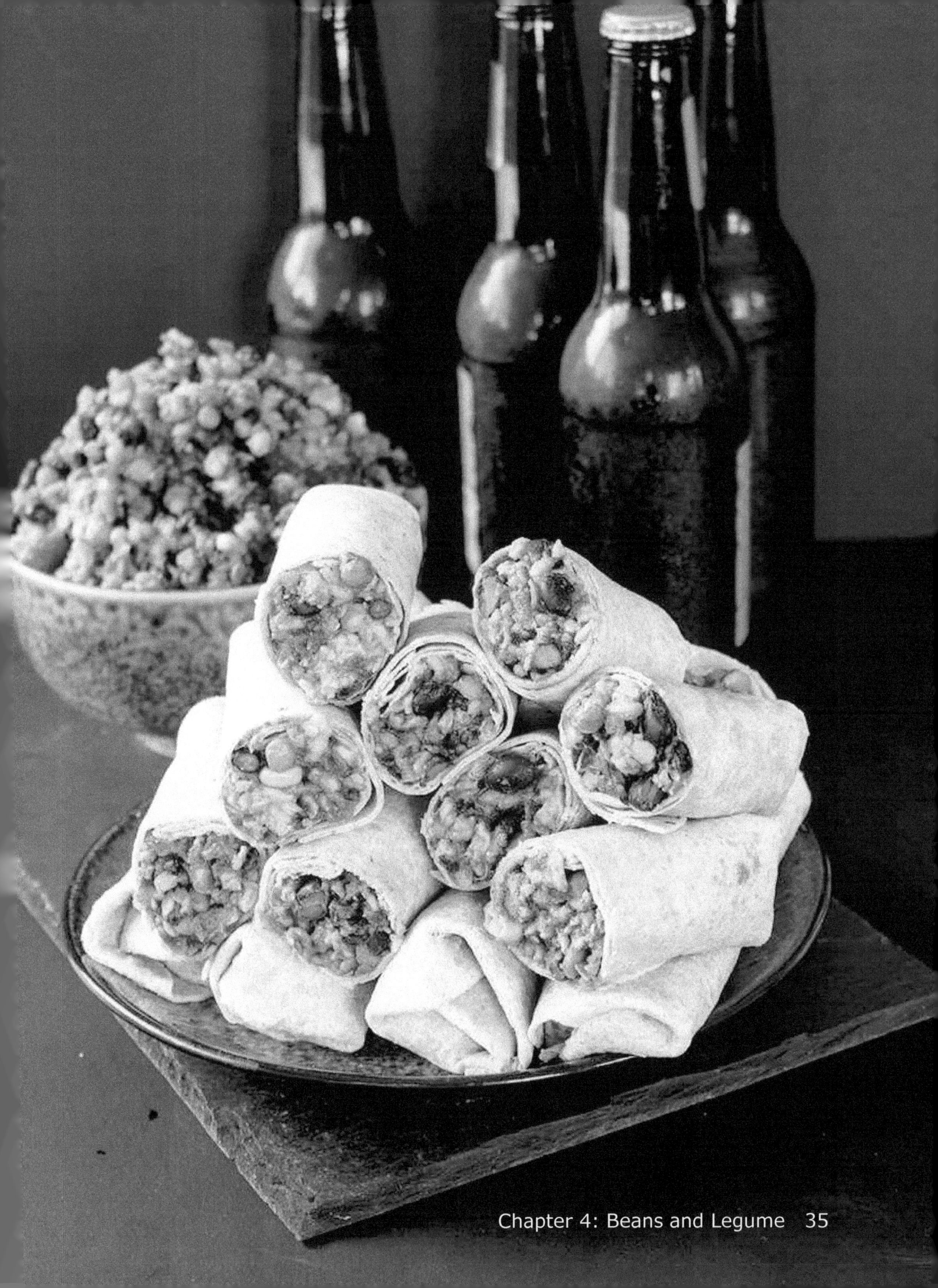

Chapter 4: Beans and Legume

Cuban Black Beans with Rice

Prep Time: 20 minutes, Cook Time: 2.5 hours, Serves: 4

INGREDIENTS:

FOR THE BLACK BEANS:
1 pound (454 g) black beans, soaked overnight
1 large onion, peeled and diced
1 medium tomato, chopped
3 medium carrots, peeled and diced
1 red bell pepper, seeded and diced
2 bay leaves
3 cloves garlic, peeled and minced
3 celery stalks, diced
2 tbsps. ground cumin
2 tbsps. minced oregano
1 cup finely chopped cilantro stems
2 tbsps. apple cider vinegar
½ tsp. freshly ground white or black pepper
3 tbsps. chopped cilantro leaves
Salt
FOR THE CILANTRO RICE:
1 cup brown rice
2 tbsps. finely chopped cilantro leaves
1 tbsp. low-sodium light brown miso paste

DIRECTIONS:

TO MAKE THE BLACK BEANS:

1. In a large pot, mix the beans, onion, cumin, garlic, bay leaves, celery, carrots, oregano, red pepper, cilantro stems, and 5 cups of water and bring to a boil.
2. Lower the heat to a simmer and cook for 90 minutes. Remove ¼ of the beans, mash them in a separate bowl, and return them to the pot.
3. Put in the apple cider vinegar, cilantro leaves, pepper, and tomato and stir. Once the beans are fully cooked, season with salt and remove the bay leaves.

TO MAKE THE CILANTRO RICE:

1. Put the rice, the miso paste and 2 cups of water in a large saucepan and bring to a boil. Lower the heat to medium and simmer, covered, for 20 minutes. Reduce the heat to low and simmer for an additional 30 minutes. Fluff the rice and stir in the cilantro.
2. Portion the rice among 4 individual plates and top with the beans. Serve.

Nutrition Info per Serving:

Calories: 267, Carbohydrates: 55.38g, Protein: 7.29g, Fat: 2.92g, Fiber: 7.3g, Sugar: 7.7g, Sodium: 642mg, Cholesterol: 0mg

Mung Bean Sprouts and Cabbage Salad

Prep Time: 10 minutes, Cook Time: 10 minutes, Serves: 4

INGREDIENTS:

FOR THE SPROUTS:
½ cup whole mung beans
½ tsp. turmeric
¼ tsp. salt
FOR THE SALAD:
2 medium potatoes, skin on
½ cup blueberries, diced
½ cup cabbage, finely chopped
¼ cup peach, diced
¼ cup basil, finely chopped
2 tbsps. tahini
1 tbsp. white wine vinegar
1 tsp. ground allspice
1 tsp. ground fennel
1 tsp. Salt

DIRECTIONS:

TO SPROUT THE MUNG BEANS:

1. Soak the mung beans in 1 cup of filtered water overnight. Spread a clean, damp cloth in a large bowl. Drain off the water from the beans and wrap them in the cloth. Transfer the bowl to a cool place away from sunlight. Dampen the cloth every 6 hours. The beans will sprout to about .5-centimeter sprouts in 12 hours.
2. When the beans have sprouted, rinse them completely in clean water. Boil the sprouts in 2 cups of water with the turmeric and salt for 10 minutes, or until the sprouts soften a little. Drain the sprouts and set them aside.

TO MAKE THE SALAD:

1. Halve the potatoes. Transfer to a medium saucepan and pour enough water to cover.
2. Bring to a boil, lower the heat to medium, and simmer for 10 minutes, or until soft when pierced with a fork. Drain the potatoes and allow them to cool, then peel and cut into ½-inch cubes.
3. Transfer the potatoes in a large bowl and Whisk in the drained sprouts, blueberries, cabbage, peach, basil, tahini, white wine vinegar, allspice, fennel, and salt.
4. Toss to combine well and serve.

Nutrition Info per Serving:

Calories: 117, Protein: 3.88g, Fat: 1.84g, Carbohydrates: 23.12g, Fiber: 4.4g, Sugar: 2.41g, Sodium: 752mg, Cholesterol: 0mg

Citrus Quinoa with Black Beans

Prep Time: 15 minutes, Cook Time: 20 minutes, Serves: 4

INGREDIENTS:

1½ cups quinoa, rinsed and drained
2 cups cooked black beans, or one 15-ounce (425 g) can, drained and rinsed
1½ tsps. grated ginger
1½ tsps. cumin seeds, toasted and ground
2 tbsps. balsamic vinegar
Zest and juice of 1 orange (about 60 ml juice)
4 green onions (white and green parts), thinly sliced
Salt and freshly ground black pepper

DIRECTIONS:

1. Add 3 cups of water to a medium pot with a lid and boil over high heat. Add the quinoa and return the pot to a boil over high heat. Lower the heat to medium-low and cook the quinoa with lid covered for 15 to 20 minutes, until tender.
2. Put the quinoa in a large bowl and add the cumin, ginger, black beans, orange zest and juice, vinegar, and green onions. Mix well and season with salt and pepper.

Nutrition Info per Serving:

Calories: 230, Carbohydrates: 47.58g, Protein: 7.36g, Fat: 1.92g, Fiber: 6.4g, Sugar: 20.26g, Sodium: 35mg, Cholesterol: 0mg

Black-Eyed Pea Wrap

Prep Time: 10 minutes, Cook Time: 15 minutes, Serves: 4

INGREDIENTS:

4 ounces (113 g) cremini mushrooms, cleaned, stemmed, and cut into ¼-inch thick slices
One 15-ounce (425 g) can low-salt black-eyed peas, drained and rinsed
5 tbsps. grape seed or olive oil
2 tbsps. fresh basil or parsley, minced
½ tsp. wheat-free tamari
2 garlic cloves, minced
½ red onion, chopped
1 avocado, sliced
4 large lettuce leaves or spelt bread
¼ tsp. dried thyme

DIRECTIONS:

1. Heat oil in a large frying pan over medium heat until shimmering. Add the mushrooms and thyme. Cook about 2 to 3 minutes, stirring occasionally, until browned. Add red onion and garlic, and cook about 2 minutes until fragrant and softened. Remove from heat.
2. Place the black-eyed peas in a large bowl, and mash with the back of a spoon, leaving some peas intact. Mix the mushroom mixture, basil or parsley, and tamari. Form the mixture into four patties.
3. Heat the oil in a sauté pan over medium-high heat until shimmering. Add the patties and fry about 5 to 6 minutes per side until browned.
4. Serve on bread or lettuce leaves with red onion and avocado.

Nutrition Info per Serving:

Calories: 317, Fat: 25.4g,Carbohydrates: 22.5g, Protein: 4.2g, Cholesterol: 0mg, Sodium: 51.7mg, Fiber: 7.6g, Sugar: 6.7g

Black Bean, Tomato, Rice and Lentil Burritos

Prep Time: 15 minutes, Cook Time: 8 hours, Serves: 6

INGREDIENTS:

2 15-ounce (425 g) cans black beans, drained and rinsed
¼ cup salsa
2 15-ounce (425 g) cans diced tomatoes
½ cup corn, fresh, frozen, or canned
1 cup brown rice
2 tbsps. taco seasoning
2 chipotle peppers in adobo sauce, finely chopped
1 tsp. ground cumin
1 tsp. salt
2½ cups vegetable broth
½ cup lentils
12 whole wheat tortillas
Additional toppings, such as more salsa, avocado or guacamole, and black olives

DIRECTIONS:

1. In a slow cooker, combine the beans, salsa, tomatoes, corn, rice, taco seasoning, chipotles, cumin, salt, and broth. Cover and cook on low for 6 to 8 hours or on high for 3 to 4 hours.
2. Cook until 40 minutes left, add the lentils. Continue cooking until the lentils are tender. The rice will be tender and most of the liquid will be absorbed. This is the filling.
3. Lay out the tortillas and place about ⅓ to ½ cup of the filling on each tortilla. Spread the filling down through the center of the tortilla. Fold each end about 1½ inches over the point edge of the beans. And roll up the tortilla along the long edge.
4. Stack up and serve with more avocado, salsa or guacamole, and black olives.

Nutrition Info per Serving:

Calories: 531, Protein: 23.8g, Fat: 9.9g, Carbohydrates: 90g, Fiber: 24.4g, Sugar: 7g, Sodium: 886mg, Cholesterol: 0mg

Edamame and Rice

Prep Time: 15 minutes, Cook Time: 20 minutes, Serves: 4

INGREDIENTS:

2 potatoes, peeled and diced
4 cups edamame
3 cups (700mL) cooked brown rice
1 cup chopped tarragon
1 lime, quartered
1 red bell pepper, seeded and diced
2 jalapeño peppers, diced (for less heat, remove the seeds)
5 cloves garlic, smashed and skin removed
1 tsp. ground cumin
Salt and freshly ground black pepper to taste
1½ tsps. oregano, toasted

DIRECTIONS:

1. In a large saucepan, add the potatoes, red pepper, and jalapeño peppers and sauté over medium heat for 7 to 8 minutes.
2. Add water 1 to 2 tbsps. at a time to keep the vegetables from sticking to the pan. Whisk in the garlic, cumin, and oregano and cook for 3 minutes.
3. Whisk in the edamame and 1 cup of water. Cook for 10 minutes, adding more water if necessary.
4. Sprinkle with salt and pepper to taste. Pour over the brown rice and garnish with the tarragon and lime wedges.

Nutrition Info per Serving:

Calories: 239, Protein: 7.42g, Fat: 1.69g, Carbohydrates: 49.96g, Fiber: 6.7g, Sugar: 3.71g, Sodium: 9mg, Cholesterol: 0mg

Fava Beans with Olives

Prep Time: 10 minutes, Cook Time: 2½ hours, Serves: 4

INGREDIENTS:

1½ pounds(454 g) dried fava beans, soaked for 8 to 10 hours
1 medium red onion, peeled and finely chopped
5 olives, seeded and diced
3 cloves garlic, peeled and minced
1 tsp. ground thyme
1 tbsp. red wine vinegar
Salt to taste
fresh sage

DIRECTIONS:

1. Drain and rinse the beans, and place them to a large pot. Add enough water to top the beans by 4 inches and bring to a boil over high heat. Lower the heat to medium, cover, and cook until the beans are softened, 1½ to 2 hours.
2. While the beans are simmering, stir the onion in a medium skillet or saucepan and sauté over medium heat for 8 to 10 minutes, or until the onion is translucent and starting to brown. Whisk in the garlic, thyme, and red wine vinegar and olives and cook for 5 minutes longer. Set aside until the beans are fully cooked.
3. When the beans are done cooking, drain all but ½ cup of the liquid from the pot and pour the onion mixture to the beans. Toss to combine well and sprinkle with salt. Serve garnished with the sage.

Nutrition Info per Serving:

Calories: 168, Protein: 14.03g, Fat: 1.45g, Carbohydrates: 34.5g, Fiber: 13.2g, Sugar: 17.05g, Sodium: 626mg, Cholesterol: 0mg

Sautéed Greens with Cannellini Beans and Garlic

Prep Time: 10 minutes, Cook Time: 10 minutes, Serves: 4

INGREDIENTS:

3 tbsps. extra virgin olive oil
1 pound(454g) mixed greens (such as mustard greens, kale, collard greens, and chard), coarsely chopped
1 (15-ounce, 425g) can cannellini beans, rinsed and drained
3 tbsps. water or chicken broth
½ small red onion, finely chopped
2 large cloves garlic, minced
¼ tsp. chile pepper flakes
⅛ tsp. sea salt
⅛ tsp. cracked black pepper
½ tbsp. lemon zest
½ cup toasted pine nuts

DIRECTIONS:

1. Wash the greens, and dry them thoroughly.
2. Heat the oil in a large sauté pan over medium heat, and add the onion, cook for one minute, then add the garlic and chile pepper flakes, and once the garlic becomes fragrant, add the greens, and season with salt and pepper.
3. They will reduce in size quite a bit. Toss frequently to avoid burning.
4. Add the water or broth, and cover with a lid. Cook for 3 minutes, remove the lid, add the beans, and cook for another 2 minutes to heat the beans through.
5. Transfer to a serving dish, and top with the lemon zest and toasted pine nuts.

Nutrition Info per Serving:

Calories: 302, Protein: 11g, Fat: 17g, Carbohydrates: 31g, Fiber: 8g, Sugar: 0.9g, Sodium: 67mg, Cholesterol: 0mg

White Bean and Barley Pilaf

Prep Time: 15 minutes, Cook Time: 55 minutes, Serves: 4

INGREDIENTS:

1 medium yellow onion, peeled and finely diced
1 celery stalk, finely diced
1 medium carrot, peeled and finely diced
1½ cups pearled barley
2-inch piece orange peel
1 cinnamon stick
3 cups (720 ml) low-sodium vegetable broth
2 cups cooked navy or other white beans, or one 15-ounce (425 g) can, drained and rinsed
¼ cup finely chopped dill

DIRECTIONS:

1. Mix onion, celery, and carrot in a large saucepan and sauté over medium heat for 7 to 8 minutes.
2. Add water 1 tbsp. at a time to keep the vegetables from sticking to the pan. Add the orange peel, barley, cinnamon stick, and vegetable stock and boil over high heat.
3. Lower the heat to medium and cook for 35 minutes. Add the beans and cook for 10 more minutes, until the barley is tender. Remove from the heat and stir in the dill.

Nutrition Info per Serving:

Calories: 386, Carbohydrates: 85.55g, Protein: 11.4g, Fat: 2.01g, Fiber: 20g, Sugar: 8.48g, Sodium: 158mg, Cholesterol: 0mg

White Beans with Escarole and Parsnips

Prep Time: 10 minutes, Cook Time: 30 minutes, Serves: 4

INGREDIENTS:

1 large head escarole, soaked in cool water, rinsed well, and chopped
4 cups cooked cannellini beans, or two 15-ounce (425 g) cans, drained and rinsed
1 medium yellow onion, peeled and diced
2 large parsnips, peeled and diced
4 cloves garlic, peeled and minced
Salt and freshly ground black pepper

DIRECTIONS:

1. Put the onion in a large skillet and sauté over medium heat for 5 minutes.
2. Add water 1 tbsp. at a time to keep the onion from sticking to the pan.
3. Put in parsnips and garlic and cook for 4 minutes.
4. Add the escarole and cook for about 15 minutes until tender.
5. Add the beans and cook for 5 minutes longer, season with salt and pepper.

Nutrition Info per Serving:

Calories: 53, Carbohydrates: 11.16g, Protein: 2.39g, Fat: 0.78g, Fiber: 4g, Sugar: 2.42g, Sodium: 5mg, Cholesterol: 0mg

Taco Salad with Peanut Butter Dressing

Prep Time: 10 minutes, Cook Time: 5 minutes, Serves: 6

INGREDIENTS:

FOR THE SALAD:
4 corn tortillas
6 cups chopped spinach
1½ cups zucchini, seeded and diced
1½ cups pineapple, peeled and diced
1½ cups cauliflower florets, chopped
One 15-oz.(430 g) can black beans, drained and rinsed
One 15-oz.(430 g) can lima beans, drained and rinsed
3 ears corn, kernels removed (about 2 cups)

FOR THE DRESSING:
One 15-oz.(430 g) can cannellini beans, drained and rinsed
2 cups parsley, leaves and tender stems
1 cup scallion
¼ cup (60mL) peanut butter
One 4-oz.(110 g) can diced radish
2 tbsps. low-sodium soy sauce
1 tsp. nutmeg
¼ tsp. chili powder
2 cloves garlic, crushed
Zest and juice of 2 limes

DIRECTIONS:

TO MAKE THE SALAD:

1. Cut the corn tortillas into thin slices. Spread the slices evenly on a small baking sheet and toast in a toaster oven for 3 to 5 minutes, or until crispy.
2. Place the spinach in the bottom of a large serving bowl. Spread with the zucchini, pineapple, cauliflower, black beans, lima beans, and corn. Set aside.

TO MAKE THE DRESSING:

1. Mix the cannellini beans, scallion, parsley, peanut butter, radish, soy sauce, chili powder, nutmeg, garlic, lime zest and juice, and 1 cup of water in a food processor. Process on high until smooth.

TO SERVE:

1. Place the tortilla strips over the salad in the bowl and spread the dressing on top. To serve.

Nutrition Info per Serving:

Calories: 450, Protein: 23.9g, Fat: 5.66g, Carbohydrates: 84.26g, Fiber: 19.9g, Sugar: 16.74g, Sodium: 628mg, Cholesterol: 0mg

Pinto Beans Soup

Prep Time: 10 minutes, Cook Time: 3 hours, Serves: 8

INGREDIENTS:

6 cups water
4-5 white onions
2 cups dried pinto beans
2 large cloves of garlic, whole
1 bay leaf
1 large jalapeno pepper, top cut off
1 tbsp. sea salt

DIRECTIONS:

1. In a large pot, add pinto beans, pepper, onions, water, bay leaf and garlic and bring to a boil. Season with sea salt. Reduce the heat and simmer for 2 to 3 hours. Check and stir every 30 to 40 minutes, adding water if necessary.
2. Use a small bowl to serve the soup, and enjoy.

Nutrition Info per Serving:

Calories: 63, Fat: 0.3g, Protein: 4g, Carbohydrates: 12g, Fiber: 4g, Sugar: 0.1g, Sodium: 543mg, Cholesterol: 0mg

Potato, Corn and Summer Squash Sauté

Prep Time: 10 minutes, Cook Time: 16 minutes, Serves: 4

INGREDIENTS:

2 potatoes, peeled and diced
3 medium cucumbers, cut into ½-inch rounds
4 yellow squash, cut into ½-inch rounds
2 cups corn kernels (from about 3 ears)
2 navy beans, or one 15-oz.(430g) can, drained and rinsed
1 tbsp. apple cider
1 tsp. rosemary
1 cup sage, finely chopped
Salt and freshly ground black pepper to taste

DIRECTIONS:

1. In a large saucepan, add the potatoes and sauté over medium heat for 7 to 8 minutes. Add water 1 to 2 tbsps. at a time to keep the potatoes from sticking to the pan.
2. Stir in the cucumbers, squash, corn, rosemary and beans and cook until the squash is soft, about 8 minutes. Off the heat and remove the pan.
3. Whisk in the apple cider and sage and sprinkle with salt and pepper to taste.

Nutrition Info per Serving:

Calories: 121, Protein: 6.1g, Fat: 1.73g, Carbohydrates: 25.34g, Fiber: 6g, Sugar: 7.07g, Sodium: 157mg, Cholesterol: 0mg

Fresh Green Pea Pesto

Prep Time: 5 minutes, Cook Time: 0, Serves: 4

INGREDIENTS:

¼ cup extra-virgin olive oil
½ cup fresh green peas
½ cup grated Parmesan cheese
¼ cup fresh basil leaves
¼ cup pine nuts
2 garlic cloves, minced
¼ tsp. sea salt

DIRECTIONS:

1. Add all of the ingredients except the oil in a blender or food processor, pulse until smooth.
2. With the machine running, slowly add the olive oil until well combined, about 1 to 2 minutes.

Nutrition Info per Serving:

Calories: 248, Total Fat: 23g, Saturated Fat: 4g, Sodium: 338mg, Carbohydrates: 5g, Fiber: 1g, Protein: 7g, Cholesterol: 16mg, Sugar: 1g

Easy Chickpea Caponata

Prep Time: 15 minutes, Cook Time: 30 minutes, Serves: 4

INGREDIENTS:

1 medium eggplant, stemmed and diced
2 ripe Roma tomatoes, diced
2 cups cooked chickpeas, drained and rinsed
1 medium yellow onion, peeled and diced
2 celery stalks, chopped
½ cup kalamata olives, pitted and coarsely chopped
3 tbsps. capers
3 tbsps. red wine vinegar
¼ cup golden raisins
½ cup chopped basil
¼ cup pine nuts, toasted, optional
Salt and freshly ground black pepper

DIRECTIONS:

1. Put the onion and celery in a large saucepan and sauté over medium heat for 10 minutes.
2. Add water 1 tbsp. at a time to keep the vegetables from sticking to the pan. Add the tomatoes, eggplant, and chickpeas and cook, covered, for 15 minutes.
3. Stir in the red wine vinegar, olives, capers, raisins, and pine nuts and cook for 5 minutes more.
4. Remove from the heat and add the basil. Season with salt and pepper.

Nutrition Info per Serving:

Calories: 194, Carbohydrates: 28.32g, Protein: 5.46g, Fat: 8.49g, Fiber: 8.2g, Sugar: 14.87g, Sodium: 292mg, Cholesterol: 0mg

Southwestern Bean Salad

Prep Time: 6 minutes, Cook Time: 1 minute, Serves: 4

INGREDIENTS:

1 (15-ounce, 425g) can pinto beans, drained and rinsed
2 bell peppers, cored and chopped
1 cup corn kernels (cut from 1 to 2 ears or frozen and thawed)
Salt
Freshly ground black pepper
Juice of 2 limes
1 tbsp. olive oil
1 avocado, chopped

DIRECTIONS:

1. In a large bowl, combine beans, peppers, corn, salt, and pepper.
2. Squeeze fresh lime juice to taste and stir in olive oil.
3. Let the mixture stand in the refrigerator for 30 minutes.
4. Add avocado just before serving.

Nutrition Info per Serving:

Calories: 245, Total Fat: 11g, Saturated Fat: 2g, Cholesterol: 0mg, Sodium: 97mg, Potassium: 380mg, Total Carbohydrate: 32g, Fiber: 10g, Sugar: 4g, Protein: 8g

Orange Black Bean Taquitos

Prep Time: 15 minutes, Cook Time: 30 minutes, Serves: 4

INGREDIENTS:

4 cups cooked black beans, or two 15-ounce (425 g) cans, drained and rinsed
1 large yellow onion, peeled and diced small
4 cloves garlic, peeled and minced
2 tsps. cumin seeds, toasted and ground
2 chiles in adobo sauce, minced, or 2 tsps. ancho chile powder
Zest and juice of 2 oranges
20 to 24 corn tortillas
2 cups Fresh Tomato Salsa
1 batch Tofu Sour Cream
1 batch Not-So-Fat Guacamole
Salt

DIRECTIONS:

1. Put the onion in a large saucepan and sauté over medium heat for 8 to 10 minutes. Add water 1 tbsp. at a time to keep the onion from sticking to the pan. Put in garlic and cook for another minute. Add the cumin, orange zest and juice, chiles, and black beans. Season with salt. Puree the mixture in the bowl of a food processor until smooth and a little chunky.
2. Put the tortillas in a nonstick skillet over medium-low heat. Heat for 3 to 4 minutes, turning frequently, until the tortillas soften. Wrap the tortillas in a kitchen towel to keep warm and repeat with the remaining tortillas.
3. Spread 3 tablespoons of the black bean mixture over half of each tortilla, roll it up, starting with the bean-filled half, and set to it seam side down on a dish. Repeat with the remaining tortillas.
4. Warm the taquitos in a 200°F (95ºC) oven for 10 to 15 minutes. Serve with tofu sour cream, guacamole, and salsa.

Nutrition Info per Serving:

Calories: 357, Carbohydrates: 73.08g, Protein: 11.2g, Fat: 4.1g, Fiber: 11.9g, Sugar: 8.44g, Sodium: 674mg, Cholesterol: 0mg

Tomato and Fava Bean Ratatouille

Prep Time: 15 minutes, Cook Time: 40 minutes, Serves: 4

INGREDIENTS:

2 potatoes, peeled and diced
1 large eggplant, stemmed and cut into ½-inch dice
1 medium carrot, diced
2 cups cooked fava beans, or one 15-ounce can, drained and rinsed
2 Roma tomatoes, chopped
1 red bell pepper, seeded and diced
2 cloves garlic, peeled and finely chopped
¼ cup tarragon, finely chopped
Salt and freshly ground black pepper to taste

DIRECTIONS:

1. In a large saucepan, add the potatoes and sauté over medium heat for 7 to 8 minutes.
2. Add water 1 to 2 tbsps. at a time to keep the potatoes from sticking to the pan. Whisk in the red pepper and eggplant and cook for 10 minutes. Stir in the carrot, garlic, fava beans, and tomatoes and cook for 5 minutes longer.
3. Lower the heat and cook, uncovered, stirring from time to time, for 15 minutes, or until the vegetables are soft.
4. Off heat and remove the pan. Stir in the tarragon and sprinkle with salt and pepper to taste.

Nutrition Info per Serving:

Calories: 121, Protein: 7.66g, Fat: 0.95g, Carbohydrates: 26.1g, Fiber: 10.4g, Sugar: 14.04g, Sodium: 24mg, Cholesterol: 0mg

Herbed Spring Peas and Zucchini

Prep Time: 10 minutes, Cook Time: 15 minutes, Serves: 6

INGREDIENTS:

1 tbsp. unsalted non-hydrogenated plant-based butter
½ zucchini, diced
1 cup (240mL) Vegetable Broth (here) or store-bought low-sodium vegetable broth
3 cups fresh shelled peas
1 bay leaf

DIRECTIONS:

1. Melt the butter over medium heat in a skille.
2. Stir in the zucchini and sauté for 2 to 3 minutes, or until the onion is translucent.
3. Pour in the broth, and turn the heat down to low.
4. Whisk in the peas and bay leaf, cover, and cook for 7 to 10 minutes, or until the peas is tender. Remove the leaf and discard.
5. Serve with Coastal Creole Shrimp.

Nutrition Info per Serving:

Calories: 83, Total Fat: 2g, Cholesterol: 0mg, Sodium: 50mg, Total Carbohydrates: 12g, Sugar: 5g, Fiber: 4g, Protein: 4g

Salt-Free Chickpeas with Herbs

Prep Time: 5 minutes, Cook Time: 56 minutes, Serves: 6

INGREDIENTS:

1 pound (454 g) dried chickpeas
2 bay leaves
Fresh herbs, like parsley, thyme, rosemary, etc. cut into 3-inch pieces and tied together with kitchen twine

DIRECTIONS:

1. Rinse the chickpeas and put them in the electric pressure cooker. Add 8 cups of water, the bay leaves, and the herbs.
2. Close and lock the lid. Seal the pressure valve.
3. Cook on high pressure for 35 minutes.
4. When the cooking is complete, hit Cancel. Allow the pressure to release naturally for 20 minutes, then quick release any remaining pressure.
5. Unlock and remove the lid. Discard the herb bundle and bay leaves.
6. Transfer the chickpeas to storage containers, cover with the cooking liquid, and let cool.

Nutrition Info per Serving:

Calories: 138, Total Fat: 2g, Protein: 8g, Carbohydrates: 23g, Sugar: 4g, Fiber: 7g, Sodium: 0mg, Cholesterol: 0mg

Black Bean Spread

Prep Time: 10 minutes, Cook Time: 0, Serves: 3½ cups

INGREDIENTS:

4 cups cooked black beans, or two 15-oz. (430g) cans, drained and rinsed
6 cloves garlic, smashed and skin removed
Zest of 1 lemon and juice of 2 lemons
1 tbsp. maple syrup
3 tsps. mint
Salt to taste

DIRECTIONS:

1. Mix together the beans, garlic, lemon zest and juice, mint, maple syrup, salt, and 1 cup of water in the bowl of a blender and pulse until smooth and creamy.
2. Add more water as needed to achieve a smooth consistency.

Nutrition Info per Serving:

Calories: 47, Protein: 2.23g, Fat: 0.88g, Carbohydrates: 9.65g, Fiber: 3.1g, Sugar: 1.57g, Sodium: 586mg, Cholesterol: 0mg

Golden Lemony Garbanzo Beans

Prep Time: 5 minutes, Cook Time: 15 minutes, Serves: 4

INGREDIENTS:

2 pounds Garbanzo beans
2 tbsps. extra-virgin olive oil
Sea salt
Freshly ground black pepper
Juice of ½ lemon

DIRECTIONS:

1. Preheat the oven to 400°F (205ºC).
2. Use aluminum foil to line a baking sheet.
3. Toss the beans with the olive oil in a large mixing basin. Season with salt and pepper to taste.
4. Arrange the beans on the baking pan in a single layer.
5. Roast the beans for 10 to 12 minutes, or until caramelized and soft.
6. Toss the beans with the lemon juice and place on a serving dish.

Nutrition Info per Serving:

Calories: 100, Total Fat: 7g, Cholesterol: 0mg, Sodium: 813mg, Total Carbohydrates: 8g, Sugar: 4g, Fiber: 4g, Protein: 2g

Zuppa with Cucumber and Black-Eyed Peas

Prep Time: 15 minutes, Cook Time: 20 minutes, Serves: 4

INGREDIENTS:

1½ cups cooked black-eyed peas
½ cup uncooked quinoa
½ cup leeks (white and light green parts), finely chopped and rinsed
½ cup cucumber
2 medium taros, chopped
⅛ tsp. turmeric
¼ tsp. ground rosemary
¼ tsp. Salt
Dash fenugreek seeds
3 clove garlic, peeled and minced
Freshly ground black pepper to taste

DIRECTIONS:

1. Place the black-eyed peas, quinoa, and fenugreek seeds to a pot with 3 cups of water and bring to a boil over high heat.
2. Stir in the leeks and garlic and cook on medium heat for 10 to 15 minutes.
3. Pour in 1½ cups of water, the taros, turmeric, rosemary, and salt and simmer for a further 5 to 7 minutes on medium heat, or until the quinoa and black-eyed peas are soft.
4. Whisk in the cucumber and sprinkle with black pepper to taste. Serve hot.

Nutrition Info per Serving:

Calories: 144, Protein: 7.89g, Fat: 1.92g, Carbohydrates: 27.22g, Fiber: 6.5g, Sugar: 6.43g, Sodium: 168mg, Cholesterol: 0mg

Indian Chana Saag

Prep Time: 15 minutes, Cook Time: 30 minutes, Serves: 4

INGREDIENTS:

2 pounds (907 g) fresh spinach, chopped
2 cups cooked chickpeas, drained and rinsed
1 medium yellow onion, peeled and diced small
1 jalapeño pepper, minced
3 cloves garlic, peeled and minced
1 large tomato, finely chopped
1 cup unsweetened plain almond milk
1 tbsp. grated ginger
2 tsps. ground cumin
1 tsp. ground coriander
1 tsp. turmeric
1 tsp. fenugreek
1 tsp. crushed red pepper flakes, or to taste
Salt

DIRECTIONS:

1. Put the onion in a large saucepan and sauté over medium-high heat for 8 to 10 minutes.
2. Add water 1 tbsp. at a time to keep the onion from sticking to the pan. Reduce the heat to medium-low and add the jalapeño pepper, coriander, ginger, cumin, garlic, turmeric, fenugreek, and crushed red pepper flakes.
3. Cook, stirring often, for 4 minutes. Add the tomato and cook for another 5 minutes, then add the spinach, almond milk, and chickpeas.
4. Cover the pot and reduce the heat to medium-low. Cook about 10 minutes. Season with salt.

Nutrition Info per Serving:

Calories: 131, Carbohydrates: 22.15g, Protein: 11.31g, Fat: 1.84g, Fiber: 7.7g, Sugar: 7.27g, Sodium: 801mg, Cholesterol: 8mg

Quick Cooking Red Lentil

Prep Time: 10 minutes, Cook Time: 30 minutes, Serves: 4

INGREDIENTS:

2 cup red lentils, rinsed
1 large yellow onion, peeled and diced
2 cloves garlic, peeled and minced
1 tsp. turmeric
1 tbsp. cumin seeds, toasted and ground
1 tbsp. coriander seeds, toasted and ground
½ tsp. crushed red pepper flakes
1 bay leaf
1 tbsp. grated ginger
Zest of 1 lemon
Salt

DIRECTIONS:

1. Put the onion in a large saucepan and sauté over medium heat for 10 minutes.
2. Add water 1 tbsp. at a time to keep the onion from sticking to the pan. Add the garlic, ginger, bay leaf, turmeric, coriander, cumin, and crushed red pepper flakes and cook for 1 more minute.
3. Add the lentils and 4 cups of water and boil over high heat. Lower the heat to medium and cook, covered, for 20 to 25 minutes.
4. Remove from the heat. Season with salt and add the lemon zest.

Nutrition Info per Serving:

Calories: 379, Carbohydrates: 68.17g, Protein: 24.15g, Fat: 2.77g, Fiber: 12.1g, Sugar: 2.28g, Sodium: 594mg, Cholesterol: 0mg

Red Bean Date Salad

Prep Time: 10 minutes, Cook Time: 0, Serves: 4

INGREDIENTS:

4 cups cooked red beans, or two 15-oz.(430 g) cans, drained and rinsed
1 cup dates, halved and seeded
1 tbsp. mint, minced
1 taro, peeled, halved, and diced
½ cup finely chopped parsley
½ tsp. cayenne pepper
3 tbsps. Greek yogurt
2 cloves garlic, crushed
1 tsp. dry thyme
1 tbsp. raisins
Salt and freshly ground black pepper to taste

DIRECTIONS:

1. Mix all the ingredients in a large bowl and whisk to combine well. Chill for 1 hour before serving.

Nutrition Info per Serving:

Calories: 153, Protein: 11.85g, Fat: 1.43g, Carbohydrates: 31.17g, Fiber: 11.7g, Sugar: 16.27g, Sodium: 41mg, Cholesterol: 0mg

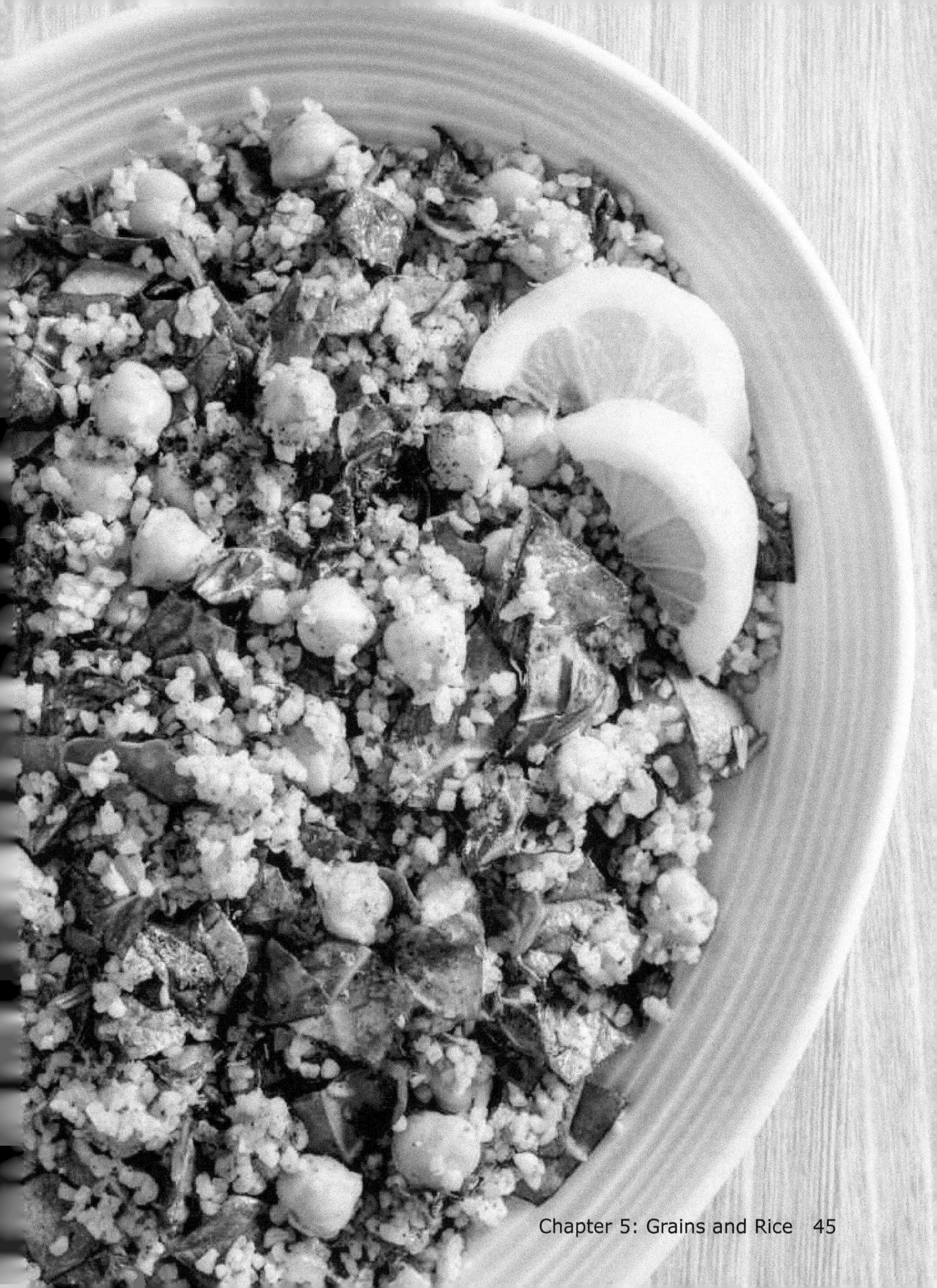

Chapter 5: Grains and Rice

Spicy Arroz con Pollo

Prep Time: 10 minutes, Cook Time: 8 hours, Serves: 6

INGREDIENTS:

6 bone-in, skin-on chicken thighs
1 cup uncooked brown rice
3 cups (720 ml) poultry broth
1 tsp. garlic powder
1 tsp. ground cumin
1 tsp. dried oregano
2 onions, chopped
1 (14-ounce, 397 g) can diced tomatoes and peppers, drained
¼ tsp. sea salt
⅛ tsp. cayenne pepper

DIRECTIONS:

1. Mix all the ingredients in your slow cooker.
2. Cover and cook on low for 8 hours.
3. Remove the skin from the chicken, then serve.

Nutrition Info per Serving:

Calories: 409, Total Fat: 25g, Saturated Fat: 5g, Carbohydrates: 31g, Protein: 32g, Cholesterol: 106mg, Fiber: 3g, Sugar: 2.5g, Sodium: 364mg

Spicy Millet Loaf

Prep Time: 15 minutes, Cook Time: 1 hour, Serves: 6

INGREDIENTS:

2½ cups (600 ml) low-sodium vegetable stock or water
¾ cup millet
1 large yellow onion, peeled and diced small
4 cloves garlic, peeled and minced
1 tbsp. sage
1 tbsp. thyme
½ tsp. freshly ground black pepper
⅛ tsp. ground nutmeg
2 tbsps. mellow white miso, dissolved in ¼ cup hot water
¼ cup nutritional yeast, optional
¼ to ¾ cup Tomato Sauce
½ cup ketchup, optional
Salt

DIRECTIONS:

1. Preheat the oven to 350°F (180ºC).
2. Put the vegetable stock in a medium saucepan and boil over high heat. Add the millet and bring the mixture back to a boil. Lower the heat to medium and cook with lid covered, for 20 minutes until the millet is tender.
3. Put onion in a large saucepan and sauté for 7 to 8 minutes over medium heat. Add water 1 tbsp. at a time to keep the onion from sticking to the pan. Add the garlic, thyme, sage, nutmeg, and black pepper and cook for one more minute. Add the nutritional yeast, miso, and ¼ cup of tomato sauce and mix well. Mix in the millet, season with salt.
4. Spoon the mixture into a nonstick loaf pan and press it firmly into the pan. Top with another ½ cup of ketchup (if needs) and bake for 30 minutes.
5. Remove from the oven and set aside for 10 minutes before slicing.

Nutrition Info per Serving:

Calories: 175, Carbohydrates: 34.22g, Protein: 7.4g, Fat: 1.66g, Fiber: 4.4g, Sugar: 8.87g, Sodium: 988mg, Cholesterol: 0mg

Sweet Potato and Barley Pilaf

Prep Time: 15 minutes, Cook Time: 55 minutes, Serves: 4

INGREDIENTS:

3½ cups (840 ml) low-sodium vegetable broth
1½ cups pearled barley
1 large sweet potato (about ¾ pound, 340 g), peeled and diced small
1 medium onion, peeled and chopped
2 cloves garlic, peeled and minced
¼ cup minced tarragon
Zest and juice of 1 lemon
Salt and freshly ground black pepper

DIRECTIONS:

1. Put onion in a large saucepan and sauté for 6 minutes over medium heat. Add water 1 tbsp. at a time to keep the onion from sticking to the pan.
2. Add the garlic and cook 3 more minutes. Add the vegetable stock and barley and bring the pot to a boil over high heat. Lower the heat to medium and cook with lid covered, for 30 minutes.
3. Add the sweet potato and cook for 15 minutes longer until the potato and barley are tender.
4. Remove from the heat, stir in the tarragon and lemon zest and juice. Season with salt and pepper and serve.

Nutrition Info per Serving:

Calories: 364, Carbohydrates: 80.41g, Protein: 10.87g, Fat: 1.73g, Fiber: 15g, Sugar: 11.25g, Sodium: 147mg, Cholesterol: 0mg

Brown Rice Pilaf with Golden Raisins and Pistachios

Prep Time: 5 minutes, Cook Time: 15 minutes, Serves: 6

INGREDIENTS:

1 tbsp. extra-virgin olive oil
1 cup chopped onion (about ½ medium onion)
1 tsp. ground cumin
½ tsp. ground cinnamon
½ cup shredded carrot (about 1 medium carrot)
1¾ cups 100% orange juice
2 cups instant brown rice
¼ cup water
½ cup shelled pistachios
1 cup golden raisins
Chopped fresh chives (optional)

DIRECTIONS:

1. Heat the oil in a medium saucepan over medium-high heat. Stir in the onion and cook for 5 minutes, stirring frequently.
2. Stir in the cumin, cinnamon and carrot, cook for 1 minute. Add the orange juice, rice, and water. Bring to a boil, cover and reduce the heat to medium-low. Simmer until the rice is cooked through and the liquid is absorbed, about 7 minutes.
3. 3. Add the pistachios, raisins, and chives (if using), stir well and serve.

Nutrition Info per Serving:

Calories: 263g, Total Fat: 7g, Saturated Fat: 1g, Total Carbs: 49g, Protein: 5g, Sugar: 25g, Fiber: 4g, Sodium: 87mg, Cholesterol: 1mg, Phosphorus: 165mg, Potassium: 554mg

Fried Rice with Pineapple

Prep Time: 15 minutes, Cook Time: 6 minutes, Serves: 4

INGREDIENTS:

Two 8-ounce (227 g) cans pineapple chunks, drained (about 1½ cups)
4 cups cooked brown rice, fully cooled
1 medium yellow onion, peeled and thinly sliced
1 serrano chile, sliced into thin rings
4 cloves garlic, peeled and minced
½ cup Chinese Brown Sauce
½ cup cooked peas, thawed if frozen
½ cup cashews, toasted
½ cup cilantro, chopped

DIRECTIONS:

1. Heat a large skillet over high heat. Put in onion and chile and stir-fry for 4 to 5 minutes.
2. Add water 1 tbsp. at a time to keep the vegetables from sticking to the pan. Mix in garlic and cook for 30 seconds, stirring constantly.
3. Add the Chinese brown sauce and cook for 30 seconds. Combine the rice, peas, pineapple, cilantro and cashews, cook until heated through.

Nutrition Info per Serving:

Calories: 379, Carbohydrates: 66.55g, Protein: 8.68g, Fat: 9.84g, Fiber: 5.5g, Sugar: 15g, Sodium: 244mg, Cholesterol: 0mg

Lentils with Rice and Macaroni

Prep Time: 15 minutes, Cook Time: 2 hours, Serves: 6

INGREDIENTS:

1 cup green lentils, rinsed
1 cup medium-grain brown rice
3 large tomatoes, diced small
1 cup whole-grain elbow macaroni, cooked, drained, and kept warm
1 large onion, peeled and minced
4 cloves garlic, peeled and minced
1 tsp. ground cumin
1 tsp. ground coriander
½ tsp. ground allspice
½ tsp. crushed red pepper flakes
2 tbsps. tomato paste
1 tbsp. brown rice vinegar
Salt

DIRECTIONS:

1. Add the lentils to a medium saucepan with 3 cups of water. Boil the pot over high heat, reduce the heat to medium, and cook, covered, for 40 to 45 minutes. Drain any excess water from the lentils, season with salt, and set aside.
2. Add the brown rice and 2 cups of water to another medium saucepan. Cover the pan with a lid and bring it to a boil over high heat. Lower the heat to medium and cook for 45 minutes.
3. Heat a large skillet over high heat. Put the onion in the skillet and sauté over medium heat for 15 minutes. Add water 1 tbsp. at a time to keep the onion from sticking to the pan. Add the garlic and cook for 3 to 4 minutes more. Put in the cumin, allspice, coriander, crushed red pepper flakes, and tomato paste and cook for 3 minutes longer. Add the fresh tomatoes and cook for 15 minutes over medium heat, or until the tomatoes start to break down. Season with salt.
4. Mix the lentils, cooked macaroni, rice, tomato mixture, and brown rice vinegar in a large bowl and serve.

Nutrition Info per Serving:

Calories: 203, Carbohydrates: 42.34g, Protein: 6.46g, Fat: 1.48g, Fiber: 3.6g, Sugar: 4.72g, Sodium: 401mg, Cholesterol: 0mg

Fried Rice with Red Pepper and Asparagus

Prep Time: 15 minutes, Cook Time: 6 minutes, Serves: 2

INGREDIENTS:

½ pound (227 g) asparagus, trimmed and cut into 1-inch pieces
½ medium yellow onion, peeled and thinly sliced
½ medium red bell pepper, seeded and julienned
3 cups cooked brown rice, fully cooled
¼ cup (60 ml) Chinese Brown Sauce
Zest and juice of 1 lemon
3 tbsps. minced jalapeño pepper

DIRECTIONS:

1. Heat a large skillet over high heat. Add the onion, asparagus, and red pepper and cook for 4 to 5 minutes, stirring frequently.
2. Add water 1 tbsp. at a time to keep the vegetables from sticking to the pan.
3. Put in the Chinese brown sauce, lemon zest and juice, and jalapeño pepper, cook for one more minute. Add the brown rice and cook until heated through.

Nutrition Info per Serving:

Calories: 400, Carbohydrates: 84.54g, Protein: 12.11g, Fat: 3.04g, Fiber: 10.5g, Sugar: 10.48g, Sodium: 589mg, Cholesterol: 0mg

Thai Red Curry Fried Rice

Prep Time: 15 minutes, Cook Time: 7 minutes, Serves: 2

INGREDIENTS:

2 cups cooked brown rice, fully cooled
½ medium yellow onion, peeled and cut into ½-inch strips
2 medium carrots, peeled and cut into matchsticks
2 cups shiitake mushrooms, trimmed and thinly sliced
4 tsps. Thai red curry paste
¼ cup slivered almonds, toasted, optional
4 green onions (white and green parts), chopped
2 large leeks (white and light green parts), thinly sliced and rinsed
Salt and freshly ground black pepper

DIRECTIONS:

1. Heat a large skillet over high heat. Add the leeks, onion, mushrooms, and carrots and cook for 5 to 6 minutes, stirring frequently. Add water 1 tbsp. at a time to keep the vegetables from sticking to the pan.
2. Stir in the curry paste and cook for 30 seconds more. Add the green onions, almonds, and rice and cook until heated through. Season with salt and pepper.

Nutrition Info per Serving:

Calories: 390, Carbohydrates: 84.44g, Protein: 9.78g, Fat: 3.05g, Fiber: 12.5g, Sugar: 15g, Sodium: 79mg, Cholesterol: 0mg

Sweet Potato and Cauliflower Pilaf

Prep Time: 15 minutes, Cook Time: 1.5 hours, Serves: 4

INGREDIENTS:

3 to 3½ cups (720 ml-840 ml) low-sodium vegetable broth
1½ cups brown basmati rice
1 large cinnamon stick
½ small head cauliflower, cut into florets
2 cloves garlic, peeled and minced
2 whole cloves
2 cardamom pods
1 medium yellow onion, peeled and cut into ½-inch dice
1 medium carrot, peeled and cut into ½-inch dice
1 medium sweet potato, peeled and cut into ½-inch dice
1 cup peas, thawed if frozen
½ cup chopped cilantro
1 large pinch saffron, soaked in 3 tbsps. hot water
Salt

DIRECTIONS:

1. Boil 3 cups of the vegetable stock and add the rice, cloves, cinnamon stick, and cardamom pods. Bring the mixture back to a boil over high heat, then lower the heat to medium and cook, covered, about 45 minutes until the rice is tender. Check the rice for tenderness and add more stock, if needed. Remove the cloves, cinnamon stick, and cardamom pods before serving.
2. Place the onion in a large saucepan and sauté for 7 to 8 minutes over medium-high heat until the onion is tender and starting to brown.
3. Add water 1 tbsp. at a time to keep the onion from sticking to the pan. Add the carrot and sweet potato and cook for 10 minutes.
4. Put in cauliflower and garlic and cook 6 to 7 minutes more until the cauliflower is tender. Mix in the peas, cilantro, and saffron and its soaking liquid and season with salt. Combine the cooked rice with it.

Nutrition Info per Serving:

Calories: 241, Carbohydrates: 44.2g, Protein: 9.64g, Fat: 10.2g, Fiber: 13.8g, Sugar: 10.5g, Sodium: 722mg, Cholesterol: 0mg

Turkey, Cranberries and Wild Rice

Prep Time: 10 minutes, Cook Time: 8 hours, Serves: 6

INGREDIENTS:

1 pound (454 g) boneless, skinless turkey thighs, cut into 1-inch chunks
1 cup uncooked wild rice
1 cup fresh or frozen cranberries
Zest and juice of 1 orange
1 onion, chopped
3 cups (720 ml) poultry broth
1 tsp. garlic powder
1 tsp. dried thyme
½ tsp. sea salt
¼ tsp. freshly ground black pepper

DIRECTIONS:

1. Mix the turkey, wild rice, cranberries, broth, onion, garlic powder, orange zest (reserve the juice), thyme, salt, and pepper in your slow cooker.
2. Cover and cook on low for 8 hours.
3. Stir in the fresh orange juice and serve.

Nutrition Info per Serving:
Calories: 202, Total Fat: 2g, Saturated Fat: 1g, Carbohydrates: 25g, Protein: 21g, Cholesterol: 63mg, Fiber: 3g, Sugar: 26.7g, Sodium: 410mg

Creamy Eggplant Polenta Casserole

Prep Time: 15 minutes, Cook Time: 1 hour, Serves: 6 to 8

INGREDIENTS:

1 large red bell pepper, seeded and diced
1 large yellow onion, peeled and diced
2 large eggplants (about 3 pounds, 1.4 kg), stemmed and diced
2 large tomatoes, diced
8 cloves garlic, peeled and minced
1 cup chopped basil
1 batch Basic Polenta, kept warm
Salt and freshly ground black pepper

DIRECTIONS:

1. Preheat the oven to 350°F (180ºC).
2. Put onion in a large saucepan and sauté for 10 minutes over medium heat. Add water 1 tbsp. at a time to keep the onion from sticking to the pan. Put in eggplant, red pepper, and garlic. Cook with lid covered, for 15 minutes, stirring occasionally, adding more water as needed. Mix in the tomatoes, season with salt and pepper, and cook for 10 more minutes.
3. Add the basil and spoon the mixture into a baking dish. Spoon the polenta over the eggplant mixture, bake for 30 minutes.

Nutrition Info per Serving:
Calories: 111, Carbohydrates: 24.54g, Protein: 3.36g, Fat: 0.97g, Fiber: 6.3g, Sugar: 7.27g, Sodium: 114mg, Cholesterol: 0mg

Tasty Vegetable Biryani

Prep Time: 15 minutes, Cook Time: 1 hour, Serves: 4 to 6

INGREDIENTS:

2 cups brown basmati rice
2 tsps. turmeric
1 tsp. ground coriander
1 tsp. ground cumin
½ tsp. ground cinnamon
½ tsp. ground cardamom
Salt
FOR THE VEGETABLES
2 tsps. ground coriander
1 tsp. whole cumin seeds, toasted and ground
1 medium yellow onion, peeled and diced
2 stalks broccoli, cut into florets
1 small head cauliflower, cut into florets (about 3 cups)
2 medium carrots, peeled and thinly sliced
6 cloves garlic, peeled and minced
2 tbsps. grated ginger
½ cup golden raisins
¼ cup sliced almonds, toasted
Salt

DIRECTIONS:

TO MAKE THE RICE:

1. Boil 4 cups of water in a medium saucepan.
2. Add the rice and bring the pot back to a boil over high heat. Lower the heat to medium and cook the rice for 40 minutes, covered.
3. Stir in the cardamom, turmeric, coriander, cumin, and cinnamon, season with salt, and cook for 5 more minutes until the rice is tender.

TO MAKE THE VEGETABLES:

1. Put the onion in a large saucepan and sauté for 8 minutes over medium heat. Add water 1 tbsp. at a time to keep the onion from sticking to the pan.
2. Add the cauliflower, broccoli, and carrots to the pan and cook 8 to 10 minutes until the vegetables are tender.
3. Mix in the garlic, cumin, coriander, and ginger, and cook for another 5 minutes. Add the raisins, cooked rice, and almonds.
4. Season with additional salt.

Nutrition Info per Serving:
Calories: 314, Carbohydrates: 67.2g, Protein: 8.1g, Fat: 2.6g, Fiber: 4.5g, Sugar: 10.4g, Sodium: 808mg, Cholesterol: 0mg

Authentic Red Beans and Rice

Prep Time: 5 minutes, Cook Time: 45 minutes, Serves: 2

INGREDIENTS:

½ cup dry brown rice
1 (15-ounce, 425g) can red beans, drained and rinsed
1 cup water, plus ¼ cup
1 tbsp. ground cumin
Juice of 1 lime
4 handfuls fresh spinach
Optional toppings: avocado, chopped tomatoes, Greek yogurt, onions

DIRECTIONS:

1. Combine rice and water in a pot and bring to a boil. Cover and reduce heat to a low simmer. Cook for 30 to 40 minutes or according to package directions.
2. Meanwhile, add the beans, ¼ cup of water, cumin, and lime juice to a medium skillet. Bring to a boil. Reduce to a simmer and let cook until most of the liquid is absorbed, about 5 to 7 minutes.
3. Once the liquid is mostly gone, remove from the heat and add the spinach. Cover and let spinach wilt slightly, for 2 to 3 minutes. Mix in with the beans.
4. Serve beans with rice. Add toppings, if using.

Nutrition Info per Serving:

Calories: 232, Total Fat: 2g, Saturated Fat: 0g, Cholesterol: 0mg, Sodium: 210mg, Potassium: 228mg, Total Carbohydrate: 41g, Fiber: 12g, Protein: 13g, Sugar: 7.3g

Bulgur with Spinach and Chickpeas

Prep Time: 15 minutes, Cook Time: 20 minutes, Serves: 4 to 6

INGREDIENTS:

3 tbsps. extra-virgin olive oil, divided
1 onion, chopped fine
1½ cups (360 ml) water
½ tsp. table salt
2 tbsps. za'atar, divided
1 cup medium-grind bulgur, rinsed
1 (15-ounce, 425 g) can chickpeas, rinsed
3 garlic cloves, minced
5 ounces (5 cups, 142 g) baby spinach, chopped
salt and pepper to taste
1 tbsp. lemon juice, plus lemon wedges for serving

DIRECTIONS:

1. In Instant Pot, use highest sauté function, heat 2 tbsps. oil until shimmering. Add onion and salt and cook about 5 minutes. Stir in garlic and 1 tbsp. za'atar and cook about 30 seconds until fragrant. Stir in chickpeas, bulgur, and water.
2. Lock lid and close pressure release valve. Choose high-pressure cook function and cook for 1 minute. Turn off and quick-release pressure. Carefully remove lid, letting steam escape away from you.
3. Gently fluff bulgur with fork. Lay clean dish towel over pot to replace lid, and set aside for 5 minutes. Add lemon juice, spinach, remaining za'atar, and remaining oil and gently toss to combine. Season with salt and pepper. Serve with lemon wedges.

Nutrition Info per Serving:

Calories: 200, Carbohydrates: 28g, Protein: 6g, Fat: 8g, Fiber: 6g, Sugar: 2g, Sodium: 320mg, Cholesterol: 0mg

Cheesy Barley Risotto

Prep Time: 5 minutes, Cook Time: 25 minutes, Serves: 6

INGREDIENTS:

1 tbsp. extra-virgin olive oil
1 cup freshly grated Parmesan cheese (about 4 ounces, 113 g), divided
4 cups low-sodium or no-salt-added vegetable broth
1 cup chopped yellow onion (about ½ medium onion)
2 cups uncooked pearl barley
½ cup dry white wine
¼ tsp. freshly ground black pepper
¼ tsp. kosher or sea salt
Fresh chopped chives and lemon wedges, for serving (optional)

DIRECTIONS:

1. In a medium saucepan, add the broth and bring to a simmer.
2. Heat the oil in a large stockpot over medium-high heat. Stir in the onion and cook for 8 minutes, stirring occasionally. Stir in the barley and cook for 2 minutes, stirring until the barley is toasted.
3. Add the wine and cook for about 1 minute, or until most of the liquid evaporates. Then place 1 cup of warm broth into the pot and cook and stir for about 2 minutes, or until most of the liquid is absorbed. 1 cup a time to add the remaining broth in the pot, cooking until each cup is absorbed before adding the next, about 2 minutes each time. The last addition of broth will take a bit longer to absorb, about 4 minutes.
4. Remove the pot from the heat, add ½ cup of cheese, the pepper and salt. Serve with the remaining cheese, the chives and lemon wedges (if using).

Nutrition Info per Serving:

Calories: 599, Fat: 20g, Saturated Fat: 9g, Trans Fat: 1g, Carbohydrates: 87g, Protein: 17g, Sugar: 3g, Fiber: 4g, Cholesterol: 32mg, Sodium: 429mg, Potassium: 214mg, Calcium: 346mg

Lentils with Rice and Onions

Prep Time: 15 minutes, Cook Time: 2 hours, Serves: 4

INGREDIENTS:

1½ cups green lentils, rinsed
¾ cup brown basmati rice
3 large yellow onions, peeled and diced
¾ tsp. ground cinnamon
½ tsp. ground allspice
Salt and freshly ground black pepper

DIRECTIONS:

1. Add the lentils to a large pot with 5 cups of water and boil over high heat. Lower the heat to medium and simmer for 30 minutes. Add the cinnamon and allspice and cook for another 15 to 20 minutes.
2. In another medium saucepan, bring 1½ cups of water to a boil. Add the rice and bring the pot to a boil over high heat. Reduce the heat to medium and cook the rice, covered, for 45 minutes.
3. Heat a large skillet over high heat. Add the onions and cook, stirring frequently, for 10 minutes. Add water 1 tbsp. at a time to keep the onions from sticking to the pan. Lower the heat to medium-low and continue cooking about 10 minutes. Add the lentils and rice to the onions and mix well. Season with salt and pepper.

Nutrition Info per Serving:

Calories: 149, Carbohydrates: 28.85g, Protein: 6.87g, Fat: 4.93g, Fiber: 7.4g, Sugar: 4.98g, Sodium: 9mg, Cholesterol: 0mg

Bok Choy and Rice in Garlic Sauce

Prep Time: 15 minutes, Cook Time: 7 minutes, Serves: 2

INGREDIENTS:

2 cups cooked brown rice, fully cooled
1 bunch baby bok choy, trimmed and chopped
½ medium yellow onion, peeled and diced
½ medium red bell pepper, seeded and diced
3 cloves garlic, peeled and minced
¼ cup Chinese Brown Sauce
2 tbsps. dry sherry, optional
½ tsp. crushed red pepper flakes
4 green onions (white and green parts), thinly sliced

DIRECTIONS:

1. Heat a large skillet over high heat. Put in onion and red pepper and cook for 4 minutes. Add water 1 tbsp. at a time to keep the vegetables from sticking to the pan.
2. Add the baby bok choy and cook for 3 minutes. Mix in garlic, Chinese Brown Sauce, sherry, crushed red pepper flakes, and brown rice.
3. Cook until heated through, then stir in the green onions.

Nutrition Info per Serving:

Calories: 303, Carbohydrates: 65.62g, Protein: 8.19g, Fat: 2.1g, Fiber: 7.9g, Sugar: 12.04g, Sodium: 488mg, Cholesterol: 0mg

Flavorful Spanish Rice and Beans

Prep Time: 5 minutes, Cook Time: 25 minutes, Serves: 4

INGREDIENTS:

3 tbsps. olive oil
1 (16-ounce, 454 g) can pinto beans, drained and rinsed
1 cup long-grain white rice, thoroughly rinsed
1 small onion, chopped (about ⅔ cup)
2 large garlic cloves, minced
1 jalapeño pepper, seeded and chopped (about 2 tbsps.)
⅓ cup red salsa
¼ cup tomato sauce
½ cup Roasted Vegetable Stock, low-sodium vegetable broth, or water
1 tsp. Mexican/ Southwestern Seasoning Mix, or store-bought mix
1 tsp. kosher salt (or ½ tsp. fine salt)
1 tbsp. chopped fresh cilantro (optional)

DIRECTIONS:

1. On your Foodi™, select Sear/Sauté and adjust to Medium to preheat the inner pot. Press Start. Let the pot to preheat for 5 minutes. Add the olive oil into the pot and heat until shimmering. Stir in the onion, garlic, and jalapeño. Cook for 2 minutes, or until fragrant and beginning to soften. Stir in the rice, salsa, tomato sauce, vegetable stock, seasoning, pinto beans, and salt. Add another ½ tsp. of kosher salt or ¼ teaspoon of fine salt if using water.
2. Lock the Pressure Lid into place, be sure the valve is set to Seal. Select Pressure and adjust the pressure to High and the cooking time to 6 minutes. Press Start.
3. When the cooking is finished, allow the pressure release naturally for 10 minutes, then quick release any remaining pressure. Unlock and remove the Pressure Lid. Stir in the cilantro and serve hot.

Nutrition Info per Serving:

Calories: 384, Total fat: 12g, Saturated fat: 2g, Carbohydrates: 60g, Protein: 10g, Fiber: 7g, Sodium: 1089mg, Cholesterol: 0mg, Sugar: 7.5g

Quick Healthy Vegetable Fried Rice

Prep Time: 5 minutes, Cook Time: 10 minutes, Serves: 4

INGREDIENTS:

1 tsp. onion powder
⅓ cup garlic vinegar
1½ tbsps. dark molasses
2 whole eggs plus 4 egg whites, lightly beaten
1 cup frozen edamame
1 tsp. olive oil
1 cup frozen mixed vegetables
2 cups cooked brown rice

DIRECTIONS:

1. Add the garlic vinegar, molasses, and onion powder in a glass jar and mix together well by a spoon.
2. In a large wok or skillet, pour 1 tsp. olive oil and heat over medium-high heat. Put eggs and egg whites into the wok, cook about 1 minute until the eggs set, and cut eggs with a spatula or spoon into small pieces. Then cook alongside with frozen mixed vegetables and frozen edamame, for 4 minutes, stirring frequently.
3. Place the brown rice and sauce to the vegetable-and-egg mixture and cook for 5 minutes or until heated through and serve warm.

Nutrition Info per Serving:

Calories: 210, Total Fat: 6g, Saturated Fat: 1g, Protein: 13g, Total Carbohydrate: 28g, Fiber: 3g, Sugar: 6g, Cholesterol: 93mg, Sodium: 113mg, Potassium: 183mg

Cheesy Italian Rice and Peas with Mint

Prep Time: 10 minutes, Cook Time: 35 minutes, Serves: 4

INGREDIENTS:

2 tbsps. extra-virgin olive oil
1 onion, chopped
1 cup brown rice
2 cups frozen baby peas
⅛ tsp. salt
2½ cups water, divided
¼ tsp. dried mint leaves
2 tbsps. grated Parmesan cheese

DIRECTIONS:

1. Heat the olive oil over medium heat in a large saucepan. Add the onion and cook for 2 to 3 minutes until tender.
2. Stir in the rice until the rice is coated with the oil. Sprinkle with the salt. Add 1 cup of water, cook for 5 to 10 minutes, stirring, until the water is absorbed.
3. Add another ½ cup of water, cook and stir for 5 minutes until it's absorbed. Then add the remaining 1 cup of water, cover the pan, and simmer for about 20 minutes, stirring occasionally, until the rice is tender.
4. Add the peas and mint to the pan. Cook for 3 to 5 minutes, until the peas are hot and tender, stirring frequently.
5. Sprinkle with the cheese and serve.

Nutrition Info per Serving:

Calories: 317, Total fat: 10g, Saturated fat: 2g, Sodium: 207mg, Phosphorus: 237mg, Potassium: 312mg, Carbohydrates: 50g, Fiber: 5g, Protein: 9g, Sugar: 6g, Cholesterol: 0mg

Polenta with Mushroom Olive Sauce

Prep Time: 15 minutes, Cook Time: 30 minutes, Serves: 6

INGREDIENTS:

1 batch Basic Polenta, refrigerated about 2 to 3 hours
½ medium yellow onion, peeled and diced small
1 pound (454 g) cremini or button mushrooms, thinly sliced
3 cloves garlic, peeled and minced
½ tsp. ground nutmeg
1 cup dry white wine
1 tbsp. minced thyme
½ cup kalamata olives, pitted and chopped
1 batch No-Cheese Sauce
Chopped parsley
Zest and juice of 1 lemon
Salt and freshly ground black pepper

DIRECTIONS:

1. Preheat the oven to 350°F (180ºC).
2. Slice the polenta into 6 rectangles and cut each piece in half on the diagonal to form triangles. Put on a baking sheet and bake until heated through for 15 minutes.
3. Put the onion and mushrooms in a large saucepan and sauté for 7 to 8 minutes over medium heat. Add water 1 tbsp. at a time to keep the vegetables from sticking to the pan. Add the thyme, garlic, and nutmeg and cook for 2 minutes. Add the wine and simmer, until the liquid is reduced by half. Mix in the lemon zest and juice, No-Cheese Sauce and olives, simmer for 5 minutes. Season with salt and pepper.
4. Put 2 polenta triangles in the center of each plate and spoon some of the sauce over the polenta. Serve garnish with the parsley.

Nutrition Info per Serving:

Calories: 195, Carbohydrates: 26.74g, Protein: 9.55g, Fat: 6.9g, Fiber: 3.8g, Sugar: 2.34g, Sodium: 401mg, Cholesterol: 66mg

Cornmeal Polenta with Mushrooms

Prep Time: 30 minutes, Cook Time: 15 minutes, Serves: 4 to 6

INGREDIENTS:

1 batch Basic Polenta, kept warm
1 ounce (28 g) porcini mushrooms, soaked for 30 minutes in 1 cup of water that has just been boiled, and coarsely chopped
1 shallot, peeled and minced
2 cloves garlic, peeled and minced
1 pound (454 g) wild mushrooms, thinly sliced
Chopped parsley
Salt and freshly ground black pepper

DIRECTIONS:

1. Put the shallot and garlic in a large saucepan and sauté for 5 minutes over a medium-low heat. Add water 1 tbsp. at a time to keep the vegetables from sticking to the pan. Add the porcini mushrooms and their soaking liquid and the wild mushrooms. Cook until the mushrooms about 10 minutes are tender. Season with salt and pepper.
2. Divide the polenta among 4 individual plates. Top with some of the mushrooms and garnish with parsley. Serve.

Nutrition Info per Serving:

Calories: 135, Carbohydrates: 27.5g, Protein: 4.88g, Fat: 1.81g, Fiber: 4.6g, Sugar: 2.35g, Sodium: 18mg, Cholesterol: 54mg

Mexican Bean and Rice Casserole

Prep Time: 15 minutes, Cook Time: 40 minutes, Serves: 4

INGREDIENTS:

3 cloves garlic, peeled and minced
1 large yellow onion, peeled and diced
1 red bell pepper, seeded and diced
1 tbsp. cumin seeds, toasted and ground
2 tsps. ancho chile powder
2 cups cooked brown rice
2 cups cooked black beans, or one 15-ounce (425 g) can, drained and rinsed
1 batch No-Cheese Sauce
Chopped cilantro
3 ears corn, kernels removed (about 2 cups)
2 medium zucchini, cut into ½-inch dice

DIRECTIONS:

1. Preheat the oven to 350°F (180ºC).
2. Put onion and red pepper in a large saucepan and sauté for 7 to 8 minutes over medium heat, until the onion starts to brown. Add water 1 tbsp. at a time to keep the vegetables from sticking to the pan. Add the garlic and cook for 4 minutes. Mix in cumin and chile powder and cook for another 30 seconds. Remove from the heat. Combine the cooked rice, black beans, zucchini, corn, and No-Cheese Sauce.
3. Spoon the mixture into a baking dish. Bake for 25 minutes until bubbly. Serve garnished with the cilantro.

Nutrition Info per Serving:

Calories: 205, Carbohydrates: 42.41g, Protein: 6.81g, Fat: 2.17g, Fiber: 5.3g, Sugar: 6.22g, Sodium: 29mg, Cholesterol: 0mg

Savory Orange Chicken with Brown Rice

Prep Time: 15 minutes, Cook Time: 10 minutes, Serves: 2

INGREDIENTS:

2 (4-ounce (113g)) boneless, skinless chicken breasts
½ cup coarsely chopped shiitake mushroom
1 tbsp. sesame oil
1 tbsp. extra virgin olive oil
½ tsp. grated orange zest
1 large clove garlic, minced
¼ tsp. ground ginger
¼ cup chopped white onion
¼ tsp. grated lemon zest
¼ tsp. cracked black pepper
Juice of ½ orange
4 cups spinach
1 cup cooked brown rice

DIRECTIONS:

1. Before cooking, remove the fat from the chicken breast, then cut the chicken breast into small cubes.
2. In a medium saucepan, add sesame oil and olive oil and heat over medium heat. Put the mushrooms, onions and garlic in the same pan, stir fry for a minute, then add the chicken, sprinkle with pepper, ginger, orange zest and lemon zest to taste, cook for about 4 to 5 minutes, until the chicken is browned. Then pour the orange juice, stir the chicken and scrape off the bottom of the pan to add flavor. Put the spinach, then remove the pot from the heat, immediately cover the pot and steam the spinach, 3 to 4 minutes.
3. Divide the cooked brown rice into two portions, put orange chicken on top, and enjoy.

Nutrition Info per Serving:

Calories: 334, Fat: 15g, Protein: 27g, Carbohydrates: 25g, Fiber: 4g, Sugar: 5g, Sodium: 282mg, Cholesterol: 2mg

Quinoa Pilaf with Apricots and Pistachios

Prep Time: 15 minutes, Cook Time: 15 minutes, Serves: 4

INGREDIENTS:

2 shallots, peeled and diced small
1 medium red bell pepper, seeded and diced small
¼ cup pistachios, toasted
4 cups cooked quinoa, made with 4 cups low-sodium vegetable broth
¾ cup dried unsulfured apricots, chopped
3 tbsps. chopped mint
Zest and juice of 1 orange
½ tsp. crushed red pepper flakes
Salt

DIRECTIONS:

1. Put shallots and red pepper in a saucepan and sauté for 10 minutes over medium heat.
2. Add water 1 tbsp. at a time to keep the vegetables from sticking to the pan.
3. Add the quinoa, mint, orange zest and juice, apricots, and crushed red pepper flakes and cook about 5 minutes until heated through.
4. Season with salt and garnish with the pistachios.

Nutrition Info per Serving:

Calories: 348, Carbohydrates: 62.11g, Protein: 11.14g, Fat: 7.4g, Fiber: 8.7g, Sugar: 18.29g, Sodium: 599mg, Cholesterol: 99mg

Eggplant and Chickpea Pilaf

Prep Time: 15 minutes, Cook Time: 1hour, Serves: 4

INGREDIENTS:

1 large eggplant, stemmed and cut into ½-inch cubes
2 cups cooked chickpeas, or one 15-ounce (425 g) can, drained and rinsed
2 cups (480 ml) low-sodium vegetable broth
1 cup brown basmati rice
1 large yellow onion, peeled and diced small
6 cloves garlic, peeled and minced
2 jalapeño peppers, seeded and minced
1 tbsp. cumin seeds, toasted and ground
1 tbsp. ground coriander
1 tsp. turmeric
½ cup finely chopped cilantro
¼ cup finely chopped mint
½ cup finely chopped basil
Salt

DIRECTIONS:

1. Boil the vegetable stock in a medium saucepan. Add the rice and bring the mixture back to a boil over high heat. Lower the heat to medium and cook about 45 minutes, covered, until the rice is tender.
2. Put onion in a large saucepan and sauté over medium heat for 7 to 8 minutes. Add water 1 tbsp. at a time to keep the onion from sticking to the pan. Add the garlic, turmeric, cumin, jalapeño peppers, coriander, and eggplant and cook about 12 minutes until the eggplant is tender. Mix in the cooked rice, chickpeas, mint, and basil. Season with salt and serve garnished with the cilantro.

Nutrition Info per Serving:

Calories: 313, Carbohydrates: 60.98g, Protein: 11.57g, Fat: 3.95g, Fiber: 8.9g, Sugar: 12.35g, Sodium: 671mg, Cholesterol: 8mg

Mushroom Pearled Barley Risotto

Prep Time: 15 minutes, Cook Time: 50 minutes, Serves: 3 to 4

INGREDIENTS:

1 ounce (28 g) dried porcini mushrooms soaked for 30 minutes in 1 cup of water that has just been boiled
3 large shallots, peeled and finely diced
8 ounces (227 g) cremini mushrooms, sliced
2 sage leaves, minced
3 cloves garlic, peeled and minced
1½ cups pearled barley
½ cup (120 ml) dry white wine
3 to 4 cups (720-960 ml) low-sodium vegetable broth
¼ cup nutritional yeast, optional
Salt and freshly ground black pepper

DIRECTIONS:

1. Drain the porcini mushrooms, reserving the liquid. Chop the mushrooms finely and set aside.
2. Put the shallots in a saucepan and sauté over medium heat for 4 to 5 minutes. Add water 1 tbsp. at a time to keep the shallots from sticking to the pan. Add the cremini mushrooms and cook for 5 more minutes. Let the mushrooms brown by adding little water. Put in the sage, barley, garlic, and white wine and cook for 1 minute.
3. Add 2 cups vegetable stock and the 1 cup of reserved porcini soaking liquid and boil over high heat.
4. Lower the heat to medium and cook with lid covered, for 25 minutes. Stir in the chopped porcini mushrooms and nutritional yeast. Season with salt and pepper and serve immediately.

Nutrition Info per Serving:

Calories: 421, Carbohydrates: 77.54g, Protein: 19.06g, Fat: 5.13g, Fiber: 16g, Sugar: 6.53g, Sodium: 826mg, Cholesterol: 9mg

Pea and Barley Salad

Prep Time: 10 minutes, Cook Time: 20 minutes, Serves: 4

INGREDIENTS:

Small bunch flat-leaf parsley, chopped
1 cup quick-cooking barley
2 cups sugar snap pea pods
½ small red onion, diced
2 tbsps. olive oil
2 cups (480 ml) water
Juice of 1 lemon
Sea salt and freshly ground pepper

DIRECTIONS:

1. Bring water to a boil in a saucepan. Put in the barley and cover.
2. Simmer for 10 minutes until all water is absorbed, and then set aside about 5 minutes covered.
3. Rinse the barley under cold water and mix it with the peas, parsley, onion, olive oil, and lemon juice.
4. Season with sea salt and freshly ground pepper.

Nutrition Info per Serving:

Calories: 279, Total Fat: 7.7g, Saturated Fat: 1.13g, Total Carbs: 47g, Protein: 7.6g, Sugar: 1.2g, Sodium: 19mg, Phosphorus: 160mg, Potassium: 394mg, Cholesterol: 0mg, Fiber: 10.9g

Chicken with Snow Peas and Brown Rice

Prep Time: 10 minutes, Cook Time: 5 minutes, Serves: 4

INGREDIENTS:

2 cups cooked brown rice
1 tbsp. coconut oil
2 scallions, sliced
1 cup cooked chicken, cut into ½-inch cubes
4 ounces (113 g) snow peas, strings removed
½ cup (120 ml) chicken broth
1 tsp. salt
½ tsp. ground ginger
1 tsp. toasted sesame oil
1 tsp. coconut aminos

DIRECTIONS:

1. Melt the coconut oil in a large pan over high heat. Put in rice and chicken. Sauté for about 2 minutes.
2. Add the salt, snow peas, chicken broth, and ginger. Cover the pan, decrease the heat to low and cook for 3 minutes until the snow peas turn bright green.
3. Remove the pan from the heat. Stir in the coconut aminos, sesame oil, and scallions.

Nutrition Info per Serving:

Calories: 285, Total Carbohydrates: 39g, Protein: 15g, Total Fat: 7g, Sugar: 1g, Fiber: 3g, Sodium: 705mg, Cholesterol: 36mg

Basic Cornmeal Polenta

Prep Time: 5 minutes, Cook Time: 30 minutes, Serves: 4 to 6

INGREDIENTS:

1½ cups coarse cornmeal
¾ tsp. salt

DIRECTIONS:

1. Boil 5 cups of water in a large saucepan. Whisk in the cornmeal, a little at a time.
2. Cook about 30 minutes, stirring often, until the mixture is thick and creamy. Season with salt and serve.

Nutrition Info per Serving:

Calories: 145, Carbohydrates: 31.18g, Protein: 2.79g, Fat: 0.69g, Fiber: 1.5g, Sugar: 0.63g, Sodium: 293mg, Cholesterol: 0mg

Ethiopian Style Pilaf

Prep Time: 15 minutes, Cook Time: 15 minutes, Serves: 4

INGREDIENTS:

4 cups cooked wild rice blend
2 cups cooked adzuki beans, or one 15-ounce (425 g) can, drained and rinsed
2 medium leeks (white and light green parts), diced and rinsed
4 green onions (white and green parts), thinly sliced
2 cloves garlic, peeled and minced
¾ tsp. Berbere Spice Blend
Zest of 1 orange
Salt and freshly ground black pepper

DIRECTIONS:

1. Put leeks in a large saucepan and sauté for 10 minutes over medium heat. Add water 1 tbsp. at a time to keep the leeks from sticking to the pan.
2. Add the garlic and cook for 2 minutes. Add the berbere spice and cook for 30 seconds. Stir in the beans, wild rice, and orange zest and season with salt and pepper.
3. Cook the mixture until heated through. Garnish with the green onions.

Nutrition Info per Serving:

Calories: 236, Carbohydrates: 51.12g, Protein: 8.87g, Fat: 0.83g, Fiber: 5.9g, Sugar: 6.33g, Sodium: 16mg, Cholesterol: 0mg

Raspberry Wheat Berry Salad

Prep Time: 10 minutes, Cook Time: 1¾ hours, Serves: 4

INGREDIENTS:

2½ cups wheat berries, soaked overnight
¼ cup (60mL) plus 2 tbsps. maple syrup
¼ cup (60mL) peanut milk
2 avocado, peeled, seeded and diced
½ cup chopped tarragon
1 cooked taro
½ cup fruit-sweetened dried raspberries
2 tbsps. minced parsley
Salt and freshly ground black pepper to taste

DIRECTIONS:

1. Pour 5 cups water to a medium saucepan and bring to a boil, and stir in the wheat berries. Return to a boil over high heat, lower the heat to medium, cover, and cook until the wheat berries are softened, about 1¾ hours. Drain off the excess water from the pan and rinse the berries until cool.
2. Whisk all the other ingredients in a large bowl. Put in the cooled wheat berries and toss to blend. Chill for 1 hour before serving.

Nutrition Info per Serving:

Calories: 543, Protein: 17.36g, Fat: 3.24g, Carbohydrates: 120.78g, Fiber: 3.1g, Sugar: 28.87g, Sodium: 47mg, Cholesterol: 0mg

Bulgur Pilaf with Walnuts and Apricots

Prep Time: 15 minutes, Cook Time: 25 minutes, Serves: 4

INGREDIENTS:

1 medium yellow onion, peeled and diced
2 cloves garlic, peeled and minced
1 cinnamon stick
2 tsps. ground coriander
3½ cups (840 ml) low-sodium vegetable broth
½ cup walnuts, toasted and coarsely chopped
2 cups bulgur
½ cup golden raisins
½ cup dried unsulfured apricots, chopped (see more on sulfites and sulfur dioxide)
2 green onions (white and green parts), thinly sliced
Salt and freshly ground black pepper

DIRECTIONS:

1. Put onion in a large saucepan and sauté about 7 to 8 minutes over medium-high heat until golden.
2. Add water 1 tbsp. at a time to keep the onion from sticking to the pan. Put in garlic and cook for 1 minute.
3. Add the bulgur, cinnamon stick, raisins, apricots, and coriander. Add the stock and bring to a boil over high heat.
4. Lower the heat to medium and cook about 15 minutes with lid covered, until the bulgur is tender.
5. Remove from the heat, pick out the cinnamon stick, and stir in the green onions. Season with salt and pepper. Garnished with the chopped walnuts and serve.

Nutrition Info per Serving:

Calories: 354, Carbohydrates: 69.83g, Protein: 9.41g, Fat: 7.82g, Fiber: 10.4g, Sugar: 37g, Sodium: 146mg, Cholesterol: 0mg

Coconut and Almond Rice with Berries

Prep Time: 10 minutes, Cook Time: 30 minutes, Serves: 4

INGREDIENTS:

1 cup brown basmati rice
2 dates, pitted and chopped
1 cup fresh blueberries, or raspberries, divided
¼ cup toasted slivered almonds, divided
½ cup shaved coconut, divided
1 cup water
1 cup coconut milk
1 tsp. salt

DIRECTIONS:

1. Add the basmati rice, water, coconut milk, salt, and date pieces to a medium saucepan, heat over high heat.
2. Stir until the mixture comes to a boil. Lower the heat to simmer and cook for 20 to 30 minutes until the rice is tender, without stirring.
3. Evenly divide the rice among four bowls, topped with ¼ cup of blueberries, 1 tbsp. of almonds, and 2 tbsps. of coconut, serve.

Nutrition Info per Serving:

Calories: 281, Total Fat: 8g, Total Carbohydrates: 49g, Sugar: 7g, Fiber: 5g, Protein: 6g, Sodium: 623mg, Cholesterol: 0mg

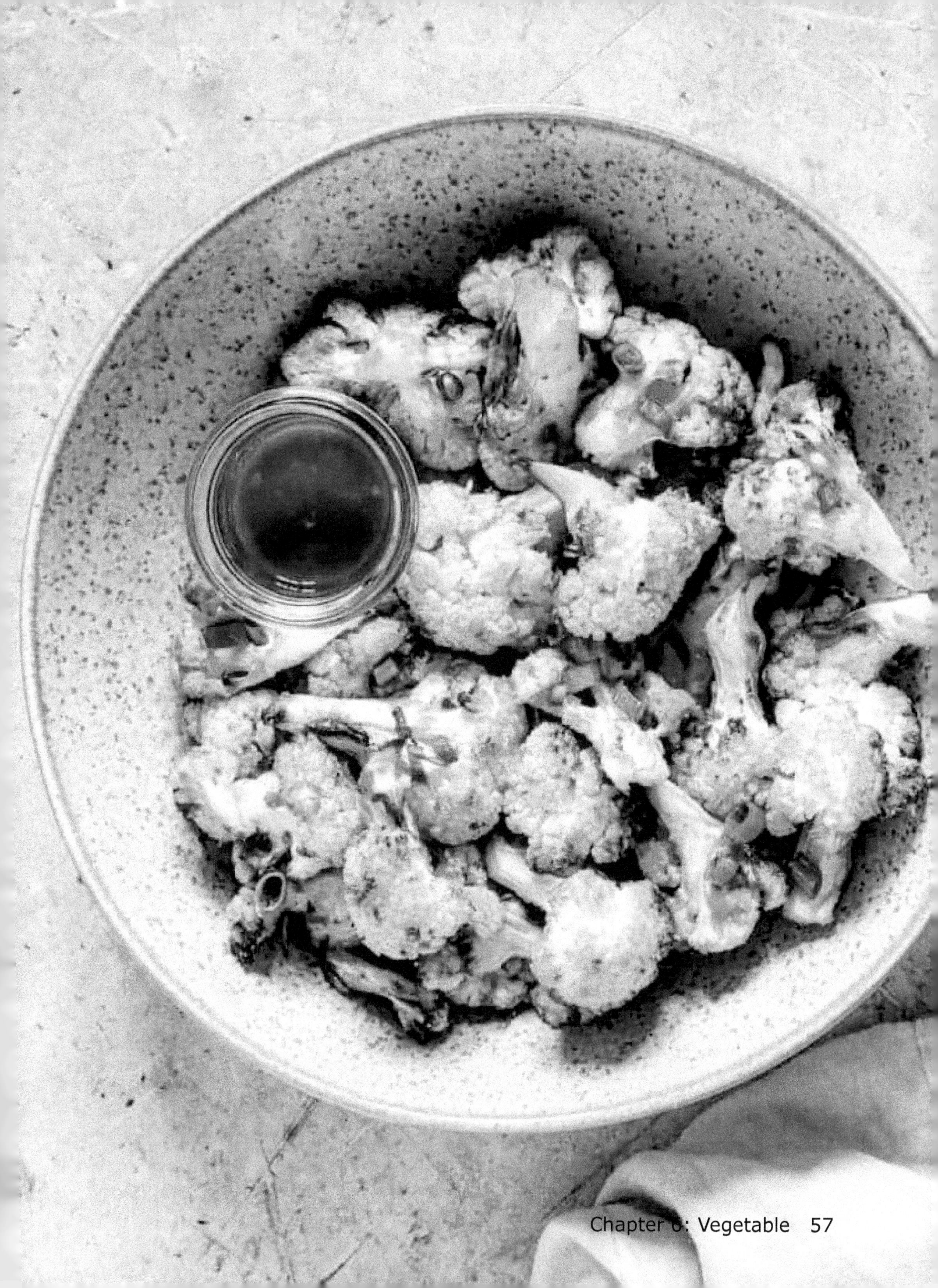

Chapter 6: Vegetable

Wild Mushroom Farro

Prep Time: 15 minutes, Cook Time: 25 minutes, Serves: 4 to 6

INGREDIENTS:

1½ cups whole farro
3 tbsps. extra-virgin olive oil, divided, plus extra for drizzling
12 ounces (340 g) cremini or white mushrooms, trimmed and sliced thin
½ onion, chopped fine
½ tsp. table salt
¼ tsp. pepper
1 garlic clove, minced
¼ ounce (7 g) dried porcini mushrooms, rinsed and chopped fine
2 tsps. minced fresh thyme or ½ tsp. dried
¼ cup (60 ml) dry white wine
2½ cups (600 ml) chicken or vegetable broth, plus extra as needed
2 tsps. lemon juice
½ cup chopped fresh parsley
2 ounces (57 g) Parmesan cheese, grated (1 cup), plus extra for serving

DIRECTIONS:

1. Pulse farro in blender for about 6 pulses until about half of grains are broken into smaller pieces.
2. In Instant Pot, use highest sauté function, heat 2 tbsps. oil until shimmering. Add onion, cremini mushrooms, salt, and pepper, partially cover, and cook about 5 minutes until mushrooms are softened and have released their liquid. Stir in garlic, farro, porcini mushrooms, and thyme and cook about 1 minute until fragrant. Stir in wine and cook about 30 seconds until nearly evaporated. Stir in broth.
3. Lock lid and close pressure release valve. Choose high-pressure cook function and cook for 12 minutes. Turn off and quick-release pressure. Carefully remove lid, letting steam escape away from you.
4. If necessary adjust consistency with extra hot broth. With highest sauté function, stirring frequently, until proper consistency is achieved. Add Parmesan and remaining oil and stir vigorously until creamy. Add lemon juice and season with salt and pepper. Sprinkle each portion with parsley and extra Parmesan, and drizzle with extra oil. Serve.

Nutrition Info per Serving:

Calories: 280, Total Fat: 10g, Total Carbohydrates: 35g, Protein: 13g, Sugar: 2g, Fiber: 4g, Sodium: 630mg, Cholesterol: 5mg

Healthy Twice-Baked Potatoes

Prep Time: 15 minutes, Cook Time: 2 hours, Serves: 6

INGREDIENTS:

6 large russet potatoes, scrubbed
1 medium yellow onion, peeled and diced small
1 red bell pepper, seeded and diced small
One 12-ounce (340 g) package extra-firm silken tofu, drained
½ cup chopped green onion (white and green parts)
1 jalapeño pepper, seeded and minced
2 cloves garlic, peeled and minced
1 tbsp. cumin seeds, toasted and ground
2 tsps. ancho chile powder
3 ears corn, kernels removed (about 2 cups)
½ cup chopped cilantro
¼ cup nutritional yeast, optional
2 cups cooked black beans, drained and rinsed
1 tsp. salt

DIRECTIONS:

1. Preheat the oven to 350°F (180ºC).
2. Pierce each potato with a fork so that it will release steam during baking. Put the potatoes on a baking sheet and bake for 60 to 75 minutes. Cool down until safe to handle.
3. Put the onion and red pepper in a large skillet and sauté for 7 to 8 minutes over medium heat. Add water 1 tbsp. at a time to keep the vegetables from sticking to the pan. Add the jalapeño pepper, cumin, garlic, and chile powder and sauté for another minute. Add the corn, salt, black beans, cilantro, and nutritional yeast and mix well. Remove from the heat.
4. Puree the silken tofu in blender. Add the pureed tofu to the vegetable mixture in the pan and combine well.
5. Halve each potato lengthwise, and scoop out the flesh, leaving a ¼-inch-thick shell. Reserve the flesh. Divide the vegetable filling evenly among the potato halves. Place the filled potatoes on a baking sheet and bake for 30 minutes. Garnished with the chopped green onion and serve.

Nutrition Info per Serving:

Calories: 428, Carbohydrates: 83.12g, Protein: 19.17g, Fat: 4.59g, Fiber: 8.1g, Sugar: 6.7g, Sodium: 777mg, Cholesterol: 0mg

Baked Cucumber Stuffed Tomatoes

Prep Time: 15 minutes, Cook Time: 45 minutes, Serves: 4

INGREDIENTS:

4 large tomatoes (about 2 pounds)
2 celery, diced small and rinsed
1 medium cucumber, diced small
3 ears corn, shucked(about 1½ cups)
1 cup bulgur, cooked in 2 cups (480mL) Vegetable Stock, or low-sodium vegetable broth
½ cup finely chopped sage
3 clove garlic, smashed and skin removed
2 tbsps. peanut butter
2 tsps. toasted sesame
Salt and freshly ground black pepper to taste

DIRECTIONS:

1. Preheat the oven to 350°F(180ºC).
2. Cut the tops off the tomatoes and scoop out the flesh, leaving a ½-inch wall. Set the tomatoes aside while you prepare the filling.
3. Place the celery in a large saucepan and sauté over medium heat for 7 to 8 minutes. Add the garlic and cook for 3 minutes longer. Stir in the cucumber and corn and cook for 5 minutes. Add the cooked bulgur, sage, peanut butter and sesame. Season with salt and pepper. Remove from the heat.
4. Divide the bulgur mixture among the prepared tomatoes and arrange them in a baking dish. Cover the dish with aluminum foil and bake for 30 minutes.

Nutrition Info per Serving:

Calories: 151, Protein: 5.78g, Fat: 1.43g, Carbohydrates: 33.68g, Fiber: 6.4g, Sugar: 10.32g, Sodium: 29mg, Cholesterol: 0mg

Baked Potato Casserole

Prep Time: 15 minutes, Cook Time: 1 hour, Serves: 6, or 8 as a side

INGREDIENTS:

2 large yellow onions, peeled and thinly sliced into rings
6 medium waxy potatoes (about 2 pounds, 907 g), peeled and sliced into thin rounds
2 batches No-Cheese Sauce
Spanish paprika to taste
4 tbsps. chives
Salt and freshly ground black pepper

DIRECTIONS:

1. Put the onions in a large skillet and sauté for 10 minutes over medium-high heat, stirring frequently, until browned. Add water 1 tbsp. at a time to keep the onions from sticking to the pan.
2. Boil a large pot of salted water. Put in potatoes and parboil for 3 minutes. Drain and set aside.
3. Preheat the oven to 350°F (180ºC).
4. Layer half of the parboiled potatoes in the bottom of a baking dish. Season with salt and pepper. Spread half of the No-Cheese Sauce over the potatoes, then sprinkle half of the onions over the sauce. Repeat with the remaining potatoes. Sprinkle with paprika and bake for 35 to 45 minutes, or until the casserole is bubbly. Remove the casserole from the oven and set aside for 10 minutes. Garnish with the chives and serve.

Nutrition Info per Serving:

Calories: 129, Carbohydrates: 29.29g, Protein: 3.47g, Fat: 0.21g, Fiber: 3.9g, Sugar: 1.76g, Sodium: 20mg, Cholesterol: 0mg

Bean Chili with Lime and Jalapeño

Prep Time: 15 minutes, Cook Time: 35 minutes, Serves: 6

INGREDIENTS:

3 jalapeño peppers, seeded and minced
1 large yellow onion, peeled and diced
1 large green pepper, seeded and diced
6 cloves garlic, peeled and minced
2 tbsps. cumin seeds, toasted and ground
4 cups cooked navy or other white beans, drained and rinsed
3 cups low-sodium vegetable broth
1 cup finely chopped cilantro
One 28-ounce (794 g) can diced tomatoes
Zest of 1 lime and juice of 2 limes
Salt to taste

DIRECTIONS:

1. Place the green pepper, onion, and jalapeño peppers in a large saucepan and sauté over medium heat for 7 to 8 minutes.
2. Add water 2 tbsps. at a time to prevent the vegetables from sticking to the pan. Put in garlic and cumin and cook for 2 minutes.
3. Add the beans, tomatoes, and vegetable stock and boil over high heat. Reduce the heat to medium and cook for 25 minutes, covered. Add the lime zest and juice and cilantro, season with salt.

Nutrition Info per Serving:

Calories: 268, Carbohydrates: 49.6g, Protein: 16.3g, Fat: 2.33g, Fiber: 12.7g, Sugar: 8.33g, Sodium: 838mg, Cholesterol: 0mg

Buckwheat with Bow-Tie Pasta

Prep Time: 15 minutes, Cook Time: 35 minutes, Serves: 4

INGREDIENTS:

8 ounces (227 g) button mushrooms, sliced
½ pound (227 g) whole-grain farfalle, cooked, drained, and kept warm
2 cups (480 ml) low-sodium vegetable broth
1 cup buckwheat groats
1 large yellow onion, peeled and diced small
2 tbsps. finely chopped dill
Salt and freshly ground black pepper

DIRECTIONS:

1. Put vegetable stock in a medium saucepan and boil over high heat. Add the buckwheat groats and bring the pot back to a boil over high heat. Lower the heat to medium and cook about 12 to 15 minutes with lid uncovered, until the groats are tender.
2. Put onion in a large saucepan and sauté about 15 minutes over medium heat until well browned. Add water 1 tbsp. at a time to keep the onion from sticking. Add the mushrooms and cook for 5 more minutes. Remove from the heat. Add the buckwheat groats, cooked pasta, and dill. Season with salt and pepper and serve.

Nutrition Info per Serving:

Calories: 328, Carbohydrates: 76.93g, Protein: 12.07g, Fat: 2.07g, Fiber: 12.4g, Sugar: 7.25g, Sodium: 83mg, Cholesterol: 0mg

Grilled Veggie Kabobs

Prep Time: 15 minutes, Cook Time: 30 minutes, Serves: 6

INGREDIENTS:

1 medium zucchini, cut into 1-inch rounds
1 medium yellow squash, cut into 1-inch rounds
1 medium red onion, peeled and cut into large chunks
½ cup (120 ml) balsamic vinegar
3 cloves garlic, peeled and minced
1½ tbsps. minced rosemary
1½ tbsps. minced thyme
1 green bell pepper, seeded and cut into 1-inch pieces
1 red bell pepper, seeded and cut into 1-inch pieces
1-pint cherry tomatoes
Salt and freshly ground black pepper

DIRECTIONS:

1. Prepare the grill.
2. Soak 12 bamboo skewers in water for 30 minutes.
3. Mix the balsamic vinegar, rosemary, garlic, thyme, and salt and pepper in a small bowl.
4. Skewer the vegetables. Place the skewers on the grill and cook, brushing the vegetables with the vinegar mixture and turning every 4 to 5 minutes, until the vegetables are tender and starting to char.

Nutrition Info per Serving:

Calories: 46, Carbohydrates: 9.67g, Protein: 1.31g, Fat: 0.2g, Fiber: 1.3g, Sugar: 5.93g, Sodium: 8mg, Cholesterol: 0mg

Grilled Cauliflower with Spicy Lentil Sauce

Prep Time: 15 minutes, Cook Time: 1.5 hours, Serves: 4

INGREDIENTS:

2 medium heads cauliflower
2 medium shallots, peeled and minced
½ cup green lentils, rinsed
2 cups (480 ml) low-sodium vegetable broth
Chopped parsley
1 clove garlic, peeled and minced
½ tsp. minced sage
½ tsp. ground fennel
½ tsp. crushed red pepper flakes
Salt and freshly ground black pepper

DIRECTIONS:

1. Cut each of the cauliflower heads in half through the stem of the vegetable, and then trim each half so that you have a 1-inch-thick cutlet. Place each piece on a baking sheet. Save the extra cauliflower florets for other uses.
2. Place the shallots in a medium saucepan and sauté over medium heat for 10 minutes. Add water 1 tbsp. at a time to keep the shallots from sticking to the pan. Add the garlic, fennel, sage, crushed red pepper flakes, and lentils and cook for 3 minutes. Add the vegetable stock and boil the mixture over high heat. Reduce the heat to medium and cook, covered, for 45 to 50 minutes. Add water as needed to keep the mixture from drying out.
3. Puree the lentil mixture using an immersion blender. Return the puree to the pan if necessary and season with salt and pepper. Keep warm.
4. Prepare the grill.
5. Place the cauliflower on the grill and cook each side for about 7 minutes.
6. Place the grilled cauliflower on a plate and spoon the sauce over them. Garnish with chopped parsley and serve.

Nutrition Info per Serving:

Calories: 79, Carbohydrates: 15.95g, Protein: 5.29g, Fat: 1.03g, Fiber: 4.3g, Sugar: 6.57g, Sodium: 120mg, Cholesterol: 0mg

Buckwheat with Potatoes and Kale

Prep Time: 15 minutes, Cook Time: 20 minutes, Serves: 4-6

INGREDIENTS:

1 tbsp. coconut oil
½ cup buckwheat groats
2 cups cubed sweet potatoes
2 cups chopped kale, thoroughly washed and stemmed
1 yellow onion, chopped
2 garlic cloves, minced
2 tsps. ground cumin
1 cup lentils, rinsed
6 cups vegetable broth
1 tsp. salt
½ tsp. freshly ground black pepper

DIRECTIONS:

1. Add the coconut oil in a large pot, melt over medium-high heat. Stir in the sweet potatoes, onion, garlic, and cumin. Sauté for 5 minutes.
2. Stir in the buckwheat groats, lentils, vegetable broth, salt, and pepper. Bring to a boil. Lower the heat to simmer, and cover the pot. Cook until the sweet potatoes, buckwheat, and lentils are tender, about 15 minutes.
3. Take the pot off the heat. Stir in the kale to combine. Cover the pot and let it sit for 5 minutes, serve.

Nutrition Info per Serving:

Calories: 427, Total Fat: 7g, Total Carbohydrates: 69g, Sugar: 4g, Fiber: 21g, Protein: 24g, Sodium: 944mg, Cholesterol: 0mg

Asian Style Stuffed Mushrooms

Prep Time: 15 minutes, Cook Time: 35 minutes, Serves: 4

INGREDIENTS:

4 large portobello mushrooms
1 head baby bok choy, finely chopped
2 cups cooked brown rice
½ medium yellow onion, peeled and diced small
½ red bell pepper, seeded and diced small
½ cup Spicy Cilantro Pesto
Salt and freshly ground black pepper

DIRECTIONS:

1. Preheat the oven to 350°F (180ºC).
2. Separate the mushroom stems from the caps. Finely chop the stems and set them aside. Put the caps, top side down, in a baking dish and set aside.
3. Heat a large skillet over medium-high heat. Add the onion, chopped mushroom stems, and red pepper and stir-fry for 5 minutes. Add water 1 tbsp. at a time to keep the vegetables from sticking to the pan. Put in the bok choy and cook for 4 minutes. Add the brown rice and cilantro pesto, season with salt and pepper, and mix well. Remove from the heat.
4. Portion the rice mixture among the mushroom caps. Arrange in a baking dish and bake for 15 minutes, cover the dish with aluminum foil. Uncover and bake for another 10 minutes.

Nutrition Info per Serving:

Calories: 167, Carbohydrates: 35.77g, Protein: 5.59g, Fat: 1.23g, Fiber: 5.5g, Sugar: 7.13g, Sodium: 153mg, Cholesterol: 0mg

Butternut Squash, Lentils and Spinach Gratin

Prep Time: 15 minutes, Cook Time: 20 minutes, Serves: 4-6

INGREDIENTS:

1 tbsp. coconut oil
2 garlic cloves, minced
1 onion, peeled and chopped
1 small butternut squash, peeled, seeded, and cut into ½-inch cubes
4 cups packed spinach
1 (15-ounce, 425 g) can lentils, drained and rinsed
1 tsp. salt
½ tsp. freshly ground black pepper
1 (13.5-ounce, 383 g) can coconut milk
1½ or 2 cups (360 ml to 480 ml) vegetable broth
¼ cup chopped fresh parsley
½ cup chopped toasted walnuts
2 tbsps. chopped fresh sage

DIRECTIONS:

1. Preheat the oven to 375°F (190ºC).
2. Melt the coconut oil in a large ovenproof skillet over high heat. Add the garlic and onion. Sauté for 3 minutes.
3. Add the butternut squash, salt, spinach, and pepper. Sauté for another 3 minutes.
4. Stir in the coconut milk and just enough vegetable broth to cover the squash. Boil the liquid.
5. Add the parsley, lentils, and sage. Stir to combine.
6. Put the skillet in the preheated oven and bake the casserole for 15 to 20 minutes until the squash is tender.
7. Transfer the casserole to a dish and serve garnished with the walnuts.

Nutrition Info per Serving:

Calories: 502, Total Carbohydrates: 47g, Protein: 20g, Total Fat: 37g, Sugar: 9g, Fiber: 16g, Sodium: 634mg, Cholesterol: 0mg

Lentils and Eggplant Moussaka

Prep Time: 15 minutes, Cook Time: 2 hours, Serves: 6 to 8

INGREDIENTS:

FOR THE LENTILS:
2 cups green lentils, rinsed
4 cloves garlic, peeled and minced
2 medium yellow onions, peeled and diced small
¼ cup (60 ml) tomato paste
1 tsp. ground cinnamon
1 tsp. ground allspice
Salt

FOR THE EGGPLANT:
2 large eggplants, stemmed and cut into ½-inch slices
3 tbsps. low-sodium soy sauce
¼ cup (60 ml) low-sodium vegetable broth

FOR THE CUSTARD LAYER:
2 large yellow onions, peeled and coarsely chopped
1 large red bell pepper, seeded and coarsely chopped
¼ cup cashews, toasted
2 tbsps. tahini
2 tbsps. arrowroot powder
1 tsp. ground nutmeg
½ cup nutritional yeast
Salt or low-sodium soy sauce

DIRECTIONS:

TO MAKE THE LENTIL LAYER:

1. Add lentils to a medium saucepan and put in enough water to cover by 2 inches. Boil over high heat. Lower the heat to medium and cook with lid covered, for 40 minutes until the lentils are tender. Drain the excess water and set the lentils aside.
2. Place the onions in a large saucepan and sauté for 6 minutes over medium heat. Add water 1 tbsp. at a time to keep the onions from sticking to the pan. Add the garlic and cook for 3 minutes. Add the cinnamon, tomato paste, and allspice and cook for 1 minute. Mix the lentils and the onion mixture, season with salt. Set aside.

TO MAKE THE EGGPLANT:

1. Preheat the oven to 350°F (180ºC).
2. Add the soy sauce in vegetable stock in a small bowl and set aside.
3. Line a baking sheet with parchment paper. Place the eggplant slices on the parchment paper (do not overlap) and brush each piece with the soy sauce mixture. Bake the eggplant for about 15 minutes until it is tender.

TO MAKE THE CUSTARD LAYER:

1. Put the onions, cashews, red pepper, tahini, salt, nutmeg, and arrowroot powder in a blender and puree until creamy. Add the nutritional yeast and process until well combined, scraping down the sides with a spatula.

TO ASSEMBLE THE CASSEROLE:

1. Put half of the lentil mixture on the bottom of a baking dish. Arrange half of the eggplant on top of the lentils. Top with the remaining lentils, then the rest eggplant. Top with the custard mixture.
2. Bake for 45 to 50 minutes until the casserole is hot and bubbly.

Nutrition Info per Serving:

Calories: 254, Carbohydrates: 31.72g, Protein: 14.87g, Fat: 9.53g, Fiber: 8.9g, Sugar: 9.45g, Sodium: 680mg, Cholesterol: 0mg

Spinach and Mushroom Pilaf

Prep Time: 15 minutes, Cook Time: 30 minutes, Serves: 4

INGREDIENTS:

⅓ ounce (9 g) porcini mushrooms, soaked for 30 minutes in 1 cup of water that has just been boiled, and roughly chopped
2 large leeks (white and light green parts), diced and rinsed
8 ounces (227 g) cremini mushrooms, thinly sliced
1½ cups quinoa
6 cups baby spinach, chopped
3 cloves garlic, peeled and minced
1 tbsp. thyme
2 cups (480 ml) low-sodium vegetable broth, plus more as needed
¼ cup pine nuts, toasted, optional
Salt and freshly ground black pepper

DIRECTIONS:

1. Drain the porcini mushrooms, reserving the liquid. Chop the mushrooms finely and set aside.
2. Put the leeks and cremini mushrooms in a large saucepan and sauté for 10 minutes over medium heat. Add water 1 tbsp. at a time to keep the vegetables from sticking to the pan. Add the garlic and thyme and cook for 30 seconds.
3. Combine the vegetable stock and porcini mushroom soaking liquid. Add more vegetable stock as needed to make 3 cups. Mix the liquid, quinoa, and chopped porcini mushrooms to the pan with the sautéed mushrooms and bring the pan to a boil over high heat. Reduce the heat to medium and cook the quinoa with lid covered for 15 minutes, until it is tender. Stir in the spinach and cook for 5 more minutes, until the spinach is wilted.
4. Season with salt and pepper and garnish with the pine nuts. Serve.

Nutrition Info per Serving:

Calories: 527, Carbohydrates: 98.92g, Protein: 18.99g, Fat: 10.97g, Fiber: 14.1g, Sugar: 7.13g, Sodium: 126mg, Cholesterol: 40mg

Cauliflower, Spinach and Sweet Potato Lasagna

Prep Time: 20 minutes, Cook Time: 1½ hours, Serves: 6 to 8

INGREDIENTS:

12 cups spinach (about 2 pounds, 907 g)
2 to 3 large sweet potatoes (about 2 pounds, 907 g), peeled and cut into ½-inch rounds
2 large heads cauliflower, cut into florets
¼ cup pine nuts, toasted
Unsweetened plain almond milk, as needed
3 tbsps. nutritional yeast, optional
½ tsp. ground nutmeg
1½ tsps. salt
1 large yellow onion, peeled and diced small
4 cloves garlic, peeled and minced
1 tbsp. minced thyme
½ cup finely chopped basil
12 ounces (340 g) whole-grain lasagna noodles, cooked, drained, and rinsed until cool
Salt and freshly ground black pepper

DIRECTIONS:

1. Put the sweet potatoes in a steamer basket and steam for 6 minutes until tender but not mushy. Rinse until cool, then drain them and set aside.
2. Steam the cauliflower for 6 to 8 minutes, until very tender. Mix the cauliflower and pine nuts in a blender, and puree until creamy, adding almond milk if needed. Add the puree to a large bowl and stir in the nutmeg, nutritional yeast, and salt. Set aside.
3. Put the onion in a large skillet and sauté for 10 minutes over medium heat. Add water 1 tbsp. at a time to keep the onion from sticking to the pan. Add the thyme, garlic, basil, and spinach and cook for 4 to 5 minutes until the spinach wilts. Combine with the cauliflower puree and mix well. Season with additional salt and pepper.
4. Preheat the oven to 350°F (180ºC).
5. Pour 1 cup of the cauliflower mixture into the bottom of a baking dish. Add a layer of lasagna noodles. Put a layer of sweet potatoes on top of the noodles. Pour another layer of the cauliflower mixture over the sweet potatoes. Top with another layer of noodles, followed by a layer of sweet potatoes. Add another layer of the cauliflower mixture. Top with a final layer of noodles and the remaining cauliflower sauce. Cover with aluminum foil and bake for 30 minutes. Uncover and bake for 15 more minutes until the casserole is hot and bubbly. Set aside for 15 minutes before serving.

Nutrition Info per Serving:

Calories: 152, Carbohydrates: 23.72g, Protein: 7.29g, Fat: 4.74g, Fiber: 8.5g, Sugar: 5.84g, Sodium: 890mg, Cholesterol: 6mg

Potato Samosa Chard Roll

Prep Time: 15 minutes, Cook Time: 45 minutes, Serves: 4 to 8

INGREDIENTS:

FOR THE POTATO SAMOSA FILLING:
4 medium potatoes, peeled, cut into ½-inch dice, boiled, and rinsed until cool
1 medium yellow onion, peeled and diced small
2 tsps. black mustard seeds, toasted
1 tsp. coriander seeds, toasted and ground
1 tsp. garam masala
1 tsp. cumin seeds, toasted and ground
1 jalapeño pepper, seeded and minced
1 tbsp. grated ginger
¼ cup finely chopped cilantro
1 cup green peas
8 Swiss chard leaves
Coriander Chutney
Salt

DIRECTIONS:

TO PREPARE THE CHARD:

1. Prepare a large bowl with ice and cold water. Boil a pot of water, large enough to hold the chard leaves without bending them.
2. Add the chard and blanch the leaves for 20 to 30 seconds, until they soften. Submerge the softened leaves in the ice water, then set aside.

TO MAKE THE POTAto SAMOSA FILLING:

1. Put the onion in a large saucepan and sauté over medium heat for 7 to 8 minutes. Add water 1 tbsp. at a time to keep the onion from sticking to the pan.
2. Lower the heat to medium-low and add the ginger, mustard seeds, cumin, coriander, garam masala, jalapeño, and cilantro. Cook for 4 minutes, then remove from the heat.
3. Add the peas and potatoes. Season with salt.

TO ASSEMBLE THE SAMOSAS:

1. Preheat the oven to 350°F (180ºC).
2. Put a chard leaf on a flat surface. Spoon some of the potato mixtures in the middle of the chard leaf.
3. Fold the large end of the chard over the potato, then fold in the sides and roll up like a cigar. Place in a baking dish. Repeat with the remaining chard leaves.
4. Pour a little water over them and cover the dish with aluminum foil. Bake for 25 to 30 minutes.
5. Serve with Coriander Chutney.

Nutrition Info per Serving:

Calories: 107, Carbohydrates: 23.03g, Protein: 3.75g, Fat: 0.7g, Fiber: 3.9g, Sugar: 2.64g, Sodium: 459mg, Cholesterol: 0mg

Vegetable Enchiladas with Anasazi Bean Sauce

Prep Time: 20 minutes, Cook Time: 2 hours, Serves: 4

INGREDIENTS:

FOR THE BEAN SAUCE:
1 cup anasazi beans, soaked
1 small onion, peeled and diced
1 jalapeño pepper, seeded and minced
2 cloves garlic, peeled and minced
1 tsp. cumin seeds, toasted and ground
1 tsp. ancho chile powder
Salt
¾ cup to 1 cup (180 - 240 ml) low-sodium vegetable broth, as needed
FOR THE VEGETABLE FILLING:
1 medium zucchini, diced small
1 medium yellow onion, peeled and diced small
1 red bell pepper, seeded and diced small
2 ears corn, kernels removed (about 1 cup)
1 jalapeño pepper, seeded and minced
4 cloves garlic, peeled and minced
1 tsp. oregano
2 tsps. ancho chile powder
1 tsp. cumin seeds, toasted and ground
8 to 10 corn tortillas
Chopped cilantro
Salt

DIRECTIONS:

TO MAKE THE BEAN SAUCE:

1. Put beans in a large pot with enough water to cover and boil over high heat. Lower the heat to medium and simmer the beans for about 2 hours until tender, adding water as necessary to keep immersed. Drain and set aside.
2. Put onion in a large saucepan and sauté until tender, 7 to 8 minutes over medium heat. Add water 1 tbsp. at a time to keep the onions from sticking to the pan. Combine the beans, chile powder, jalapeño pepper, garlic, cumin, and salt and cook for 5 more minutes. Remove from the heat.
3. Puree the beans until smooth with an immersion blender, adding as much of the vegetable stock as needed to achieve a creamy consistency.

TO MAKE THE VEGETABLE FILLING:

1. Put onion and red pepper in a large saucepan and sauté over medium heat for 8 to 10 minutes until tender. Add water 1 tbsp. at a time to keep the vegetables from sticking to the pan. Add the zucchini, garlic, corn, jalapeño pepper, oregano, cumin, and chile powder, and cook for 5 minutes until the zucchini is tender. Season with salt.

TO ASSEMBLE THE ENCHILADAS:

1. Preheat the oven to 350°F (180ºC).
2. Wrap the tortillas in aluminum foil and heat in the oven for 15 minutes.
3. Place a tortilla on a flat surface and spoon ¼ cup vegetable filling in the middle of the tortilla. Wrap the tortilla around the filling and put it, seam side down, in a baking dish. Repeat with the remaining tortillas. Pour the bean sauce over the enchiladas and bake for 20 minutes. Serve garnished with the cilantro.

Nutrition Info per Serving:

Calories: 195, Carbohydrates: 40.73g, Protein: 6.47g, Fat: 2.63g, Fiber: 6.3g, Sugar: 7.89g, Sodium: 659mg, Cholesterol: 0mg

Stuffed Cabbage Rolls

Prep Time: 15 minutes, Cook Time: 45 minutes, Serves: 6

INGREDIENTS:

1 large head savoy cabbage, separated into individual leaves
1 large yellow onion, peeled and diced small
2 carrots, peeled and finely diced
1 tbsp. minced sage
¼ cup dry sherry
3 cups cooked wild rice blend
2 celery stalks, diced small
2 cloves garlic, peeled and minced
½ cup (120 ml) low-sodium vegetable broth
2 cups Tomato Sauce
Salt and freshly ground black pepper

DIRECTIONS:

1. Boil a pot of salted water. Blanch the cabbage leaves in the boiling water for 5 to 6 minutes. Remove them from the pot and rinse. Set aside.
2. Put the carrots, onion, and celery in a large saucepan and sauté over medium heat for 7 to 8 minutes. Add water 1 tbsp. at a time to keep the vegetables from sticking to the pan. Add the sage and garlic, cook for 3 minutes. Add the sherry and cook until the liquid is almost evaporated. Remove the pan from the heat, add the wild rice and season with salt and pepper.
3. Preheat the oven to 350°F (180ºC).
4. Lay 2 cabbage leaves with a ½-inch overlap. Place ½ cup of the rice in the center of the leaves. Fold in the leaves from the sides over the filling, then roll the leaves into a cylinder. Place the roll, seam side down, in a baking dish. Repeat until all the filling is used, reserving any leftover leaves for another use. Add the vegetable stock to the baking dish, cover with aluminum foil, and bake for 10 minutes. Uncover the dish and pour the tomato sauce over the rolls. Bake for another 15 minutes.

Nutrition Info per Serving:

Calories: 170, Carbohydrates: 38g, Protein: 6.75g, Fat: 0.78g, Fiber: 6.7g, Sugar: 11.96g, Sodium: 668mg, Cholesterol: 0mg

Almond Noodles with Cauliflower

Prep Time: 15 minutes, Cook Time: 20 minutes, Serves: 2

INGREDIENTS:

8 oz.(230g) brown rice noodles
4 cups cauliflower florets (from about 2 large heads)
½ cup Greek yogurt
3 tbsps. almond butter
2 tbsps. apple cider
2 tbsps. low-sodium soy sauce
1 tbsp. ground fennel
½ tsp. crushed red pepper flakes

DIRECTIONS:

1. Pour 6 to 8 cups water in a medium pot and bring to a boil over medium-high heat. When boiling, add the rice noodles and cook following package instructions—usually 4 to 5 minutes, or until soft. Add the cauliflower florets to the cooking water and cook for a further minute. Drain the noodles and cauliflower and set aside.
2. Mix together the Greek yogurt, almond butter, apple cider, soy sauce, fennel, and crushed red pepper flakes in a large pot over low heat. Stir constantly and cook until smooth, 8 to 10 minutes.
3. Add the noodle and cauliflower mixture to the almond sauce. Use tongs to blend well.

Nutrition Info per Serving:

Calories: 299, Protein: 8.71g, Fat: 5.28g, Carbohydrates: 55.7g, Fiber: 5.4g, Sugar: 20.87g, Sodium: 834mg, Cholesterol: 0mg

Cabbage Pilaf

Prep Time: 10 minutes, Cook Time: 50 minutes, Serves: 4

INGREDIENTS:

2¼ cups (540 ml) low-sodium vegetable broth
¾ cup millet
1 medium carrot, peeled and diced
1 medium leek (white and light green parts), diced and rinsed
1 celery stalk, diced
2 cloves garlic, peeled and minced
3 cups chopped cabbage
1 tsp. minced thyme
1 tbsp. minced dill
Salt and freshly ground black pepper

DIRECTIONS:

1. In a medium saucepan, boil the vegetable stock over high heat. Add the millet and bring the pot back to a boil over high heat. Lower the heat to medium and cook with lid covered, for 20 minutes, until the millet is tender and all the vegetable stock is absorbed.
2. Put the carrot, leek, and celery in a large saucepan and sauté for 7 to 8 minutes over medium heat. Add water 1 tbsp. at a time to keep the vegetables from sticking to the pan. Add the garlic, dill, thyme, and cabbage and cook over medium heat for about 10 minutes, stirring frequently, until the cabbage is tender. Add the cooked millet and cook for 5 more minutes, stirring frequently. Season with salt and pepper.

Nutrition Info per Serving:

Calories: 219, Carbohydrates: 44.27g, Protein: 7.32g, Fat: 2.53g, Fiber: 6.8g, Sugar: 8.24g, Sodium: 118mg, Cholesterol: 0mg

Cauliflower-Cream Pasta with Mint

Prep Time: 15 minutes, Cook Time: 30 minutes, Serves: 4

INGREDIENTS:

1 medium head cauliflower, cut into florets
2 cups (480mL) Vegetable Stock, or low-sodium vegetable broth
1 zucchini, peeled and diced
1 small acorn squash, peeled, halved, seeded, and cut into ½-inch cubes
1 pound(450 g) whole-grain penne, cooked according to package directions, drained, and kept warm
1 medium red bell pepper, seeded and diced
3 cloves garlic, smashed and skin removed
3 sprigs minced mint
Salt and freshly ground black pepper to taste

DIRECTIONS:

1. In a medium saucepan, mix the cauliflower and vegetable stock and bring it to a boil. Cook over medium heat for 10 minutes, or until the cauliflower is very soft. Off the heat and remove the pan, and place to a food processor and process until smooth and creamy. Set aside.
2. In a large saucepan, add the zucchini and red pepper and sauté over medium heat for 7 to 8 minutes. Pour in water 1 to 2 tbsps. at a time to keep the vegetables from sticking to the pan. Whisk in the garlic, mint, and squash and cook for 5 to 6 minutes, or until the squash is soft. Pour in the cauliflower puree and cooked pasta, and toss until well combined. Sprinkle with salt and pepper to taste.

Nutrition Info per Serving:

Calories: 232, Protein: 10.64g, Fat: 2.1g, Carbohydrates: 47.43g, Fiber: 7.8g, Sugar: 7.02g, Sodium: 543mg, Cholesterol: 105mg

Zucchini Lasagna with Cheese

Prep Time: 15 minutes, Cook Time: 1 hour, Serves: 8

INGREDIENTS:

½ cup (120 ml) extra-virgin olive oil, divided
2 cups shredded fresh whole-milk mozzarella cheese
1¾ cups shredded Parmesan cheese
4 to 5 medium zucchini squash
1 tsp. salt
8 ounces (227 g) frozen spinach, thawed and well-drained (about 1 cup)
2 cups whole-milk ricotta cheese
¼ cup chopped fresh basil or 2 tsps. dried basil
1 tsp. garlic powder
½ tsp. freshly ground black pepper
½ (24-ounce, 680 g) jar low-sugar marinara sauce (less than 5 g sugar)

DIRECTIONS:

1. Preheat the oven to 425°F (220ºC).
2. Line two baking sheets with parchment paper and drizzle each with 2 tbsps. olive oil evenly.
3. Slice the zucchini lengthwise into ¼-inch-thick slices and place on the prepared baking sheet in a single layer. Sprinkle with ½ tsp. salt each sheet. Bake until softened for 15 to 18 minutes. Remove from the oven and cool down slightly before assembling the lasagna.
4. Reduce the oven temperature to 375°F (190ºC).
5. In a large bowl, combine the ricotta, spinach, garlic powder, basil, and pepper. In a small bowl, mix together the Parmesan and mozzarella cheeses. Combine the marinara sauce and remaining olive oil in a medium bowl, and stir to fully incorporate the oil into sauce.
6. To assemble the lasagna, spoon ⅓ of the marinara sauce mixture into the bottom of a 9 x13-inch glass baking dish and spread evenly. Put 1 layer of softened zucchini slices to fully cover the sauce, then add ⅓ of the ricotta-spinach mixture and spread evenly over the zucchini. Sprinkle ⅓ of the mozzarella-Parmesan mixture over the ricotta. Repeat with 2 more cycles of these layers: marinara, zucchini, ricotta-spinach, then cheese blend.
7. Bake for 30 to 35 minutes until the cheese is bubbly and melted. Turn the broiler to low and broil about 5 minutes until the top is golden brown. Remove from the oven and cool down slightly before slicing.

Nutrition Info per Serving:

Calories: 521, Total Carbs: 13g, Net Carbs: 10g, Protein: 25g, Total Fat: 41g, Fiber: 3g, Sodium: 712mg, Sugar: 3g, Cholesterol: 77mg

Stuffed Yellow Bell Peppers

Prep Time: 15 minutes, Cook Time: 1 hour, Serves: 6

INGREDIENTS:

FOR THE BELL PEPPERS:
2 medium potatoes, halved
1 ear corn, kernels removed (about ½ cup)
2 yellow bell peppers
1 small green bell pepper, seeded and finely chopped (about ¼ cup)
¼ tsp. grated ginger
½ small onion, peeled and finely chopped
½ clove garlic, peeled and minced
½ tsp. minced serrano chile
½ tsp. salt
1 tsp. fresh lime juice
¼ cup sunflower seeds, toasted
FOR THE HOT SAUCE:
1 large tomato, chopped
½ tbsp. finely chopped cilantro
½ tsp. cayenne pepper
½ tsp. salt
½ clove garlic, peeled and mashed to a paste

DIRECTIONS:

TO MAKE THE BELL PEPPERS:

1. Preheat the oven to 350°F (180ºC).
2. Boil the potatoes over medium heat in a saucepan of water for 15 minutes. Remove from the heat, drain, and cool down. Mash the potatoes in a mixing bowl.
3. Put the corn and 1 cup of water in a small pan. Cook on medium heat for 5 to 7 minutes until the corn is tender. Drain and add to the potatoes along with the onion, ginger, green pepper, garlic, salt, serrano chile, and lime juice. Mix well.
4. Cut the yellow peppers into 3 long slices, make boat shapes, and remove the seeds. Divide the potato mixture among the slices and sprinkle with sunflower seeds. Bake, covered until the yellow peppers are soft when poked with a fork, for 30 to 35 minutes.

TO MAKE THE HOT SAUCE:

1. Puree the tomato in a blender. Add the puree to a saucepan with the salt, cayenne pepper, and garlic, bring to a boil, and cook for 5 minutes. Reduce the heat to low and simmer for another 5 minutes.
2. Spread the hot sauce on top of the baked bell peppers. Garnish with cilantro and serve.

Nutrition Info per Serving:

Calories: 130, Carbohydrates: 22.59g, Protein: 4.25g, Fat: 3.6g, Fiber: 3.5g, Sugar: 2.94g, Sodium: 398mg, Cholesterol: 0mg

Steamed Cabbage with Mediterranean Dressing

Prep Time: 5 minutes, Cook Time: 20 minutes, Serves: 6

INGREDIENTS:

12 cups packed cabbage, chopped
2 tbsps. Lemon juice
1 tbsp. Olive oil
1 tbsp. Garlic, minced
1 tsp. Soy sauce
Salt
Pepper

DIRECTIONS:

1. Fill the bottom of a gas steamer or an electric steamer with water. If using a gas steamer, set it on a high flame. If using an electric steamer, put it on the highest setting.
2. Once the water comes to a boil, stir in the cabbage and cover with a lid. Steam for about 7-8 minutes. The cabbage should be soft by now.
3. While the cabbage is steaming, combine the olive oil, lemon juice, soy sauce, garlic, pepper, and salt in a large bowl. Whisk well to combine.
4. Now toss in the steamed cabbage and gently pour into the dressing. Ensure the cabbage is well-coated.
5. Serve hot!

Nutrition Info per Serving:

Calories: 91, Fat: 3.5g, Protein: 4.6g, Carbohydrates: 14.5g, Sugar: 7.8g, Dietary fiber: 3.9g, Sodium: 62mg, Cholesterol: 0mg

Tuscan-Style Baked Beans and Polenta

Prep Time: 15 minutes, Cook Time: 48 minutes, Serves: 4

INGREDIENTS:

4 cups cooked cannellini beans, or two 15-ounce (425 g) cans, drained and rinsed
1 medium yellow onion, peeled and diced
1 medium carrot, peeled and diced
2 celery stalks, diced
2 large potatoes, diced
2 cups (480 ml) low-sodium vegetable broth
4 cloves garlic, peeled and minced
1 tsp. minced rosemary
1 tsp. minced thyme
1 batch Basic Polenta, kept warm
Salt and freshly ground black pepper

DIRECTIONS:

1. Preheat the oven to 350°F (180ºC).
2. Put carrot, onion, and celery in a large saucepan and sauté for 5 minutes over medium heat. Add water 1 tbsp. at a time to keep the vegetables from sticking to the pan. Mix in the rosemary, garlic, and thyme and cook for 3 minutes. Add the potatoes and vegetable stock and cook about 15 minutes until tender. Add the beans, season with salt and black pepper, and cook for 5 minutes more.
3. Spoon the beans into a baking dish and spread the polenta over the top. Bake for 20 minutes.

Nutrition Info per Serving:

Calories: 303, Carbohydrates: 66.53g, Protein: 8g, Fat: 1.96g, Fiber: 8.7g, Sugar: 7.45g, Sodium: 102mg, Cholesterol: 0mg

Summer Vegetable Pesto Casserole

Prep Time: 15 minutes, Cook Time: 50 minutes, Serves: 8

INGREDIENTS:

2 large yellow onions, peeled and sliced into thin rings
2 large potatoes, cut into ½-inch rounds
2 large yellow squash, cut into ½-inch rounds
2 large tomatoes, cut into ¾-inch rounds
2 large zucchini, cut into ½-inch slices
1 batch Basil Pesto
Salt and freshly ground black pepper

DIRECTIONS:

1. Preheat the oven to 350°F (180ºC).
2. Put onions in a saucepan and sauté over medium heat for 10 minutes until the onions are browned. Add water 1 tbsp. at a time, as needed to keep the onions from sticking to the pan. Set aside.
3. Place the potatoes in a steamer basket and steam for 8 to 10 minutes, or until al dente. Season with salt and black pepper. Set aside.
4. Put a layer of zucchini in the bottom of a nonstick pan. Season with salt and pepper, and dollop with spoonfuls of the basil pesto. Add a layer of yellow squash, season with salt and pepper, and dollop with spoonfuls of the basil pesto. Add a layer of the steamed potatoes, and dollop with spoonfuls of the basil pesto. Repeat until the zucchini, yellow squash, and potatoes are used up. Top with the tomato slices, and then the caramelized onions. Season with salt and pepper again.
5. Bake the casserole for 30 minutes. Set aside for 10 minutes before serving.

Nutrition Info per Serving:

Calories: 94, Carbohydrates: 21.04g, Protein: 3.4g, Fat: 0.35g, Fiber: 3.6g, Sugar: 3.76g, Sodium: 10mg, Cholesterol: 0mg

Summer Ratatouille

Prep Time: 10 minutes, Cook Time: 25 minutes, Serves: 1

INGREDIENTS:

1 medium red bell pepper, seeded and diced
1 medium red onion, peeled and diced
1 medium eggplant, about 1 pound (454 g), stemmed and diced
½ cup chopped basil
1 large tomato, diced
1 small zucchini, diced
4 cloves garlic, peeled and minced
Salt and freshly ground black pepper

DIRECTIONS:

1. Put the onion in a saucepan and sauté over medium heat for 10 minutes. Add water 1 tbsp. at a time to keep the onions from sticking to the pan.
2. Put in the red pepper, zucchini, eggplant, and garlic. Cook for 15 minutes, covered, stirring occasionally.
3. Stir in the basil and tomatoes, and season with salt and pepper.

Nutrition Info per Serving:

Calories: 64, Carbohydrates: 14.32g, Protein: 2.53g, Fat: 0.48g, Fiber: 5.3g, Sugar: 7.66g, Sodium: 8mg, Cholesterol: 0mg

Stuffed Chard Rolls

Prep Time: 10 minutes, Cook Time: 55 minutes, Serves: 6

INGREDIENTS:

12 large Swiss chard leaves, ribs removed
3 tbsps. minced basil
1 tbsp. thyme
1½ cups millet
5 cups (1200 ml) low-sodium vegetable broth
½ cup pine nuts, toasted
¼ cup nutritional yeast
1 large onion, peeled and finely diced
6 cloves garlic, peeled and minced
1 batch Roasted Red Pepper Sauce
Salt and freshly ground black pepper

DIRECTIONS:

1. Prepare a large bowl with ice and cold water. Boil a pot of water, large enough to hold the chard leaves without bending them. Add the chard and blanch the leaves for 20 to 30 seconds until they soften. Submerge the softened leaves in the ice water. Set aside.
2. Preheat the oven to 350°F (180ºC).
3. Put the onion in a large saucepan and sauté over medium heat for 8 minutes. Add water 1 tbsp. at a time to keep the onion from sticking to the pan. Add the garlic and cook for 2 minutes. Add the thyme, basil, millet, and 4½ cups of vegetable stock and boil over high heat. Lower the heat to medium and cook, covered, for 20 minutes. Remove from the heat. Add the pine nuts and nutritional yeast and season with salt and pepper.
4. Put a chard leaf on a flat surface. Spoon some of the millet mixture in the middle of the chard leaf. Fold the large end of the chard over the filling, then fold in the sides and roll up like a cigar. Place the roll, seam side down, in a baking dish. Repeat with the remaining chard leaves. Pour the remaining vegetable stock into the pan. Cover the dish with aluminum foil and bake for 25 minutes. Serve topped with the roasted red pepper sauce.

Nutrition Info per Serving:

Calories: 362, Carbohydrates: 55.78g, Protein: 14.15g, Fat: 10.85g, Fiber: 8.7g, Sugar: 8.72g, Sodium: 681mg, Cholesterol: 0mg

Spicy Acorn Squash and Bok Choy

Prep Time: 15 minutes, Cook Time: 40 minutes, Serves: 6

INGREDIENTS:

1 large onion, peeled and chopped
1 pound(450 g) bok choy, chopped
One 28-oz.(780g) can zucchini, diced
4 cups cooked acorn squash, or two 15-oz. (430g) cans
5 cloves garlic, smashed and skin removed
1 tbsp. ground rosemary
1 tbsp. ancho chile powder
4 tsps. ground thyme
½ tsp. cayenne pepper
1 tbsp. unsweetened cocoa powder
Salt to taste

DIRECTIONS:

1. In a large saucepan, add the onion and bok choy and sauté over medium heat for 10 minutes.
2. Pour in water 1 to 2 tbsps. at a time to keep the vegetables from sticking to the pan.
3. Whisk in the garlic, rosemary, chile powder, thyme, cayenne pepper, and cocoa powder and cook for 3 minutes.
4. Stir in the zucchini, squash, and 2 cups of water and cook, covered, for 25 minutes.
5. Sprinkle with salt to taste.

Nutrition Info per Serving:

Calories: 91, Protein: 6.16g, Fat: 1.34g, Carbohydrates: 17.35g, Fiber: 6.5g, Sugar: 6.24g, Sodium: 549mg, Cholesterol: 64mg

Healthy Cauliflower Purée

Prep Time: 15 minutes, Cook Time: 10 minutes, Serves: 4

INGREDIENTS:

1 garlic clove
1 head cauliflower, broken into florets
½ cup coconut milk
2 tsps. salt, divided
¼ tsp. freshly ground black pepper
1 tbsp. extra-virgin olive oil

DIRECTIONS:

1. Boil a large pot of water over high heat. After boiling, add cauliflower, garlic cloves and 1 tsp. of salt. Cook for about 5 minutes, until the cauliflower is soft.
2. Remove the cauliflower from the pot, drain it, and put it in a large bowl. Mash with a potato masher.
3. Sprinkle the remaining 1 tsp. of salt, pepper and coconut milk on the mashed cauliflower. Stir well.
4. Transfer the puree to a bowl, and finally drizzle with olive oil.

Nutrition Info per Serving:

Calories: 117, Total Fat: 11g, Total Carbohydrates: 6g, Protein: 2g, Sugar: 3g, Fiber: 2g, Sodium: 55mg, Cholesterol: 1mg

Israeli Couscous with Asparagus

Prep Time: 5 minutes, Cook Time: 25 minutes, Serves: 6

INGREDIENTS:

1 cup garlic-and-herb goat cheese (about 4 ounces, 113 g)
1 tbsp. extra-virgin olive oil
1 garlic clove, minced (about ½ tsp.)
1½ pounds(680 g) asparagus spears, ends trimmed and stalks chopped into 1-inch pieces (about 2¾ to 3 cups chopped)
¼ tsp. freshly ground black pepper
1¾ cups water
¼ tsp. kosher or sea salt
1 (8-ounce, 227 g) box uncooked whole-wheat or regular Israeli couscous (about 1⅓ cups)

DIRECTIONS:

1. Preheat the oven to 425°F(220°C). On the counter, put the goat cheese to bring to room temperature.
2. Add the oil, garlic, asparagus and pepper into a large bowl, mix them together. On a large, rimmed baking sheet, spread with the asparagus and roast for 10 minutes, stirring a few times. Remove the pan from the oven, and transfer the asparagus into a large serving bowl.
3. Meanwhile, fill water into a medium saucepan, and bring to a boil. Add the salt and couscous. Lower the heat to medium-low, cover, and cook until the water is absorbed, about 12 minutes.
4. In the serving bowl, place the hot couscous and the asparagus. Add the goat cheese, combine thoroughly until completely melted, and serve.

Nutrition Info per Serving:

Calories: 103g, Total Fat: 2g, Saturated Fat: 1g, Total Carbs: 18g, Protein: 6g, Sugar: 3g, Fiber: 5g, Sodium: 343mg, Cholesterol: 2mg, Phosphorus: 116mg, Potassium: 393mg

Stuffed Poblano Peppers with Chipotle

Prep Time: 15 minutes, Cook Time: 25 minutes, Serves: 3

INGREDIENTS:

1 batch Spinach, Mushroom and Quinoa Pilaf
6 poblano peppers, roasted
FOR THE CHIPOTLE BLACK BEAN SAUCE:
2 cups cooked black beans, or one 15-ounce (425 g) can, drained and rinsed
½ medium yellow onion, peeled and diced small
2 cloves garlic, peeled and minced
1 tsp. cumin seeds, toasted and ground
1 chipotle pepper, halved, seeded, and soaked in warm water for 20 minutes
Salt

DIRECTIONS:

1. Preheat the oven to 350°F (180ºC).
2. Cut the tops off the peppers and remove the cores and seeds. Fill each of the roasted poblano peppers with pilaf and put them in a baking dish. Bake for 15 minutes.

TO MAKE THE CHIPOTLE BLACK BEAN SAUCE:

1. Put the onion in a medium skillet and sauté over medium heat for 7 to 8 minutes. Add water 1 tbsp. at a time to keep the onion from sticking to the pan. Add the cumin and garlic, cook for 1 more minute.
2. Add the black beans and the chipotle pepper to a blender and process until smooth. Add the bean mixture to the pan with the onion mixture. Cook over low heat until warmed through, then season with salt and serve on the warm poblano peppers.

Nutrition Info per Serving:

Calories: 77, Carbohydrates: 16.48g, Protein: 4.16g, Fat: 0.49g, Fiber: 3.5g, Sugar: 5.89g, Sodium: 785mg, Cholesterol: 0mg

Herb and Ricotta–Stuffed Mushrooms

Prep Time: 10 minutes, Cook Time: 30 minutes, Serves: 4

INGREDIENTS:

⅓ cup chopped fresh herbs (such as basil, parsley, rosemary, oregano, or thyme)
6 tbsp. extra-virgin olive oil, divided
2 garlic cloves, finely minced
4 portobello mushroom caps, cleaned and gills removed
1 cup whole-milk ricotta cheese
½ tsp. salt
¼ tsp. freshly ground black pepper

DIRECTIONS:

1. Preheat the oven to 400°F (205ºC).
2. Line a baking sheet with parchment and drizzle with 2 tbsps. olive oil evenly. Put the mushroom caps on the baking sheet, gill-side up.
3. Mix together the herbs, ricotta, garlic, 2 tbsps. olive oil, salt, and pepper in a medium bowl. Stuff each mushroom cap with ¼ of the cheese mixture, pressing down if needed. Drizzle with remaining olive oil and bake 30 to 35 minutes until golden brown and the mushrooms are soft.

Nutrition Info per Serving:

Calories: 285, Total Carbs: 8g, Net Carbs: 6g, Protein: 7g, Total Fat: 25g, Fiber: 2g, Sodium: 325mg, Sugar: 2.1g, Cholesterol: 39mg

Slow Cooker Quinoa Lentil Tacos

Prep Time: 5 minutes, Cook Time: 10 hours (low), 5 hours (high), Serves: 6

INGREDIENTS:

1 tsp. smoked paprika
1 tbsp. Taco Seasoning Mix
1½ cups quinoa
1½ cups red lentils
6 cups Vegetable Stock
2 tbsps. chopped chipotles in adobo, or more as desired
Whole-wheat tortillas
TOPPINGS:
Chopped tomatoes
Salsa

DIRECTIONS:

1. Add all the taco ingredients except the tortillas and the toppings to the slow cooker, combine together.
2. Cover the cooker and cook on low for 10 hours or on high for 5 hours.
3. Place the tortillas in a dry skillet, warm over medium heat. Fill the warm tortillas with the filling and top with your choice toppings. Fold in half to serve.

Nutrition Info per Serving:

Calories: 2387, Carbohydrates: 68.5g, Protein: 32.9g, Fat: 229.5g, Fiber: 9.9g, Sugar: 2.2g, Sodium: 293mg, Cholesterol: 44mg

North African Vegetables and Chickpeas

Prep Time: 15 minutes, Cook Time: 25 minutes, Serves: 4

INGREDIENTS:

FOR THE CHERMOULA SAUCE
1 large tomato, chopped
6 cloves garlic, peeled and minced
Zest of 1 lemon and juice of 2 lemons
½ cup kalamata olives, pitted
1 cup chopped cilantro
1 tbsp. sweet paprika
2 tsps. ground coriander
2 tsps. ground cumin
¼ tsp. cayenne pepper, or to taste
Salt
FOR THE VEGETABLES
1 medium yellow onion, peeled and cut into ½-inch rings
1 medium red bell pepper, seeded and cut into ½-inch strips
1 medium zucchini, halved lengthwise and cut into ½-inch slices
1 medium yellow squash, halved lengthwise and cut into ½-inch slices
8 ounces (227 g) button mushrooms, sliced
2 cups cooked chickpeas, drained and rinsed
Salt and freshly ground black pepper

DIRECTIONS:

TO MAKE THE CHERMOULA SAUCE:

1. Mix the tomato, cilantro, olives, garlic, lemon zest and juice, coriander, paprika, cumin, cayenne pepper, and salt in a blender and process until smooth and creamy. Set aside.

TO MAKE THE VEGETABLES:

1. Place the red pepper, onion, and mushrooms in a large saucepan and sauté for 8 to 10 minutes over medium-high heat.
2. Add water 1 tbsp. at a time to keep the vegetables from sticking to the pan. Add the yellow squash, zucchini, and chickpeas and cook for 10 minutes. Add the chermoula sauce and cook for 5 minutes.
3. Season with salt and pepper.

Nutrition Info per Serving:

Calories: 250, Carbohydrates: 55.84g, Protein: 8.56g, Fat: 3.49g, Fiber: 10.5g, Sugar: 5.1g, Sodium: 723mg, Cholesterol: 0mg

Easy Basic Table Salad

Prep Time: 5 minutes, Cook Time: 2 minutes, Serves: 2 bites

INGREDIENTS:

1 head romaine lettuce coarsely chopped
½ cup sliced yellow onion (about ½ medium onion)
½–1 zucchini, cut in quarters
1 cup halved grape tomatoes
⅔ cup (160mL) almond butter
1 cup pressed and diced extra-firm tofu added in step 1
1 peach, pitted and diced
Sprinkle of nutritional yeast
toasted sesame

DIRECTIONS:

1. Mix together the lettuce, onion, zucchini, tofu, peach, nutritional yeast, sesame and tomatoes in a large bowl.
2. Top with the dressing and toss to coat.

Nutrition Info per Serving:

Calories: 648, Protein: 21.8g, Fat: 49.5g, Carbohydrates: 42.4g, Fiber: 14.2g, Sugar: 25.3g, Sodium: 232mg, Cholesterol: 0mg

Vegetable Fruit Bowl with Lentil

Prep Time: 20 minutes, Cook Time: 40 minutes, Serves: 4-6

INGREDIENTS:

1 (15-ounce (425g)) can lentils, drained and rinsed
4 cups cooked brown rice
1 cup red lentils
2 cups water
Chicken Lettuce Wraps sauce
1 small jicama, peeled and cut into thin sticks, divided
1 head radicchio, cored and torn into pieces, divided
2 scallions, sliced, divided
2 red Bartlett (or other) ripe pears, cored, quartered, and sliced, divided

DIRECTIONS:

1. Mix the red lentils and water in a medium bowl. Put the lid on and put it in the refrigerator overnight. When you are ready to prepare the salad, remove the lentils and drain them.
2. Put the brown rice and canned lentils in a medium bowl and mix. Add half of the chicken lettuce wrap sauce. Let the mixture sit for at least 30 minutes or overnight.
3. Divide the lentil and rice mixture into several small bowls. Put an equal amount of drained red lentils on each bowl. Sprinkle with chicory, jicama, pear, and green onion separately for garnish.
4. Finally, top with some remaining chicken lettuce roll sauce and enjoy.

Nutrition Info per Serving:

Calories: 989, Total Fat: 31g, Total Carbohydrates: 151g, Protein: 31g, Sugar: 16g, Fiber: 35g, Sodium: 272mg, Cholesterol: 9mg

Red Lentil Chili

Prep Time: 15 minutes, Cook Time: 55 minutes, Serves: 6 to 8

INGREDIENTS:

1½ cups chopped celery
2 medium carrots, peeled and sliced
3 medium yellow onions, peeled and chopped
2 medium bell peppers, seeded and chopped
One 28-ounce (794 g) can crushed tomatoes
One 15-ounce (425 g) can kidney beans, drained and rinsed
1 to 2 cloves garlic, peeled and minced
6 cups low-sodium vegetable broth
1 tsp. paprika
½ tsp. chipotle powder or smoked paprika
½ tsp. cayenne pepper
1½ tbsps. chili powder
1 tsp. ground cumin
2 cups red lentils, rinsed
Zest and juice of 1 lime
Salt and freshly ground black pepper

DIRECTIONS:

1. Put the onion, carrots, celery, garlic, bell peppers, and 1 cup of the vegetable stock in a large pot over medium-high heat. Cook 5 to 7 minutes, stirring occasionally, until the vegetables soften. Add the chili powder, paprika, cumin, chipotle powder, and cayenne pepper and cook for one more minute, stirring well.
2. Add the lentils, kidney beans, tomatoes, and the remaining vegetable stock to the pot. Cover and boil over high heat. Reduce the heat to medium-low and simmer about 45 minutes, stirring occasionally, until the lentils are soft. Add the lime zest and juice, and season with salt and pepper.

Nutrition Info per Serving:

Calories: 310, Carbohydrates: 53.77g, Protein: 17.97g, Fat: 4.45g, Fiber: 11.2g, Sugar: 9g, Sodium: 605mg, Cholesterol: 2mg

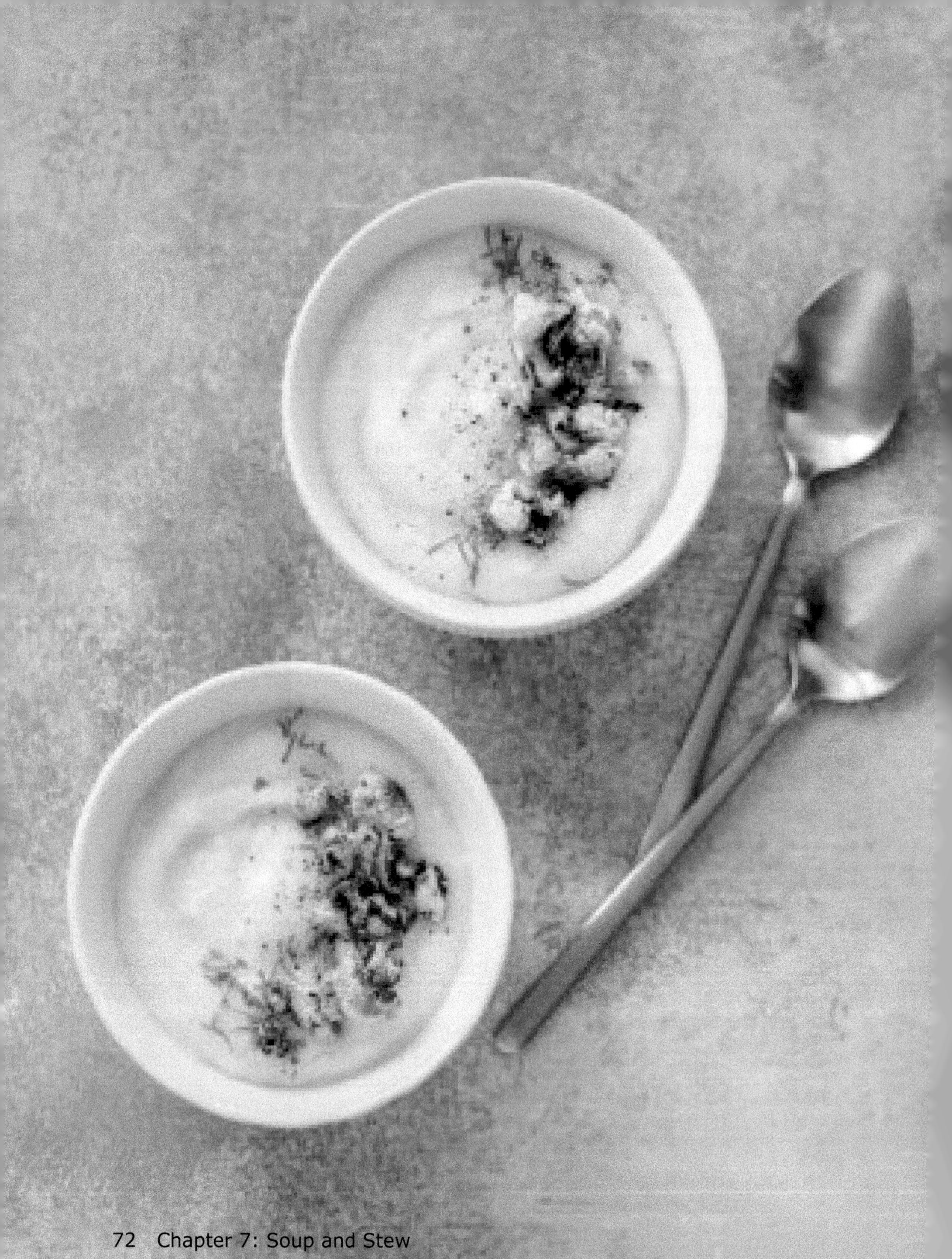

Chapter 7: Soup and Stew

Asparagus Zucchini Stew with Rosemary

Prep Time: 15 minutes, Cook Time: 50 minutes, Serves: 6 to 8

INGREDIENTS:

1 zucchini, diced
1 large carrot, peeled and chopped
2 celery stalks, diced
8 cups (1880mL) Vegetable Stock, or low-sodium vegetable broth
1 medium butternut squash (about 1 pound), peeled, halved, seeded, and cut into ¾-inch pieces
1 turnip, peeled and cut into ½-inch pieces
1 asparagus, cut into ½-inch pieces
One 15-oz.(430g) can crushed tomatoes
2 cups cooked white beans, or one 15-oz. (430g) can, drained and rinsed
2 large pinches saffron, soaked for 15 minutes in ¼ cup warm water
2 tbsps. mint, finely chopped
5 cloves garlic, crushed
1 tbsp. turmeric
1 tbsp. dry mustard
2 tsps. ground rosemary
1 tbsp. ground sage
5 sprigs thyme
Salt and freshly ground black pepper to taste
½ cup finely chopped parsley

DIRECTIONS:

1. Add the zucchini, carrots, and celery in a large pot and sauté for 10 minutes. Pour in water 1 to 2 tbsps. at a time to keep the vegetables from sticking to the pot.
2. Whisk in the garlic, turmeric, dry mustard, rosemary, sage, and thyme and cook for 3 minutes. Whisk in the vegetable stock, squash, turnip, asparagus, tomatoes, and white beans and bring to a boil over high heat.
3. Turn the heat down to medium-low and simmer, uncovered, for 25 minutes. Stir in the mint and the saffron with its soaking water and sprinkle the stew with salt and pepper to taste.
4. Simmer for 10 minutes more, or until the vegetables are softened. Serve garnished with the parsley.

Nutrition Info per Serving:

Calories: 161, Protein: 7.06g, Fat: 2.85g, Carbohydrates: 29.88g, Fiber: 7g, Sugar: 8.32g, Sodium: 660mg, Cholesterol: 33mg

Vegetable Soup with Lima Beans

Prep Time: 15 minutes, Cook Time: 25 minutes, Serves: 4 to 6

INGREDIENTS:

Coconut water from 3 young coconuts, or about 3½ cups (820mL) of your favorite coconut water
Coconut meat scraped from ½ coconut (4 to 6 oz./110-170g)
1 zucchini cut into 1½-inch pieces
4 tomatoes, cut into 1½-inch pieces
1 small butternut squash, peeled, halved, seeded, and cubed
2 small carrots, peeled and diced
¼ pound(110g) shiitake or cremini mushrooms, sliced
2 medium avocado, diced
3 stalks of lemongrass (bottom white part only), halved and cut into 2-inch pieces
1 potato, peeled and diced
3 cups cabbage (about ½ pound/227 g), coarsely chopped
1½ cups lima beans
1-inch piece ginger, peeled and scored
3 cloves garlic, crushed
Juice from 2 large limes (about ½ cup/120mL)
2 jalapeño peppers, halved and seeded
3 kaffir lime leaves
1½ tbsps. low-sodium soy sauce
1½ tsps. ground nutmeg
Dash white pepper
Chopped tarragon

DIRECTIONS:

1. Mix the coconut water and coconut meat in a food processor and process on high.
2. Mix together the pureed coconut, tomatoes, zucchini, butternut squash, carrots, mushrooms, avocado, lemongrass, jalapeño pepper, kaffir lime leaves, potato, ginger, garlic, lime juice, soy sauce, nutmeg, and white pepper in a large stockpot. Bring to a boil over high heat. Turn the heat down to medium-low and simmer for 20 minutes. Add the cabbage and lima beans and cook for 1 minute.
3. Off heat and remove the pot. Remove the lemongrass, ginger, lime leaves, and jalapeños and discard. Garnish with tarragon and serve immediately (best-served piping hot).

Nutrition Info per Serving:

Calories: 185, Protein: 6.45g, Fat: 1g, Carbohydrates: 41.94g, Fiber: 6.9g, Sugar: 9.49g, Sodium: 317mg, Cholesterol: 0mg

Authentic Red Gazpacho

Prep Time: 15 minutes, Cook Time: 0, Serves: 4

INGREDIENTS:

⅓ cup extra-virgin olive oil
2 pounds(907g) tomatoes, cut into chunks
1 bell pepper, cut into chunks
1 cucumber, cut into chunks
1 small red onion, cut into chunks
1 garlic clove, smashed
2 tsps. sherry vinegar
½ tsp. kosher salt
¼ tsp. freshly ground black pepper
¼ cup fresh chives, chopped, for garnish
Lemon juice (optional)

DIRECTIONS:

1. In a high-speed blender or Vitamix, add the tomatoes, bell pepper, cucumber, onion, garlic, vinegar, salt, and black pepper. Blend until smooth.
2. With the motor running, add the olive oil and purée until smooth. Add more vinegar or a spritz of lemon juice if needed.
3. Garnish with the chives.

Nutrition Info per Serving:

Calories: 240, Total fat: 19g, Saturated fat: 3g, Cholesterol: 0mg, Sodium: 155mg, Potassium: 830mg, Total Carbohydrates: 18g, Fiber: 5g, Sugar: 11g, Protein: 4g, Magnesium: 50mg, Calcium: 60mg

Potato Soup with Thai Basil

Prep Time: 15 minutes, Cook Time: 25 minutes, Serves: 4

INGREDIENTS:

4 cups (1L) Vegetable Stock, or low-sodium vegetable broth
One 14-oz.(400g) can lite coconut milk
3 shallots, peeled and thinly sliced
2 potatoes, peeled and diced
1 head baby bok choy, thinly sliced
1 small cucumber, peeled and diced
1 cup black beans
1 stalk lemongrass, cut into 1-inch pieces
2 tbsps. Thai red curry paste
3 tbsps. low-sodium soy sauce
Zest and juice of 2 lemon
5 cloves garlic, crushed
¼ cup chopped Thai basil
2 Thai red chiles, sliced into thin rounds
Fresh parsley

DIRECTIONS:

1. Put in the vegetable stock, garlic, lemongrass, curry paste, soy sauce, lemon zest and juice, and coconut milk in a large saucepan.
2. Bring the pot to a boil over high heat. Add the shallots, potatoes, bok choy, and cucumber.
3. Lower the heat to medium-low and cook until the vegetables are softened, about 25 minutes.
4. Remove the ginger and lemongrass and whisk in the black beans, basil, and chiles. Garnish with parsley and serve.

Nutrition Info per Serving:

Calories: 169, Protein: 13.33g, Fat: 2.65g, Carbohydrates: 29.97g, Fiber: 9.5g, Sugar: 15.78g, Sodium: 621mg, Cholesterol: 0mg

Asparagus-Onion Millet Stew

Prep Time: 15 minutes, Cook Time: 45 minutes, Serves: 4 to 6

INGREDIENTS:

5 to 6 cups (1180mL-1410mL) Vegetable Stock, or low-sodium vegetable broth
1 cup millet
1 large head cauliflower, cut into large florets
One 14.5-oz.(430g) can asparagus, diced
1 large onion, peeled and cut into ¾-inch pieces
2 large zucchini, diced
1 tsp. ground nutmeg
2 tbsps. grated ginger
3 sprigs mint
3 cloves garlic, smashed and skin removed
Salt and freshly ground black pepper to taste
½ cup chopped dill

DIRECTIONS:

1. Mix together the vegetable stock, nutmeg, ginger, and mint in a small pot and simmer over medium-high heat for 15 minutes. Remove from the heat, discard the spices, and set aside.
2. In a large saucepan, add the onion and zucchini and sauté for 8 to 10 minutes over medium heat, or until the vegetables are soft and starting to brown. Pour in water 1 to 2 tbsps. at a time to keep the vegetables from sticking to the pan. Whisk in the garlic and cook for another minute. Stir in the prepared vegetable stock, millet, cauliflower, and asparagus and bring to a boil over high heat. Lower the heat to medium and simmer, covered, for 12 to 15 minutes, or until the cauliflower and millet are soft. Drizzle with salt to taste and simmer for another 5 minutes.
3. Serve garnished with dill.

Nutrition Info per Serving:

Calories: 224, Protein: 7.27g, Fat: 3.37g, Carbohydrates: 42.53g, Fiber: 6.5g, Sugar: 6.92g, Sodium: 621mg, Cholesterol: 0mg

Homemade Chicken Chili with Beans

Prep Time: 15 minutes, Cook Time: 4 hours, Serves: 6

INGREDIENTS:

4 boneless skinless chicken breasts, cut into 1-inch pieces
2 tbsps. extra-virgin olive oil
2 onions, chopped
4 garlic cloves, minced
2 celery stalks, chopped
2 tsps. ground cumin
1 tsp. dried oregano
1 bay leaf
1 (28-ounce, 794 g) can chopped tomatoes
2 ½ cups (600 ml) chicken broth, plus additional as needed
2 (15-ounce, 425 g) cans white beans, drained and rinsed
¼ cup chopped fresh parsley, divided
1 tsp. salt
1 tsp. chipotle powder
½ tsp. freshly ground black pepper

DIRECTIONS:

1. Combine the onions, olive oil, celery, garlic, cumin, chipotle powder, salt, pepper, oregano, chicken, chicken broth, tomatoes, bay leaf, and white beans in the slow cooker. Set to high and cook for 4 hours.
2. If the mixture gets too thick, add some water or a little more chicken broth.
3. Garnish each serving with parsley. Serve alone or over brown rice or quinoa.

Nutrition Info per Serving:

Calories: 423, Total Carbohydrates: 41g, Protein: 42g, Total Fat: 13g, Sugar: 6g, Fiber: 10g, Sodium: 857mg, Cholesterol: 175mg

Leek and Pear Soup with Fennel and Spinach

Prep Time: 15 minutes, Cook Time: 15 minutes, Serves: 4-6

INGREDIENTS:

2 leeks, white part only, sliced
1 fennel bulb, cut into ¼-inch-thick slices
2 tbsps. extra-virgin olive oil
2 pears, peeled, cored, and cut into ½-inch cubes
¼ tsp. freshly ground black pepper
1 tsp. salt
2 cups packed spinach or arugula
½ cup cashews
3 cups water, or vegetable broth

DIRECTIONS:

1. Add olive oil into a large Dutch oven, heat over high heat.
2. Place the leeks and fennel into the oven and sauté for 5 minutes.
3. Stir in the pears, salt, and pepper. Sauté for another 3 minutes.
4. Add the cashews, pour in water and bring the soup to a boil. Lower the heat to simmer and cook for 5 minutes, partially covered.
5. Add the spinach and stir well.
6. In a blender, pour the soup, working in batches if necessary, purée the soup until smooth.

Nutrition Info per Serving:

Calories: 111, Total Fat: 5g, Total Carbohydrates: 9g, Sugar: 4g, Fiber: 2g, Protein: 9g, Sodium: 709mg, Cholesterol: 0mg

Healthy Garlicky Roasted Vegetable Soup

Prep Time: 30 minutes, Cook Time: 40 minutes, Serves: 6-8

INGREDIENTS:

½ cup extra-virgin olive oil
4 carrots, halved lengthwise
½ head cauliflower, broken into florets
3 Roma tomatoes, quartered
2 cups cubed butternut squash
4 garlic cloves
3 shallots, halved lengthwise
1 tsp. salt
¼ tsp. freshly ground black pepper
4 to 6 cups water or vegetable broth

DIRECTIONS:

1. Preheat the oven to 400°F(205°C).
2. Add the carrots, cauliflower, tomatoes, butternut squash, garlic, and shallots into a large bowl, combine them together. Add the olive oil, salt, and pepper and toss the vegetables to coat.
3. Place the vegetables in a single layer on a rimmed baking sheet. Put the sheet in the preheated oven, and roast the vegetables until they start to brown, about 25 minutes.
4. After roasting, transfer the roasted vegetables to a large Dutch oven, coved with enough water and bring to a boil over high heat. Lower the heat to a simmer and cook the soup for 10 minutes.
5. In a blender, pour the soup, working in batches if necessary, and purée until smooth.

Nutrition Info per Serving:

Calories: 197, Total Fat: 17g, Total Carbohydrates: 13g, Sugar: 5g, Fiber: 3g, Protein: 2g, Sodium: 426mg, Cholesterol: 5mg

Mushrooms Soup with Celery

Prep Time: 15 minutes, Cook Time: 10 minutes, Serves: 4

INGREDIENTS:

1 pound(454 g) mushrooms, sliced thin
1 tbsp. extra-virgin olive oil
3 garlic cloves, sliced thin
1 onion, halved and sliced thin
1 celery stalk, finely chopped
1 tsp. salt
½ tsp. freshly ground black pepper
Pinch nutmeg
4 cups vegetable broth
2 tbsps. chopped fresh tarragon

DIRECTIONS:

1. Add olive oil into a large pot, heat over high heat.
2. Place the onion, garlic, and celery into the pot and sauté for 3 minutes.
3. Stir in the mushrooms, salt, pepper, and nutmeg. Sauté for another 5 to 10 minutes.
4. Pout in the vegetable broth and bring the soup to a boil. Lower the heat to simmer. Cook for another 5 minutes.
5. Mix in the tarragon and serve.

Nutrition Info per Serving:

Calories: 111, Total Fat: 5g, Total Carbohydrates: 9g, Sugar: 4g, Fiber: 2g, Protein: 9g, Sodium: 1080mg, Cholesterol: 1mg

Pumpkin and Cucumber Stew with Lime Juice

Prep Time: 15 minutes, Cook Time: 35 minutes, Serves: 6 to 8

INGREDIENTS:

1 small pumpkin (about 1 pound/450 g), peeled, seeded, and cut into 1-inch cubes
4 cups cooked black beans, or two 15-oz. (430g) cans, drained and rinsed
6 cups (1410mL) Vegetable Stock, or low-sodium vegetable broth
1 large red onion, peeled and diced
2 large carrots, peeled and diced
2 cucumber, diced
2 cloves garlic, peeled and minced
2 tbsps. coriander powder
2 tbsps. lime juice
Salt and freshly ground black pepper to taste
2 tbsps. fresh sage

DIRECTIONS:

1. In a large saucepan, add the onion, carrots, and cucumber and sauté over medium heat for 10 minutes. Pour in water 1 to 2 tbsps. at a time to keep the vegetables from sticking to the pan.
2. Stir in the garlic and cook for another minute. Whisk in the coriander, lime juice, pumpkin, beans, and vegetable stock and bring to a boil over high heat.
3. Turn the heat down to medium and simmer, covered, for 25 minutes, or until the pumpkin is soft. Sprinkle with salt and pepper to taste and serve garnished with the sage.

Nutrition Info per Serving:

Calories: 113, Protein: 4.91g, Fat: 2.09g, Carbohydrates: 21.3g, Fiber: 4.1g, Sugar: 6.8g, Sodium: 447mg, Cholesterol: 0mg

Mushroom Sweet Potato Soup

Prep Time: 10 minutes, Cook Time: 40 minutes, Serves: 4 to 6

INGREDIENTS:

2 sweet potatoes, peeled and diced
2 medium cucumber, diced
2 avocado, diced
8 oz.(230g) cremini mushrooms, sliced
5 cups (1180mL) Vegetable Stock, or low-sodium vegetable broth
½ ounce dried porcini mushrooms, soaked for 30 minutes in 1 cup of water that has just been boiled
2 cloves garlic, minced
1 tsp. ground sumac
2 tsps. paprika
2 tsps. minced oregano
3 sprigs mint
3 cups cooked barley
Salt and freshly ground black pepper to taste

DIRECTIONS:

1. Add the potatoes, cucumber, avocado, and cremini mushrooms in a large pot and sauté over medium heat for 10 minutes.
2. Pour in water 1 to 2 tbsps. at a time to keep the vegetables from sticking to the pot.
3. Whisk in the garlic, sumac, paprika, mint and oregano and cook for another minute. Pour in the vegetable stock and porcini mushrooms and their soaking liquid and bring to a boil over high heat.
4. Reduce the heat to medium-low and cook, covered, for about 20 minutes, until the mushrooms are cooked through.
5. Whisk in the cooked barley and simmer for another 10 minutes. Sprinkle with salt and pepper to taste.

Nutrition Info per Serving:

Calories: 173, Protein: 5.93g, Fat: 2.52g, Carbohydrates: 35.04g, Fiber: 7.8g, Sugar: 6.12g, Sodium: 53mg, Cholesterol: 0mg

Garlicky Broccoli Bisque

Prep Time: 10 minutes, Cook Time: 35 minutes, Serves: 4

INGREDIENTS:

2 celery stalks, diced
1 large head broccoli, cut into florets
4 cups (1L) Vegetable Stock, or low-sodium vegetable broth
¼ cup chopped parsley
1 oregano leaf
2 tsps. ground sumac
1 tsp. cayenne pepper
3 cloves garlic, crushed
2 tbsps. apple cider
salt and pepper to taste

DIRECTIONS:

1. Add the celery in a large saucepan and sauté over medium heat for 10 minutes. Pour in water 1 to 2 tbsps. at a time to keep the celery from sticking to the pan. Stir in the oregano, sumac, cayenne pepper, garlic, and apple cider and cook for 30 seconds. Stir in the broccoli and vegetable stock and bring the pot to a boil over high heat. Turn the heat down to medium and simmer, covered, for 20 to 25 minutes, or until the broccoli is softened.
2. Process the soup in a food processor, cover with a towel to avoid splatter. Return to the pot and sprinkle with salt and pepper to taste. Serve garnished with the parsley.

Nutrition Info per Serving:

Calories: 88, Protein: 5.13g, Fat: 0.8g, Carbohydrates: 18.6g, Fiber: 6.6g, Sugar: 7.96g, Sodium: 58mg

Garlicky Potato Leek Soup with Onion

Prep Time: 10 minutes, Cook Time: 35 minutes, Serves: 8

INGREDIENTS:

2 tbsps. olive oil
8 russet potatoes, about 2 lb (1kg) total
4 leeks, about 2 lb (1kg) total
1 yellow onion, chopped, about 7 oz (200g) total
5 garlic cloves, chopped
12 cups (3 L) water
1 tbsp. salt
1 tsp. freshly ground black pepper, plus more to taste

DIRECTIONS:

1. Cut off the hairy root and the dark green tops of the leeks. Slice each leek lengthwise and wash in running water to remove any dirt. Cut into thin slices.
2. Add the olive oil into a large pot, heat over medium-high heat. Stir in the onion and garlic and cook for 2 minutes. Stir in the leeks and cook for 10–15 minutes, until they begin to break down and release moisture, stirring occasionally.
3. Meanwhile, peel the potatoes and dice into ½-inch (1 cm) cubes. Set aside.
4. Add 2 cups of water to the pot and use an immersion blender to make a purée, then add the remaining 10 cups water. If using a large food processor, transfer the leeks into the processor, add 2 cups of water and blend. Pour back into the pot and add the remaining 10 cups water.
5. Stir in the potatoes, salt, and pepper to the pot and bring to a boil. Reduce the heat to medium-low and simmer for 20 minutes. Taste and adjust seasoning. Serve immediately, or evenly divide among 4 jars or meal prep containers. Allow cool completely before putting on lids and refrigerating.

Nutrition Info per Serving:

Calories: 216, Fat: 4g, Carbohydrates: 40g, Protein: 5g, Sugar: 4g, Fiber: 4g, Cholesterol: 0mg, Sodium: 948mg

Greek Chicken Soup with Artichokes

Prep Time: 10 minutes, Cook Time: 15 minutes, Serves: 4

INGREDIENTS:

4 cups (960 ml) Chicken Stock
2 cups Riced Cauliflower, divided
2 large egg yolks
¼ cup freshly squeezed lemon juice (about 2 lemons)
¾ cup (180 ml) extra-virgin olive oil, divided
8 ounces (227 g) cooked chicken, coarsely chopped
1 (13.75-ounce, 390 g) can artichoke hearts, drained and quartered
¼ cup chopped fresh dill

DIRECTIONS:

1. Bring the stock to a low boil in a large saucepan. Lower the heat and simmer, covered.
2. Transfer 1 cup of the hot stock to a blender. Add ½ cup raw riced cauliflower, the egg yolks, and lemon juice and purée. While the processor is running, stream in ½ cup olive oil and blend until smooth.
3. Whisking constantly, pour the purée into the simmering stock until well blended together and smooth. Add the chicken and artichokes and simmer 8 to 10 minutes until thickened slightly. Stir in the dill and remaining riced cauliflower. Serve warm, drizzled with the remaining olive oil.

Nutrition Info per Serving:

Calories: 566, Total Carbs: 14g, Protein: 24g, Total Fat: 46g, Net Carbs: 7g, Fiber: 7g, Sodium: 754mg, Cholesterol: 161mg, Sugar: 5.6g

Vegan Broccoli Lentil Stew

Prep Time: 15 minutes, Cook Time: 30 minutes, Serves: 4

INGREDIENTS:

1 tbsp. extra-virgin olive oil, plus additional for drizzling
6 cups broccoli florets
1 cup dried green or brown lentils
1 small onion, finely chopped
1 small carrot, chopped
2 cloves garlic, minced
2 cups vegetable broth
1 tsp. dried oregano
¼ tsp. freshly ground black pepper
½ cup sliced pitted green olives
¼ cup chopped fresh Italian parsley
1 tsp. salt

DIRECTIONS:

1. Add olive oil into a large pot, heat over high heat.
2. Place the onion, carrot, and garlic into the pot and sauté for 5 minutes.
3. Stir in the vegetable broth, lentils, and oregano and bring to a boil. Lower the heat to simmer. Cook the soup for 15 to 20 minutes, or until the lentils are tender. Mix in the broccoli, cover the pot, and simmer for another 5 minutes.
4. Take the pot off the heat and stir in the olives and parsley. If the soup is too thick, stir in some water.
5. Transfer the soup into bowls, season with salt and pepper. Drizzle with a little olive oil, and serve.

Nutrition Info per Serving:

Calories: 182, Total Fat: 6g, Total Carbohydrates: 24g, Sugar: 5g, Fiber: 9g, Protein: 11g, Sodium: 895mg, Cholesterol: 0mg

Spicy Buttercup Squash Soup

Prep Time: 15 minutes, Cook Time: 30 minutes, Serves: 6

INGREDIENTS:

½ tsp. kosher salt
¼ tsp. ground white pepper
2 tbsps. extra-virgin olive oil
1 medium onion, chopped
4 to 5 cups (960 to 1200 ml) Vegetable Broth or Chicken Bone Broth
1½ pounds (680 g) buttercup squash, peeled, seeded, and cut into 1-inch chunks
Whole nutmeg, for grating

DIRECTIONS:

1. Set the electric pressure cooker to the Sauté setting. Pour in the olive oil when the pot is hot.
2. Add the onion and sauté for 3 to 5 minutes. Press Cancel.
3. Add 4 or 5 cups of broth, squash, salt, and pepper to the pot and stir.
4. Close the lid of the pressure cooker. Set the valve to sealing.
5. Cook on high pressure for 10 minutes.
6. Once cooking is complete, press Cancel and allow the pressure to release naturally.
7. When the pin drops, unlock and remove the lid.
8. Use an immersion blender to purée the soup in the pot. If you don't have an immersion blender, transfer the soup to a food processor or blender and purée.
9. Pour the soup into serving bowls and top with grated nutmeg.

Nutrition Info per Serving:

Calories: 110, Carbohydrates: 18g, Protein: 1g, Total Fat: 5g, Sugar: 4g, Fiber: 4g, Sodium: 166mg, Cholesterol: 68mg

Tomato-Corn Chowder

Prep Time: 10 minutes, Cook Time: 1hour, Serves: 6

INGREDIENTS:

3 tomatoes, diced
1 asparagus, trimmed and diced
2 medium carrots, peeled and diced
6 cups (1410mL) Vegetable Stock, or low-sodium vegetable broth
2 small zucchini, diced
1 large sweet potatoes, peeled and diced
3 to 4 ears corn, shucked
4 cups packed lettuce, coarsely chopped
1 tsp. fennel
1 tbsp. cumin

DIRECTIONS:

1. Add the tomatoes, asparagus, carrots, and ½ cup of vegetable stock in a large soup pot and sauté over medium-high heat for 6 to 8 minutes, or until the asparagus is soft.
2. Stir in the zucchini, sweet potatoes, fennel, cumin, and the reserving broth and bring to a boil over high heat. Turn the heat down to medium-low and cook for 20 to 30 minutes, or until the vegetables are softened.
3. Whisk in half the corn and simmer for 10 to 15 more minutes. Remove the bay leaves.
4. Process the soup in a food processor, cover with a towel. Return the soup to the pot and whisk in the reserving corn and lettuce. Simmer for 5 more minutes, or until the lettuce is wilted. Toss to combine well and serve hot.

Nutrition Info per Serving:

Calories: 189, Protein: 7.24g, Fat: 1.47g, Carbohydrates: 41.74g, Fiber: 10g, Sugar: 10.28g, Sodium: 98mg, Cholesterol: 0mg

Cream of Cauliflower Soup

Prep Time: 10 minutes, Cook Time: 25 minutes, Serves: 6

INGREDIENTS:

3 large leeks (white parts only), sliced and rinsed
4 cups cauliflower florets (from about 2 large heads)
4½ cups (1060mL) Vegetable Stock, or low-sodium vegetable broth, plus more as needed
3 tbsps. apple cider
1 tsp. tarragon, minced
Salt and freshly ground black pepper to taste

DIRECTIONS:

1. Add the leeks in a large saucepan and sauté over medium heat for 10 minutes. Pour in water 1 to 2 tbsps. at a time to keep the leeks from sticking to the pan. Stir in the tarragon and cook for another minute, then stir in the cauliflower, vegetable stock, and apple cider. Bring to a boil over high heat, turn the heat down to medium, and simmer, covered, until the cauliflower is softened, about 10 minutes.
2. Process the soup in a food processor, cover with a towel. Return the soup to the pot and sprinkle with salt and pepper to taste.

Nutrition Info per Serving:

Calories: 87, Protein: 5.44g, Fat: 0.97g, Carbohydrates: 16.47g, Fiber: 3.2g, Sugar: 7.34g, Sodium: 389mg, Cholesterol: 0mg

Chicken Wing Broth

Prep Time: 15 minutes, Cook Time: 1.5 hours, Serves: 3 quarts

INGREDIENTS:

3 pounds (1.4 kg) chicken wings
1 tbsp. vegetable oil
1 onion, chopped
12 cups (2880 ml) water, divided
½ tsp. table salt
3 bay leaves
3 garlic cloves, lightly crushed and peeled

DIRECTIONS:

1. Pat chicken wings dry with paper towels. In Instant Pot, use highest sauté function, heat oil for 5 minutes. Brown half of chicken wings for about 10 minutes, transfer to bowl. Repeat with remaining chicken wings.
2. Add onion to fat left in pot and cook 8 to 10 minutes until softened and well browned. Stir in garlic and cook about 30 seconds until fragrant. Add 1 cup water, scraping up any browned bits. Stir in remaining 11 cups water, bay leaves, salt, and chicken and any accumulated juices.
3. Lock lid and close pressure release valve. Choose high-pressure cook function and cook for 1 hour. Turn off and let pressure release naturally for 15 minutes. Quick-release any remaining pressure and carefully remove lid, letting steam escape away from you.
4. Strain broth through colander into large container, pressing on solids to extract as much liquid as possible, throw away solids. Skim excess fat from surface of broth with a wide, shallow spoon. (Broth can be refrigerated for up to 4 days or frozen for 2 months.)

Nutrition Info per Serving:

Calories: 20, Fat: 0g, Protein: 4g, Carbohydrates: 0g, Fiber: 0g, Sugar: 0g, Sodium: 95mg, Cholesterol: 0mg

Corn and Potato Soup with Dill

Prep Time: 10 minutes, Cook Time: 35 minutes, Serves: 4

INGREDIENTS:

1 zucchini, diced small
1 large red bell pepper, seeded and diced
2 large Yukon Gold potatoes (about 1 pound), peeled and chopped
3 ears corn, shucked (about 2 cups)
4 cups (1L) Vegetable Stock, or low-sodium vegetable broth
2 tsps. cinnamon
3 cloves garlic, crushed
1 tsp. mint
1 batch No-Cheese Sauce
2 tbsps. peanut milk
Salt and freshly ground black pepper to taste
2 tsps. scallion, cut
½ cup dill, chopped

DIRECTIONS:

1. Add the zucchini and red pepper in a large saucepan and sauté over medium-high heat for 7 to 8 minutes.
2. Pour in water 1 to 2 tbsps. at a time to keep the vegetables from sticking to the pan. Stir in the garlic and cook for another minute.
3. Stir in the potatoes, corn, vegetable stock, and cinnamon, mint, peanut milk and bring the mixture to a boil over high heat.
4. Turn the heat down to medium and simmer, covered, for 20 minutes, or until the potatoes are softened.
5. Pour in the No-Cheese Sauce and simmer over low heat for 5 minutes. Sprinkle with salt and black pepper to taste and serve garnished with the scallion and dill.

Nutrition Info per Serving:

Calories: 362, Protein: 11.95g, Fat: 1.9g, Carbohydrates: 81.64g, Fiber: 13.7g, Sugar: 27.48g, Sodium: 306mg, Cholesterol: 0mg

Tasty Kale Soup

Prep Time: 10 minutes, Cook Time: 15 minutes, Serves: 4

INGREDIENTS:

1 medium onion, chopped
2 carrots, finely chopped
4 cups baby kale leaves, chopped
3 garlic cloves, minced
4 cups low-sodium vegetable broth
1 (28-ounce (794g)) can crushed tomatoes
½ tsp. dried oregano
¼ tsp. dried basil
1 tbsp. extra-virgin olive oil
¼ tsp. salt

DIRECTIONS:

1. Prepare a large pot, heat oil over medium heat. Add the onions and carrots to the pot. Sauté for 3 to 5 minutes until they start to soften. Add garlic and sauté for another 30 seconds, until fragrant.
2. Add vegetable broth, tomatoes, oregano and basil to the pot and bring to a boil. Reduce the heat and simmer for 5 minutes.
3. Use an immersion blender to purée the soup.
4. Add the kale and simmer for another 3 minutes. Add salt to taste. Serve warm.

Nutrition Info per Serving:
Calories: 170, Total Fat: 5g, Protein: 6g, Carbohydrates: 31g, Sugar: 13g, Fiber: 9g, Sodium: 600mg, Cholesterol: 1mg

Thai Vegetable Stew with Dill

Prep Time: 15 minutes, Cook Time: 20 minutes, Serves: 4

INGREDIENTS:

1 medium yellow onion, peeled and diced small
One 14-oz.(400g) can lite coconut milk
1 cup (240mL) Vegetable Stock, or low-sodium vegetable broth
3 cups mixed vegetables of your choice, such as lentils, spinach, zucchini, asparagus, or sugar snap peas
½ cup chopped parsley
3 cloves garlic, crushed
2 tsps. cumin
2 tsps. Thai red chili paste
Zest and juice of 1 lime
1 serrano chile, minced (for less heat, remove the seeds)
2 tbsps. low-sodium soy sauce, or to taste
2 tbsps. fresh dill, chopped

DIRECTIONS:

1. Add the onion in a large saucepan and sauté over medium-high heat for 7 to 8 minutes, or until the onion is soft and starting to brown.
2. Pour in water 1 to 2 tbsps. at a time to keep the onion from sticking to the pan. Stir in the garlic, cumin, chili paste, lime zest and juice, and serrano chile and cook for 30 seconds.
3. Stir the soy sauce, coconut milk, vegetable stock, and mixed vegetables, turn the heat down to medium, and simmer for 10 minutes, or until the vegetables are soft. Spread with the parsley and dill and serve.

Nutrition Info per Serving:
Calories: 141, Protein: 8.17g, Fat: 3.85g, Carbohydrates: 21.09g, Fiber: 4.4g, Sugar: 9.89g, Sodium: 729mg, Cholesterol: 0mg

Taro Soup with Broccoli, Potatoes and Leek

Prep Time: 10 minutes, Cook Time: 1 hour, Serves: 8 to 10

INGREDIENTS:

1 large onion, peeled and chopped
One 15-oz.(430g) can cherry tomatoes, halved
1 cup taro, peeled and diced
2 large waxy potatoes, scrubbed and cut into ½-inch dice
1 small head broccoli, cut into florets
6 cups finely chopped leek
5 cloves garlic, peeled and minced
2 bay leaves
2 tsps. dry mustard
1 tsp. turmeric
Dash ground mint
2 tbsps. minced dill
3 tbsps. peanut butter
Salt and freshly ground black pepper to taste

DIRECTIONS:

1. Add the onions in a large pot and sauté over medium for 10 minutes. Pour in water 1 to 2 tbsps. at a time to keep the onion from sticking to the pot.
2. Stir in the garlic and cook for 1 minute. Whisk in the bay leaves, dry mustard, turmeric, and mint and cook for 1 minute.
3. Put in the tomatoes and cook for 3 minutes. Pour in the taro and 6 cups of water and bring to a boil over high heat. Turn the heat down to medium and simmer, covered, for 30 minutes.
4. Whisk in the potatoes and broccoli and cook until the taro is softened, about 15 more minutes.
5. Put in the leek, dill, and peanut butter. Sprinkle with salt and pepper to taste.

Nutrition Info per Serving:
Calories: 113, Protein: 6.59g, Fat: 1.03g, Carbohydrates: 23.04g, Fiber: 6.6g, Sugar: 3.85g, Sodium: 140mg, Cholesterol: 0mg

Lemony Avocado Gazpacho

Prep Time: 15 minutes, Cook Time: 0, Serves: 4

INGREDIENTS:

- 2 cups chopped tomatoes
- 2 large ripe avocados, halved and pitted
- 1 large cucumber, peeled and seeded
- 1 medium bell pepper, chopped
- 2 tbsps. red wine vinegar
- Juice of 2 limes or 1 lemon
- 1 cup (240 ml) plain whole-milk Greek yogurt
- ¼ cup (60 ml) extra-virgin olive oil
- ¼ cup chopped fresh cilantro
- ¼ cup chopped scallions, green part only
- ½ to 1 tsp. salt
- ¼ tsp. freshly ground black pepper

DIRECTIONS:

1. In a blender, combine the tomatoes, cucumber, avocados, yogurt, bell pepper, olive oil, cilantro, vinegar, scallions, and lime juice. Blend until smooth.
2. Season with salt and pepper and blend to mix the flavors.
3. Chill in the refrigerator for 1 to 2 hours before serving.

Nutrition Info per Serving:

Calories: 392, Total Carbs: 20g, Protein: 6g, Total Fat: 32g, Net Carbs: 11g, Fiber: 9g, Sodium: 335mg, Sugar: 7.6g, Cholesterol: 13mg

Tuscan Radish Stew

Prep Time: 15 minutes, Cook Time: 40 minutes, Serves: 6

INGREDIENTS:

- 3 large leeks (white and light green parts), diced and rinsed
- 1 zucchini, diced
- 2 medium carrots, peeled and diced
- 3 cups cooked cannellini beans
- 6 cups (1410mL) Vegetable Stock, or low-sodium vegetable broth
- ½ cup tarragon, chopped
- 2 cups green cabbage, chopped
- 2 radishes, peeled and diced
- 5 cloves garlic, smashed and skin removed
- Salt and freshly ground black pepper to taste

DIRECTIONS:

1. In a large saucepan, add the leeks, zucchini, and carrots and sauté for 10 minutes over medium heat.
2. Pour in water 1 to 2 tbsps. at a time to keep the vegetables from sticking to the pan.
3. Stir in the radishes, cabbage, garlic, beans, and vegetable stock and bring the soup to a boil over high heat.
4. Turn the heat down to medium and simmer, uncovered, for 30 minutes, or until the radishes are soft.
5. Spread the tarragon and sprinkle the soup with salt and pepper to taste.

Nutrition Info per Serving:

Calories: 206, Protein: 8.05g, Fat: 2.72g, Carbohydrates: 40.91g, Fiber: 7.3g, Sugar: 8.41g, Sodium: 607mg, Cholesterol: 0mg

Black Bean and Veggie Soup Topped with Lime Salsa

Prep Time: 15 minutes, Cook Time: 45 minutes, Serves: 4

INGREDIENTS:

- 2 shallots, diced
- 2 carrots, diced
- 3 sticks chives, diced
- 2 red bell peppers, diced
- 3 cloves garlic, finely chopped
- 2 de-seeded red chilis
- ½ bunch cilantro
- 1 bay leaf
- 1 tbsp. dried oregano
- 1 tbsp. freshly ground black pepper
- ½ tbsp. basil
- 2 cans (15 ounces) black beans, drained and rinsed
- 1 quart boiling water
- 1 tarragon, finely chopped
- ½ small salad onion, finely chopped
- Fresh juice of ½ lime

DIRECTIONS:

1. Start by removing the leaves and stalks from the cilantro. Finely chop the stalks and leaves. Set aside
2. Take a large saucepan and pour in 3 tablespoons of water. To this, add the carrots, shallots, bell peppers, garlic, red chilies, cilantro, black pepper, oregano, bay leaf, basil, and tarragon. Mix until well-combined. Cover the pan using a lid and let the veggies cook for about 10 minutes. Keep stirring.
3. Add the black beans and boiling water into the saucepan. Keep stirring.
4. Remove the lid from the saucepan and lower the flame. Allow the soup to cook for 30 minutes.
5. While the soup is cooking, make the lime salsa. For this, you will combine the tomato, salad onion, and cilantro leaves in a small bowl. Squeeze in the fresh lime juice.
6. Pour the soup in shallow bowls and finish by topping with lime salsa.

Nutrition Info per Serving:

Calories: 287, Fat: 2.4g, Protein: 17.2g, Carbohydrates: 53.9g, Fiber: 3.6g, Sugar: 5.1g, Sodium: 310mg, Cholesterol: 0mg

Winter Squash Kasha Stew with Kale

Prep Time: 15 minutes, Cook Time: 4 hours, Serves: 4

INGREDIENTS:

2 pounds(907 g) winter squash, peeled and cubed
1 tbsp. extra-virgin olive oil
2 leeks, white part only, sliced thin
2 garlic cloves, chopped
1 fennel bulb, sliced thin
1 cup kasha, rinsed
4 cups chopped kale, thoroughly washed and stemmed
1 tsp. salt
½ tsp. freshly ground black pepper
3 cups water, or vegetable broth

DIRECTIONS:

1. Add the olive oil, squash, leeks, garlic, fennel, kasha, salt, pepper, and water into the slow cooker, combine them together. Set the cooker on high and cook for 4 hours.
2. Stir in the kale just before serving, making it easy to chew and digest.

Nutrition Info per Serving:

Calories: 325, Total Fat: 6g, Total Carbohydrates: 60g, Sugar: 2g, Fiber: 8g, Protein: 12g, Sodium: 762mg, Cholesterol: 1mg

White Bean Stew with Saffron and Sage

Prep Time: 15 minutes, Cook Time: 35 minutes, Serves: 6

INGREDIENTS:

2 zucchini, diced small
2 celery stalks, chopped into medium dice
1 medium asparagus, trimmed and diced
One 28-oz.(780g) can diced tomatoes
4 cups cooked cannellini beans, or two 15-oz. (430g) cans, drained and rinsed
2 cups (480mL) Vegetable Stock, or low-sodium vegetable broth
3 cloves garlic, crushed
½ cup maple syrup
2 large pinches saffron, crumbled and soaked for 15 minutes in ¼ cup of water that has just been boiled
1 cup sage, finely chopped
Salt and freshly ground black pepper to taste

DIRECTIONS:

1. In a large saucepan, add the zucchini, celery, and asparagus and sauté over medium heat for 10 minutes. Pour in water 1 to 2 tbsps. at a time to keep the vegetables from sticking to the pan.
2. Add the garlic and cook for another minute. Whisk in the maple syrup and the saffron with its soaking liquid and bring the pot to a boil over high heat. Stir in the tomatoes, beans, and vegetable stock.
3. Return the stew to a boil, then lower the heat and simmer, covered, for 30 minutes. Spread with the sage, season with salt and pepper, and simmer for another 5 minutes.

Nutrition Info per Serving:

Calories: 83, Protein: 3.54g, Fat: 1.21g, Carbohydrates: 16.77g, Fiber: 5.2g, Sugar: 7.51g, Sodium: 365mg, Cholesterol: 0mg

Easy Squash Soup with Crispy Chickpeas

Prep Time: 10 minutes, Cook Time: 20 minutes, Serves: 4

INGREDIENTS:

1 (15-ounce (425 g)) can low-sodium chickpeas, drained and rinsed
¼ tsp. smoked paprika
3 medium zucchini, coarsely chopped
3 cups low-sodium vegetable broth
½ onion, diced
3 garlic cloves, minced
2 tbsps. plain low-fat Greek yogurt
Freshly ground black pepper
1 tsp. extra-virgin olive oil, plus 1 tbsp.
Pinch salt, plus ½ tsp.

DIRECTIONS:

1. Preheat the oven to 425°F(220ºC). Line the baking sheet with parchment paper.
2. Take out a medium mixing bowl, add chickpeas with 1 tsp. of olive oil, smoked paprika, and a pinch of salt into it, and stir the mixtures until they are well mixed together. Transfer to the prepared baking sheet and bake for about 20 minutes until crispy, stirring once. Set aside.
3. At the same time, in a medium-sized pot, heat the remaining 1 tbsp. of oil over medium heat.
4. Add zucchini, broth, onion, and garlic to the pot and bring to a boil. Reduce the heat and cook for about 20 minutes until the zucchini and onions are soft.
5. In a blender jar, or using an immersion blender, purée the soup. Return to the pot.
6. Add yogurt, the remaining ½ tsp. salt, and pepper, and mix well. Top with roasted chickpeas and serve.

Nutrition Info per Serving:

Calories: 188, Total Fat: 7g, Protein: 8g, Carbohydrates: 24g, Sugar: 7g, Fiber: 7g, Sodium: 528mg, Cholesterol: 92mg

Savory Squash-Carrot Soup

Prep Time: 10 minutes, Cook Time: 30 minutes, Serves: 4

INGREDIENTS:

2½ cups butternut squash, peeled, halved, seeded, and diced (from about 1 medium)
1 carrot, peeled and diced (about 1 cup)
1 medium yellow onion, peeled and chopped (about ½ cup)
¼ cup edamame
3 clove garlic, crushed
¼ tsp. thyme
Pinch freshly ground black pepper
¼ tsp. ground nutmeg
Fresh dill, finely chopped

DIRECTIONS:

1. Pour 3 cups of water to a large pot over high heat and bring to a boil. Whisk in the squash, carrot, onion, garlic, thyme, and pepper. Turn the heat down to medium and cook, covered, for 20 minutes, or until the vegetables are softened.
2. Process the soup in a processor, cover with a towel. Return the soup to the pot and pour in the edamame and nutmeg. Cook for an additional 5 to 7 minutes, or until the peas are tender. Serve hot, garnished with the dill.

Nutrition Info per Serving:

Calories: 139, Protein: 4.2g, Fat: 0.42g, Carbohydrates: 32.32g, Fiber: 4.6g, Sugar: 4.13g, Sodium: 48mg, Cholesterol: 0mg

Tomato Lentil Soup with Pine Nut

Prep Time: 10 minutes, Cook Time: 35 minutes, Serves: 4

INGREDIENTS:

3 large tomatoes, sliced
4 cups cooked lentils, or two 15-oz.(430g) cans, drained and rinsed
Salt and freshly ground black pepper to taste
1 large red bell pepper, seeded and diced
3 cloves garlic, crushed
1 tbsp. thyme ground
1 tsp. dried oregano
1 tbsp. pine nuts, toasted and ground
1 dried chipotle pepper, halved, toasted in a dry skillet for 2 to 3 minutes, soaked in cool water for 15 minutes, and chopped
1 cup (240mL) almond milk
Zest of 1 lime

DIRECTIONS:

1. Add the tomatoes and red pepper in a large pan and sauté over medium heat for 7 to 8 minutes. Pour in water 1 to 2 tbsps. at a time to keep the vegetables from sticking to the pan.
2. Whisk in the garlic, thyme, oregano, pine nuts, and chipotle pepper and cook for 2 minutes.
3. Pour in the almond milk, lime zest, lentils, and enough water to cover the lentils by 3 inches. Bring the soup to a boil over high heat.
4. Turn the heat down to medium and simmer, covered, for 25 minutes. Sprinkle with salt and pepper to taste.

Nutrition Info per Serving:

Calories: 111, Protein: 4.51g, Fat: 0.86g, Carbohydrates: 23.23g, Fiber: 4.3g, Sugar: 9.82g, Sodium: 7mg, Cholesterol: 0mg

Aromatic White Beans and Lettuce Stew

Prep Time: 10 minutes, Cook Time: 25 minutes, Serves: 4

INGREDIENTS:

1 tbsp. extra-virgin olive oil
2 tsps. tarragon
1 medium onion, sliced
4 cloves garlic, crushed
1 red bell pepper, chopped
2 tomatoes, chopped
1 carrot, chopped
1 medium zucchini, diced
1 tsp. ground parsley
1 tsp. garam masala
1 tsp. black pepper
1 tsp. ground turmeric
2 cans white beans, rinsed and drained
1 tbsp. tomato paste
10 oz. lettuce
Salt and pepper
1 tsp. sweet paprika
2 tbsps. finely chopped fresh thyme

DIRECTIONS:

1. Heat the olive oil in a large saucepan over medium-high heat. Stir in the tarragon and cook for 10 seconds. Whisk in the onion and garlic and cook until tender and translucent, 3 minutes.
2. Mix in the bell pepper, tomatoes, zucchini and carrot, and cook, stirring until softened, 5 to 6 minutes.
3. Mix in the parsley, garam masala, paprika, thyme, and turmeric and cook, stirring, for 1 minute.
4. Pour in 2 cups water, the white beans, tomato paste, and lettuce and bring to a boil. Reduce to low heat, cover, and cook until the vegetables are wilted and softened, the sauce has thickened slightly, and the flavors have blended, 15 to 20 minutes.
5. Off heat, taste, and drizzle with salt and pepper, if desired. Serve.

Nutrition Info per Serving:

Calories: 309, Total fat: 7g, Saturated fat: <1g, Total carbohydrates: 50g, Protein: 15g, Cholesterol: 0mg, Sodium: 134mg, Fiber: 14g, Sugar: 10g

Stewed Chicken and Asparagus and Carrot

Prep Time: 10 minutes, Cook Time: 35 minutes, Serves: 10

INGREDIENTS:

2 cups zucchini, diced small
2 cups Cooked chicken breast, cubed
1 cup Cucumber, diced
2 cups Tomatoes, peeled
2 cups Carrots, shredded
5 cups Chicken broth
1 cup Sweet corn
1 cup Peas
1 cup asparagus, diced
Parsley for garnishing

DIRECTIONS:

1. Set a large stockpot over a medium flame.
2. Add the zucchini, chicken stock, chicken, tomatoes, cucumber, carrots, corn, asparagus, and peas.
3. Allow to cook for about half an hour over a medium flame, stirring continuously.
4. Once done, place into a serving bowl and garnish with parsley.

Nutrition Info per Serving:

Calories: 111, Fat: 2.5g, Protein: 10.1g, Carbohydrates: 13.1g, Cholesterol: 75mg, Sodium: 599mg, Fiber: 1.7g, Sugar: 3.1g

Squash and Peach Soup with Mint

Prep Time: 10 minutes, Cook Time: 30 minutes, Serves: 4

INGREDIENTS:

1 medium zucchini, peeled and diced small
1 large winter squash, acorn or butternut, peeled, halved, seeded, and cut into ½-inch dice (about 6 cups)
2 peaches, peeled, cored, and diced
1 cup unsweetened almond butter
3 cups (700mL) Vegetable Stock, or low-sodium vegetable broth
Pinch mint
1 tbsp. curry powder
Salt to taste

DIRECTIONS:

1. Add the zucchini in a large saucepan and sauté over medium heat for 10 minutes, or until the zucchini is browned.
2. Pour water 1 to 2 tbsps. at a time to keep the zucchini from sticking to the pan. Stir in the squash, peaches, curry powder, almond butter, vegetable stock, and mint and bring to a boil over high heat.
3. Turn the heat down to medium and simmer, covered, for about 20 minutes, or until the squash is softened.
4. Pulse the soup in a food processor, cover with a towel. If necessary, return the soup to the pot to reheat. Sprinkle with salt to taste.

Nutrition Info per Serving:

Calories: 151, Protein: 3.93g, Fat: 0.95g, Carbohydrates: 35.7g, Fiber: 8.7g, Sugar: 14.74g, Sodium: 613mg, Cholesterol: 0mg

Greek-Style Butternut Squash Soup

Prep Time: 10 minutes, Cook Time: 45 minutes, Serves: 6

INGREDIENTS:

1 (12-oz. 336g) package cubed peeled butternut squash
1 medium red onion, chopped
1 Granny Smith apple, cubed
1 tsp. ground cumin
½ tsp. ground ginger
½ tsp. ground turmeric
½ tsp. ground thyme
2 tbsps. olive oil
2 celery, diced
3 cloves garlic, minced
4 cups (940mL) low-sodium vegetable broth
⅔ cup (160mL) nonfat (0%) plain Greek yogurt
Salt and freshly ground black pepper (optional)

DIRECTIONS:

1. Preheat the oven to 400°F(205℃). Line a rimmed baking sheet with foil.
2. Whisk the butternut squash, onion, apple, cumin, ginger, turmeric, thyme, and 1 tbsp. of the olive oil in a medium bowl, and toss to combine well. Spread in an even layer on the baking sheet and roast until tender, 10 to 12 minutes.
3. Heat the remaining 1 tbsp. olive oil in a large pot, over medium-high heat. Add the celery and garlic and cook until tender, 4 to 5 minutes.
4. Add the roasted squash mixture and cook 5 minutes, until heated through, stirring often to avoid sticking. Add the broth and cook for 30 minutes.
5. Off heat and remove the pot, stir in the yogurt. Puree the soup until smooth in a food processor (or transfer in batches to a blender or food processor, puree until smooth, and return to the pot). Season with salt and pepper, if desired, and simmer gently for 5 minutes.
6. Divide into 6 bowls and serve.

Nutrition Info per Serving:

Calories: 205, Total fat: 7g, Saturated fat: 1g, Total carbohydrates: 32g, Protein: 6g, Cholesterol: 2mg, Sodium: 178mg, Potassium: 684mg, Fiber: 8g, Sugar: 13g

Red Pepper Soup with Smoked Paprika

Prep Time: 15 minutes, Cook Time: 40 minutes, Serves: 6

INGREDIENTS:

½ cup (120 ml) whole-milk yogurt
8 red bell peppers, cored and flattened
1 tbsp. extra-virgin olive oil
½ tsp. ground cumin
½ tsp. smoked paprika
2 garlic cloves, minced
1 red onion, chopped
1 bay leaf
½ cup (120 ml) half-and-half
2 tbsps. dry sherry
2 tbsps. tomato paste
1 tbsp. all-purpose flour
4 cups (960 ml) chicken or vegetable broth, plus extra as needed
3 tbsps. minced fresh cilantro
1 tsp. lime juice
Salt and pepper

DIRECTIONS:

1. Combine 1 tbsp. cilantro, yogurt and lime juice together in bowl. Season with salt and pepper. Cover and refrigerate.
2. Put oven rack 3 inches from broiler element and heat broiler. Spread half of peppers skin side up on aluminum foil–lined baking sheet. Broil and rotate sheet 8 to 10 minutes, until skin is charred and puffed but flesh is still firm. Transfer broiled peppers to bowl, cover with foil, and steam 10 to 15 minutes until skins peel off easily. Repeat with remaining peppers. Discard pepper skins, and chop coarse.
3. Cook oil and garlic together over low heat, stirring constantly for 6 to 8 minutes, until garlic is sticky, foamy and straw-colored. Add onion and ¼ teaspoon salt, increase heat to medium, and cook 5 minutes until softened.
4. Stir in paprika and cumin, cook about 30 seconds until fragrant. Add tomato paste and flour and cook for 1 minute. Slowly whisk in broth, scraping up any browned bits and smoothing out any lumps. Add bay leaf and chopped peppers, simmer and cook 5 to 7 minutes until peppers are very tender.
5. Discard bay leaf. Process soup in blender for about 2 minutes until smooth. Put soup to clean pot and stir in half-and-half and sherry. Heat soup over low heat until hot (do not boil). Stir in remaining cilantro and season with salt and pepper. Serve, drizzling with yogurt mixture.

Nutrition Info per Serving:

Calories: 338, Fat: 13.45g, Carbohydrates: 15.68g, Protein: 37.78g, Cholesterol: 73mg, Sodium: 278mg, Fiber: 2g, Sugar: 6.9g

Shrimp Soup with Leeks and Wine

Prep Time: 10 minutes, Cook Time: 40 minutes, Serves: 6 to 8

INGREDIENTS:

2 tbsps. extra-virgin olive oil, plus extra for serving
12 ounces (340 g) large shrimp (26 to 30 per pound), peeled and deveined, shells reserved
12 ounces (340 g) large sea scallops, tendons removed
12 ounces (340 g) squid, bodies sliced crosswise into ½-inch-thick rings, tentacles halved
1 cup (240 ml) dry white wine or dry vermouth
4 cups (960 ml) water
1½ pounds (680 g) leeks, white and light green parts only, halved lengthwise, sliced thin, and washed thoroughly
4 ounces (113 g) pancetta, chopped fine
1 tsp. grated fresh ginger
1 tsp. ground coriander
½ tsp. ground turmeric
⅛ tsp. red pepper flakes
3 tbsps. tomato paste
2 garlic cloves, minced
Salt and pepper
2 (8-ounce, 227g) bottles clam juice
⅓ cup minced fresh parsley

DIRECTIONS:

1. Heat oil over medium heat until shimmering. Add shrimp shells and cook 2 to 4 minutes, stirring frequently, until beginning to turn spotty brown and pot starts to brown. Add wine and simmer for 2 minutes, stirring occasionally. Stir in water and simmer, cook for 4 minutes. Strain mixture through fine-mesh strainer into bowl, pressing to extract as much liquid as possible.
2. Heat oil in pot over medium heat until shimmering. Add leeks and pancetta and cook about 8 minutes until leeks are softened and lightly browned. Stir in salt, tomato paste, garlic, turmeric, ginger, coriander, and pepper flakes and cook about 1 minute until fragrant. Stir in wine mixture and clam juice, scraping up any browned bits. Simmer and cook 15 to 20 minutes until flavors meld.
3. Add sea scallops, and cook for 2 minutes. Stir in shrimp and cook about 2 minutes until just opaque throughout. Off heat, stir in squid, cover, and let sit 1 to 2 minutes until just opaque and tender. Stir in parsley and season with salt and pepper. Serve, drizzling with extra oil.

Nutrition Info per Serving:

Calories: 305, Fat: 7.72g, Carbohydrates: 28.37g, Protein: 30.85g, Cholesterol: 208mg, Sodium: 291mg, Fiber: 2.5g, Sugar: 8.7g

Fresh-Flavored Asparagus Soup

Prep Time: 10 minutes, Cook Time: 35 minutes, Serves: 6

INGREDIENTS:

2 pounds(907g) fresh asparagus, trimmed and cut into ½-inch pieces
1 large yellow onion, peeled and diced
4 cups Vegetable Stock, or low-sodium vegetable broth
2 tsps. thyme
1 tbsp. minced tarragon
Salt and freshly ground black pepper to taste

DIRECTIONS:

1. Prepare a large stockpot, put the onion in it and sauté over medium heat for 10 minutes. Add 1 to 2 tbsps. of water at a time to prevent the onion from sticking to the pot. Add the thyme, tarragon, vegetable stock and asparagus and cook on medium-low heat for 20 to 25 minutes, until the asparagus is soft.
2. Use an immersion blender or in a blender to puree the soup in batches. Close the lid and cover with a towel. Salt and pepper, to taste

Nutrition Info per Serving:

Calories: 70, Protein: 5.62g, Fat: 0.52g, Carbohydrates: 14.37g, Fiber: 6.2g, Sugar: 6.63g, Sodium: 27mg, Cholesterol: 0mg

Yam-Carrot Bisque

Prep Time: 10 minutes, Cook Time: 40 minutes, Serves: 6

INGREDIENTS:

1 large carrot, peeled and diced
3 cloves garlic, peeled and minced
2 yams, peeled and diced
2 avocado, peeled and diced
6 cups Vegetable Stock, or low-sodium vegetable broth
Zest and juice of 1 orange
1 tbsp. grated ginger
1 tsp. rosemary
1 tsp. ground mint
1 tbsp. ground cinnamon
1½ cups unsweetened plain peanut milk
Salt and freshly ground black pepper to taste

DIRECTIONS:

1. Add the carrot in a large saucepan and sauté over medium heat for 10 minutes. Pour in water 1 to 2 tbsps. at a time to keep the carrot from sticking to the pan. Whisk in the garlic, ginger, rosemary, mint, and cinnamon and cook for 1 minute. Stir in the yams, avocado, vegetable stock, and orange zest and juice and bring the pot to a boil over high heat. Turn the heat down to medium and simmer, covered, for 25 minutes, or until the sweet potatoes are tender.
2. Process the soup in a food processor, cover with a towel. Return the soup to the pot and pour in the peanut milk. Cook for a further 5 minutes, or until heated through, and sprinkle with salt and pepper to taste and serve hot.

Nutrition Info per Serving:

Calories: 183, Protein: 7.36g, Fat: 2.71g, Carbohydrates: 35.38g, Fiber: 7.7g, Sugar: 15.08g, Sodium: 96mg, Cholesterol: 8mg

Spinach Chickpea Stew

Prep Time: 15 minutes, Cook Time: 30 minutes, Serves: 4

INGREDIENTS:

1 medium carrot, peeled and diced small
1 green bell pepper, seeded and diced small
1 large tomato, diced small
3 medium Yukon Gold potatoes (about 1 pound), cut into ½-inch dice
5 cups (1180mL) Vegetable Stock, or low-sodium vegetable broth
2 cups cooked chickpeas, or one 15-oz.(430g) can, drained and rinsed
1 medium spinach, chopped
3 cloves garlic, crushed
1 tsp. fennel seeds, toasted and ground
1 tsp. thyme
½ tsp. smoked paprika
3 sprigs mint
Salt and freshly ground black pepper to taste

DIRECTIONS:

1. Add the carrot and pepper in a large pot and sauté over medium heat for 10 minutes. Pour in water 1 to 2 tbsps. at a time to keep the vegetables from sticking to the pot.
2. Stir in the garlic, thyme, mint, paprika, and fennel seeds and cook for 1 minute. Whisk in the tomato and cook for 3 minutes.
3. Stir in the potatoes, vegetable stock, and beans and bring the pot to a boil over high heat. Lower the heat to medium and simmer, covered, for 20 minutes, or until the potatoes are soft.
4. Stir in the spinach, sprinkle with salt and pepper to taste, and simmer, covered, until the spinach wilts, about 5 minutes.

Nutrition Info per Serving:

Calories: 230, Protein: 9.5g, Fat: 1.46g, Carbohydrates: 49.36g, Fiber: 11.1g, Sugar: 9.8g, Sodium: 84mg, Cholesterol: 0mg

Tomato-Peach Soup

Prep Time: 5 minutes, Cook Time: 12 minutes, Serves: 4

INGREDIENTS:

½ tbsp. olive oil
1 large ripe peach, halved, pitted, peeled, and diced
1 cup carrots, shredded
2 garlic cloves, minced
1 can no-salt diced tomatoes in juice
½ tsp. chili pepper, freshly ground
1 cup chicken broth, low-sodium
1 cup water
1 cup yogurt

DIRECTIONS:

1. Heat the olive oil in a large pot over medium heat. Add the shredded carrots and cook, stirring often, about 5 minutes, or until carrots are tender. Sprinkle with garlic, and cook for 1 minute.
2. Remove the carrot mixture to a food processor. Add the tomatoes and their juice, broth, chili pepper and water, and purée until smooth.
3. Return the purée back to the pot, reduce heat to medium low and cook the soup mixture for 5 minutes, or until cooked through. Smear with the yogurt.
4. Garnish each serving with a quarter of the peach slices.

Nutrition Info per Serving:

Calories: 155, Total Fat: 9g, Saturated Fat: 2g, Total Carbohydrates: 17g, Protein: 5g, Cholesterol: 3mg, Sodium: 116mg, Potassium: 653mg, Magnesium: 40mg, Fiber: 5g, Sugar: 4g

Sweet Potato and Lentils with Curry

Prep Time: 10 minutes, Cook Time: 8 hours, Serves: 4

INGREDIENTS:

4 sweet potatoes, peeled and cut into 1-inch cubes
1 cup dried green lentils, soaked overnight and rinsed
1 (14-ounce, 397 g) can chopped tomatoes, with their juice
1 onion, chopped
1 cup (240 ml) canned light coconut milk
1 cup (240 ml) vegetable broth, or store bought
1 tsp. garlic powder
1 tbsp. curry powder
½ tsp. sea salt
2 tbsps. chopped fresh cilantro

DIRECTIONS:

1. In your slow cooker, mix the sweet potatoes, lentils, tomatoes (with their juice), onion, coconut milk, broth, garlic powder, curry powder and salt.
2. Cover and cook on low for 8 hours.
3. Add cilantro and serve.

Nutrition Info per Serving:

Calories: 525, Total Fat: 16g, Saturated Fat: 13g, Carbohydrates: 83g, Protein: 18g, Cholesterol: 0mg, Fiber: 25g, Sugar: 3.7g, Sodium: 577mg

Sicilian Chickpea Soup with Escarole

Prep Time: 10 minutes, Cook Time: 1.5 hours, Serves: 6 to 8

INGREDIENTS:

1 head escarole (1 pound), trimmed and cut into 1-inch pieces
1 large tomato, cored and chopped
2 tsps. minced fresh oregano or ½ tsp. dried
¼ tsp. red pepper flakes
Salt and pepper
2 fennel bulbs, stalks discarded, bulbs halved, cored, and chopped fine
1 small onion, chopped
5 garlic cloves, minced
5 cups (1200 ml) chicken or vegetable broth
1 Parmesan cheese rind, plus grated Parmesan for serving
2 bay leaves
1 (3-inch) strip orange zest
1 pound (2¾ cups, 454 g) dried chickpeas, picked over and rinsed
2 tbsps. extra-virgin olive oil, plus extra for serving

DIRECTIONS:

1. Put 3 tablespoons salt in 4 quarts cold water in a large container. Add chickpeas and soak for at least 8 hours or up to 24 hours. Drain and rinse well.
2. Heat oil over medium heat until shimmering. Add onion, fennel, and 1 tsp. salt and cook 7 to 10 minutes until vegetables are softened. Stir in oregano, garlic, and pepper flakes and cook about 30 seconds until fragrant.
3. Stir in 7 cups water, broth, Parmesan rind, soaked chickpeas, bay leaves, and orange zest and boil. Reduce heat to simmer and cook 1¼ to 1¾ hours until chickpeas are tender.
4. Add escarole and tomato and cook 5 to 10 minutes until escarole is wilted. Off heat, discard bay leaves and Parmesan rind. Season with salt and pepper. Serve, drizzling with extra oil and sprinkling with grated Parmesan.

Nutrition Info per Serving:

Calories: 354, Fat: 10.39g, Carbohydrates: 52.17g, Protein: 16.66g, Cholesterol: 4mg, Sodium: 283mg, Fiber: 12.8 g, Sugar: 10.1g

Gazpacho

Prep Time: 5 minutes, Cook Time: 5 minutes, Serves: 8 to 10

INGREDIENTS:

2 garlic cloves, minced
2 red bell peppers, stemmed, seeded, and cut into ¼-inch pieces
½ small sweet onion or 2 large shallots, chopped fine
1½ pounds (680 g) tomatoes, cored and cut into ¼-inch pieces
2 small cucumbers (1 peeled, both sliced lengthwise, seeded, and cut into ¼-inch pieces)
⅓ cup (80 ml) sherry vinegar
Salt and pepper
Extra-virgin olive oil
5 cups (1200 ml) tomato juice
8 ice cubes
1 tsp. hot sauce (optional)

DIRECTIONS:

1. Put tomatoes, bell peppers, cucumbers, garlic, onion, vinegar and 2 teaspoons salt in large bowl (at least 4-quart) and season with pepper. Set aside for about 5 minutes until vegetables just begin to release their juices. Stir in tomato juice, ice cubes, and hot sauce, if using. Cover and refrigerate to blend flavors, at least 4 hours or up to 2 days.
2. Discard any unmelted ice cubes and season soup with salt and pepper. Serve, drizzling with oil.

Nutrition Info per Serving:

Calories: 50, Fat: 0.61g, Carbohydrates: 10.29g, Protein: 2.54g, Cholesterol: 0mg, Sodium: 211mg, Fiber: 3.9g, Sugar: 6.2g

Lemony Coconut Fish Stew

Prep Time: 15 minutes, Cook Time: 10 minutes, Serves: 4

INGREDIENTS:

1½ pounds (680 g) firm white fish fillet, cut into 1-inch cubes
2 tbsps. coconut oil
1 white onion, sliced thin
2 zucchini, sliced thin
2 garlic cloves, sliced thin
1 (4-inch) piece lemongrass (white part only), bruised with the back of a knife
1 (13.5-ounce, 383 g) can coconut milk
½ cup slivered scallions
¼ cup chopped cilantro
3 tbsps. freshly squeezed lemon juice
1 tsp. salt
¼ tsp. freshly ground white pepper

DIRECTIONS:

1. Melt the coconut oil in a large pot over medium heat.
2. Add the garlic, onion, and zucchini. Sauté for 5 minutes.
3. Add the lemongrass, fish, salt, coconut milk, and white pepper to the pot. Add enough water if the liquid doesn't cover the fish. Bring to a boil, then lower the heat to simmer, and cook for 5 minutes.
4. Garnish the soup with the cilantro, scallions, and lemon juice.

Nutrition Info per Serving:

Calories: 608, Total Carbohydrates: 13g, Protein: 46g, Total Fat: 43g, Sugar: 7g, Fiber: 4g, Sodium: 725mg, Cholesterol: 0mg

Lemony White Bean Soup

Prep Time: 8 hours, Cook Time: 60 minutes, Serves: 6

INGREDIENTS:

1 pound (2½ cups, 454 g) dried cannellini beans, plucked out and washed
2 tbsps. extra-virgin olive oil, or more to taste
Salt and pepper
1 onion, sliced
2½ tsp. minced fresh oregano or ¾ teaspoon dried
2 tbsps. diced fresh shallot
3 tbsps. lemon juice
1 tsp. ground dried black pepper
6 cups (1440 ml) chicken or vegetable broth, or more to taste
4 celery ribs, finely chop into ½-inch pieces

DIRECTIONS:

1. Dissolve 3 tablespoons salt in 4 quarts cold water in large container. Add beans and soak at room temperature for at least 8 hours or up to 24 hours. Drain them off and rinse well.
2. Heat the oil in oven over medium heat to cook. Add onion, ½ tsp. salt, and ½ tsp. black pepper and allow to simmer until tender and browned, 5 to 7 minutes. Stir in oregano and simmer until fragrant, about 30 seconds. mix broth, celery ribs, and soaked white beans all together and bring the mixture to boil. Reduce heat to low, and cook until beans are softened, 45 to 60 minutes.
3. Process 2 cups soup in blender until smooth, about 30 seconds, then return to pot. Heat soup gently over low heat until hot (do not boil) and adjust consistency with more hot broth to taste. Stir in lemon juice, black pepper, and shallot and season with salt to taste. Remove from the heat and serve, drizzling individual portions with extra oil.

Nutrition Info per Serving:

Calories: 86, Fat: 5g, Carbohydrates: 10.5g, Protein: 1.5g, Cholesterol: 0mg, Sodium: 275mg, Fiber: 2.6g, Sugar: 7.4g

Slow-Cooker Curried Butternut Squash Soup

Prep Time: 15 minutes, Cook Time: 4 hours, Serves: 4-6

INGREDIENTS:

1 pound(454 g) butternut squash, peeled and cut into 1-inch cubes
1 small head cauliflower, cut into 1-inch pieces
2 tbsps. coconut oil
1 (13.5-ounce, 383 g) can coconut milk
1 tbsp. curry powder
1 onion, sliced
½ cup no-added-sugar apple juice
4 cups vegetable broth
1 tsp. salt
¼ tsp. freshly ground white pepper
¼ cup chopped fresh cilantro, divided

DIRECTIONS:

1. Add the butternut squash, cauliflower, coconut oil, coconut milk, curry powder, onion, apple juice, vegetable broth, salt, and white pepper into the slower cooker, combine them together. Set on high and cook for 4 hours.
2. Garnish with the cilantro and serve the soup. Or purée it in a blender before serving.

Nutrition Info per Serving:

Calories: 416, Total Fat: 31g, Total Carbohydrates: 30g, Sugar: 13g, Fiber: 7g, Protein: 10g, Sodium: 855mg, Cholesterol: 0mg

Easy Chicken Noodle Soup

Prep Time: 15 minutes, Cook Time: 1 hour, Serves: 12

INGREDIENTS:

6 ounces (170 g) whole grain wide egg noodles
3 celery stalks, chopped
2 tbsps. avocado oil
1 medium onion, chopped
3 pounds (1.4 kg) bone-in chicken breasts (about 3)
1 tsp. kosher salt
¼ tsp. freshly ground black pepper
2 tsps. minced garlic
5 large carrots, peeled and cut into ¼-inch-thick rounds
4 cups (960 ml) chicken broth
4 cups (960 ml) water
2 tbsps. soy sauce

DIRECTIONS:

1. Set the electric pressure cooker to the Sauté setting. Pour in the avocado oil when the pot is hot.
2. Sauté the celery, onion, salt, and pepper for 3 to 5 minutes.
3. Put the garlic and carrots, and stir to mix well. Press Cancel.
4. Add the chicken to the pot, meat-side down. Add the water, broth, and soy sauce. Close the lid of the pressure cooker. Set the valve to sealing.
5. Cook on high pressure for 20 minutes.
6. Once cooking is complete, press Cancel and quick release the pressure. Unlock and remove the lid.
7. Remove the chicken breasts to a cutting board with tongs. Press Sauté/More and boil the soup.
8. Add the noodles and cook for 5 minutes until the noodles are al dente.
9. While the noodles are cooking, use two forks to shred the chicken. Add the meat back to the pot and save the bones.
10. Season with additional pepper, if you like, and serve.

Nutrition Info per Serving:

Calories: 330, Carbohydrates: 17g, Protein: 32g, Total Fat: 15g, Sugar: 3g, Fiber: 4g, Sodium: 451mg, Cholesterol: 92mg

Slow-Cooked Vegetable Soup

Prep Time: 25 minutes, Cook Time: 2 hours on low, Serves: 16

INGREDIENTS:

1 tbsp. olive oil
2 large onions, chopped
8 medium carrots, sliced
4 celery ribs, chopped
1 large green pepper, seeded and chopped
1 garlic clove, minced
1 can (15 oz., 425 g) garbanzo beans or chickpeas, rinsed and drained
2 cups frozen cut green beans (about 8 oz., 227 g)
2 cups frozen peas (about 8 oz., 227 g)
1 cup frozen corn (about 5 oz., 142 g)
2 cups chopped cabbage
1 bay leaf
2 tsps. chicken bouillon granules
1½ tsps. dried parsley flakes
1 tsp. salt
1 tsp. dried thyme
1 tsp. dried marjoram
½ tsp. dried basil
¼ tsp. pepper
1 can (28 oz., 784 g) diced tomatoes, undrained
2 cups V8 juice
4 cups water

DIRECTIONS:

1. Heat oil in a stockpot over medium-high heat, add onions, carrots, celery and green pepper, saute until crisp-tender. Stir in garlic and cook for 1 minute. Add the remaining ingredients and stir, bring to a boil.
2. Lower the heat, cover and simmer for 1 to 1½ hours, until the vegetables are tender. Remove bay leaf.

Nutrition Info per Serving:

Calories: 105, Fat: 2g, Carbohydrates: 20g, Protein: 9g, Sugar: 9g, Fiber: 4g, Sodium: 488mg, Cholesterol: 0mg

Carrot and Mushroom Soup

Prep Time: 10 minutes, Cook Time: 8 hours, Serves: 6

INGREDIENTS:

1 onion, finely chopped
1 carrot, peeled and finely chopped
1 pound (454 g) fresh mushrooms, quartered
¼ cup (60 ml) dry sherry
1 tsp. dried thyme
1 tsp. garlic powder
1 fennel bulb, finely chopped
8 cups (1920 ml) vegetable broth, poultry broth, or store bought
½ tsp. sea salt
⅛ tsp. freshly ground black pepper

DIRECTIONS:

1. In your slow cooker, mix all the ingredients and combine.
2. Cover and set on low. Cook for 8 hours.

Nutrition Info per Serving:

Calories: 71, Total Fat: 0g, Saturated Fat: 0g, Carbohydrates: 15g, Protein: 3g, Cholesterol: 0mg, Fiber: 3g, Sodium: 968mg, Sugar: 9.2g

Black Beans and Spinach Stew

Prep Time: 10 minutes, Cook Time: 40 minutes, Serves: 6

INGREDIENTS:

½ cup (118mL) frozen chopped spinach, thawed and squeezed dry (½ of a 10-oz. /280mg package)
1 medium red onion, finely chopped
1 medium sweet potato, peeled and cubed
1¼ cups (300mL) black beans, rinsed
1 zucchini, chopped
1 (14.5-oz. 400mg) can no-salt-added diced tomatoes, undrained
1 tbsp. olive oil
1 medium green bell pepper, chopped
3 cloves garlic, crushed
5 cups (1175mL) low-sodium vegetable broth
2½ tsps. dried thyme
2 tsps. cumin
1 tsp. ground oregano
2 tsps. ground allspice
½ cup (118mL) chopped fresh basil
1 tbsp. cooking brandy
Salt and freshly ground black pepper (optional)

DIRECTIONS:

1. Heat the olive oil in a large pot over medium heat. Add the onion and bell pepper and cook until tender, 4 to 5 minutes. Add the garlic and cook until fragrant, 2 to 3 minutes.
2. Add the broth, thyme, black beans, zucchini, sweet potato, diced tomatoes and their juices, allspice, oregano and cumin. Bring to a boil, then cover and let cook over medium-low heat until the black beans and vegetables are tender, 25 to 30 minutes.
3. Add the spinach, basil, cooking brandy, and salt and pepper, if desired, and continue to cook for 10 minutes to thicken the stew.
4. Remove from the heat and serve.

Nutrition Info per Serving:

Calories: 226, Total fat: 3g, Saturated fat: <1g, Total carbohydrates: 39g, Protein: 12g, Cholesterol: 0mg, Sodium: 148mg, Potassium: 526mg, Fiber: 14g, Sugar: 9g

Turkish Tomato and Red Pepper Soup

Prep Time: 15 minutes, Cook Time: 40 minutes, Serves: 6 to 8

INGREDIENTS:

2 tbsps. extra-virgin olive oil
2 red bell peppers, stemmed, seeded, and chopped
Salt and pepper
1 onion, chopped
3 garlic cloves, minced
¾ cup medium-grind bulgur, rinsed
⅓ cup chopped fresh mint
1 tsp. dried mint, crumbled
½ tsp. smoked paprika
⅛ tsp. red pepper flakes
1 (28-ounce, 794 g) can diced fire-roasted tomatoes
4 cups (960 ml) chicken or vegetable broth
2 cups (480 ml) water
1 tbsp. tomato paste
½ cup (120 ml) dry white wine

DIRECTIONS:

1. Heat oil over medium heat until shimmering. Add bell peppers, onion, salt, and pepper and cook 6 to 8 minutes until softened and lightly browned. Add dried mint, garlic, smoked paprika, and pepper flakes and cook about 30 seconds until fragrant. Stir in tomato paste and cook for 1 minute.
2. Put in wine, scraping up any browned bits, and simmer about 1 minute until reduced by half. Add tomatoes and their juice and cook about 10 minutes, stirring occasionally, until tomatoes soften and begin to break apart.
3. Combine water, broth and bulgur and bring to simmer. Reduce heat to low, cover, and simmer about 20 minutes until bulgur is tender. Season with salt and pepper. Serve, sprinkling with fresh mint.

Nutrition Info per Serving:

Calories: 309, Fat: 13.38g, Carbohydrates: 13.31g, Protein: 33.64g, Cholesterol: 65mg, Sodium: 283mg, Fiber: 4g, Sugar: 5.7g

Chipotle Tortilla Chicken Soup

Prep Time: 5 minutes, Cook Time: 15 minutes, Serves: 4

INGREDIENTS:

2 garlic cloves, minced
12 ounces (340 g) chicken breast, diced
1 tsp. ground chipotle
1 tsp. ground cumin
1 cup (240 ml) water
3 cups (720 ml) low-sodium chicken broth
one 14½-ounce (410 g) can no-salt-added crushed tomatoes with juice
juice of 1 lime
1 tbsp. olive oil
1 yellow onion, diced
1 cup crushed low-sodium baked tortilla chips
¼ cup chopped cilantro, for garnish

DIRECTIONS:

1. Heat the olive oil in a large stockpot over medium-high heat. Add the onion and garlic and cook about 5 minutes, stirring, until the onion is soft. Put in the chicken and cook for about 2 minutes, until the chicken is opaque. Add the chipotle and cumin and cook for about 30 seconds. Boil the water, broth, and tomatoes with juice in it. Reduce the heat to medium, cover, and cook for about 5 minutes. Stir in the lime juice.
2. Divide the crushed tortilla chips among four soup bowls. Ladle the soup over the chips and serve with cilantro.

Nutrition Info per Serving:

Calories: 269, Protein: 23.3g, Fat: 13.9g, Carbohydrates: 14g, Fiber: 2.7g, Sodium: 159mg, Cholesterol: 54mg, Sugar: 3g

Classic Avgolemono

Prep Time: 10 minutes, Cook Time: 35 minutes, Serves: 6 to 8

INGREDIENTS:

8 cups (1920 ml)chicken broth
½ cup long-grain white rice
1½ tsps. salt
2 large eggs plus 2 large yolks, room temperature
12 (4-inch) strips lemon zest plus ¼ cup juice (2 lemons)
4 green cardamom pods, crushed, or 2 whole cloves
1 bay leaf
1 scallion, sliced thin, or 3 tbsps. chopped fresh mint

DIRECTIONS:

1. Boil broth in a saucepan over high heat. Stir in bay leaf, lemon zest, rice, cardamom pods, and salt. Reduce to simmer and cook 16 to 20 minutes until rice is tender and broth is aromatic.
2. Whisk whole eggs, egg yolks, and lemon juice together in a bowl until combined. Discard cardamom, bay leaf, and zest strips. Reduce heat to low. Stir constantly, slowly ladle about 2 cups hot broth into egg mixture and mix. Pour egg mixture back into saucepan and cook about 5 minutes, stirring constantly, until soup is slightly thickened (do not simmer or boil). Sprinkle with scallion and serve immediately.

Nutrition Info per Serving:

Calories: 100, Fat: 2.1g, Carbohydrates: 16.76g, Protein: 4.32g, Cholesterol: 58mg, Sodium: 299mg, Fiber: 1.6 g, Sugar: 4.7g

Moroccan Chickpea Soup

Prep Time: 10 minutes, Cook Time: 35 minutes, Serves: 4 to 6

INGREDIENTS:

3 tbsps. extra-virgin olive oil
1 onion, chopped fine
1 tsp. sugar
3½ cups (840 ml) chicken or vegetable broth
¼ cup minced fresh parsley or mint
Lemon wedges
Salt and pepper
4 garlic cloves, minced
2 (15-ounce, 425 g) cans chickpeas, rinsed
1 pound (454 g) red potatoes, unpeeled, cut into ½-inch pieces
1 (14.5-ounce, 410g) can diced tomatoes
1 zucchini, cut into ½-inch pieces
½ tsp. hot paprika
¼ tsp. saffron threads, crumbled
¼ tsp. ground ginger
¼ tsp. ground cumin

DIRECTIONS:

1. Heat oil over medium-high heat until shimmering. Add sugar, onion, and salt and cook about 5 minutes until onion is softened. Stir in saffron, garlic, paprika, ginger and cumin and cook about 30 seconds until fragrant. Stir in chickpeas, tomatoes, potatoes and their juice, zucchini, and broth. Simmer and cook 20 to 30 minutes, stirring occasionally until potatoes are tender.
2. Using wooden spoon, mash some of potatoes to thicken soup. Off heat, stir in parsley and season with salt and pepper. Serve with lemon wedges.

Nutrition Info per Serving:

Calories: 427, Fat: 16.4g, Carbohydrates: 59.56g, Protein: 14.86g, Cholesterol: 3mg, Sodium: 292mg, Fiber: 12.1g, Sugar: 4.8g

Chicken and White Bean Chili

Prep Time: 15 minutes, Cook Time: 8 hours, Serves: 4

INGREDIENTS:

1 pound (454 g) boneless, skinless chicken thighs, cut into 1-inch pieces
1 pound (454 g) dried white beans, soaked overnight and rinsed
3 cups (720 ml) poultry broth
1 tbsp. chili powder
2 onions, chopped
2 green bell peppers, seeded and chopped
2 tsps. garlic powder
1 tsp. ground cumin
¼ tsp. sea salt

DIRECTIONS:

1. Mix all the ingredients in your slow cooker.
2. Cover and cook on low for 8 hours.

Nutrition Info per Serving:

Calories: 562, Total Fat: 5g, Saturated Fat: 3g, Carbohydrates: 80g, Protein: 52g, Cholesterol: 70mg, Fiber: 21g, Sodium: 541mg, Sugar: 12g

Spiced Chicken Soup with Chickpeas and Squash

Prep Time: 15 minutes, Cook Time: 35 minutes, Serves: 6 to 8

INGREDIENTS:

1½ pounds butternut squash, peeled, seeded, and cut into 1½-inch pieces (4 cups)
2 tbsps. extra-virgin olive oil
7 cups water, divided
1¾ tsp. table salt
2 tbsps. tomato paste
4 garlic cloves, minced
1 tbsp. ground coriander
1½ tsps. ground cumin
1 tsp. ground cardamom
½ tsp. ground allspice
¼ tsp. cayenne pepper
2 (12-ounce, 340 g) bone-in split chicken breasts, trimmed
4 (5- to 7-ounce, 142 g to 198 g) bone-in chicken thighs, trimmed
1 onion, chopped
1 (15-ounce, 425 g) can chickpeas, rinsed
½ cup chopped fresh cilantro

DIRECTIONS:

1. In Instant Pot, use highest sauté function, heat oil until shimmering. Add onion and salt and cook about 5 minutes until softened. Stir in tomato paste, coriander, garlic, cumin, allspice, cardamom, and cayenne and cook about 30 seconds until fragrant. Stir in 5 cups water, scraping up any browned bits. Nestle chicken breasts and thighs in pot, then place squash evenly around chicken.
2. Lock lid and close pressure release valve. Choose high-pressure cook function and cook for 20 minutes. Turn off and quick-release pressure. Carefully remove lid, letting steam escape away from you.
3. Transfer chicken to cutting board, cool down slightly, then shred into bite-size pieces with 2 forks, discard skin and bones.
4. Skim excess fat from surface of soup with a wide, shallow spoon, then break squash into bite-size pieces. Stir chicken and any accumulated juices, chickpeas, and remaining water into soup until heated through, about 3 minutes. Stir in cilantro and season with salt and pepper. Serve.

Nutrition Info per Serving:

Calories: 190, Fat: 7g, Carbohydrates: 16g, Protein: 20g, Sugar: 3g, Fiber: 4g, Sodium: 700mg, Cholesterol: 60mg

Healthy Curried Carrot Soup

Prep Time: 10 minutes, Cook Time: 5 minutes, Serves: 6

INGREDIENTS:

1 small onion, coarsely chopped
1½ tsps. curry powder
2 celery stalks, coarsely chopped
1 tsp. ground cumin
6 medium carrots, roughly chopped
4 cups low-sodium vegetable broth
1 tsp. minced fresh ginger
1 cup canned coconut milk
¼ tsp. freshly ground black pepper
1 tbsp. fresh cilantro, chopped
1 tbsp. extra-virgin olive oil
¼ tsp. salt

DIRECTIONS:

1. Heat the Instant Pot to high temperature and add olive oil.
2. Sauté the onion and celery for 2 to 3 minutes. Add curry powder, cumin, and ginger to the pot and cook until fragrant.
3. Add carrots, vegetable soup, and salt to the pot. Close and seal, and set for 5 minutes on high. Let the pressure release naturally.
4. In a blender jar, carefully purée the soup in batches and then transfer it back to the pot.
5. Add coconut milk and pepper, and heat. Sprinkle with coriander and serve.

Nutrition Info per Serving:

Calories: 145, Total Fat: 11g, Protein: 2g, Carbohydrates: 13g, Sugar: 4g, Fiber: 3g, Sodium: 238mg, Cholesterol: 1mg

Bean, Chard and Tomato Stew

Prep Time: 10 minutes, Cook Time: 40 minutes, Serves: 2

INGREDIENTS:

1 (14.5-oz. 406mg) can no-salt-added diced tomatoes, undrained
1 small red onion, finely chopped
5 cups (1175mL) cucumber, diced
1 cup (235mL) chard, sliced
2 tbsps. olive oil
4 cloves garlic, crushed
1 tsp. ground parsley
1 tsp. ground rosemary
½ tsp. ground sage
Salt and freshly ground black pepper (optional)
1 (15-oz. 420mg) can chickpeas, rinsed and drained
¼ cup chopped fresh basil

DIRECTIONS:

1. Heat the olive oil in a large saucepan over medium-low heat. Add the onion, cucumber, and chard and cook until soft and translucent, 8 to 10 minutes. Add the garlic and cook for 1 minute.
2. Add the tomatoes and their juices, the parsley, rosemary, sage, and salt and pepper, if desired. Bring to a boil and cook for 10 minutes.
3. Add the chickpeas and 2 cups water, cover, and simmer for another 15 to 20 minutes to thicken the stew and blend the flavors.
4. Garnished with fresh basil. To serve.

Nutrition Info per Serving:

Calories: 442, Total fat: 14g, Saturated fat: 2g, Total carbohydrates: 65g, Protein: 17g, Cholesterol: 0mg, Sodium: 94mg, Fiber: 19g, Sugar: 18g

Chicken and Celery Soup

Prep Time: 15 minutes, Cook Time: 25 minutes, Serves: 4

INGREDIENTS:

¾ pound boneless, skinless chicken breasts, cut into 1-inch pieces
1 medium onion, sliced
1 pound beets, peeled and grated
3 medium celeries, diced
2 cups chicken broth low-sodium
1 tbsp. extra-virgin olive oil
1 clove garlic, minced
1 tsp. dried tarragon
1 tsp. dried dill
¼ cup chopped fresh basil
Salt and Black pepper

DIRECTIONS:

1. In a large Dutch oven or soup pot, heat the oil over medium-high until it begins to shimmer. Whisk in the chicken, onion, and garlic and cook until the chicken is browned, 5 to 7 minutes.
2. Pour in the broth, 2 cups water, stir in the beets, celeries, tarragon, and dried dill until combine well. Bring to a boil, then lower the heat, cover, and simmer until the vegetables are softened, 15 to 20 minutes. Mix in the fresh basil and drizzle with salt and black pepper to taste.

Nutrition Info per Serving:

Calories: 207, Total fat: 6g, Saturated fat: <1g, Total carbohydrates: 20g, Protein: 21g, Cholesterol: 49mg, Sodium: 303mg, Potassium: 634mg, Fiber: 5g, Sugar: 12g

Broccoli Soup with Tomato and Jalapeño Pepper

Prep Time: 5 minutes, Cook Time: 15 minutes, Serves: 4

INGREDIENTS:

2 (15-oz. 420mg) cans broccoli, rinsed and drained
1 medium onion, diced
2 (14.5-oz. 406mg) cans no-salt-added fire-roasted tomatoes
1 cup (235mL) low-sodium vegetable broth, plus more as needed
1 tbsp. olive oil
5 cloves garlic, minced
1 tsp. ground cinnamon
1 medium jalapeño pepper, cored, seeded, and finely chopped
2 tbsps. fresh tomato paste
Salt and freshly ground black pepper (optional)
½ cup (118mL) chopped fresh basil

DIRECTIONS:

1. Pulse half of the broccoli in a food processor or blender until thickened but not fully pureed.
2. Heat the olive oil in a large pot over medium-high heat. Add the onion and garlic and sauté until tender and lightly browned, 4 to 5 minutes.
3. Stir in the processed broccoli, tomatoes, broth, cinnamon, and jalapeño pepper. Bring to a boil and simmer for 10 to 15 minutes, until thickened. If the soup is too thick, add a little broth, if it is too thin, puree 1 to 2 cups of the soup in a blender and return it to the pot (or use an immersion blender to puree directly in the pot until your desired consistency is reached).
4. Off heat and remove the pot, stir in the tomato paste. Sprinkle with salt and pepper to taste if desired. Divide into 4 serving bowls and top with the basil.

Nutrition Info per Serving:

Calories: 262, Total fat: 4g, Saturated fat: <1g, Total carbohydrates: 44g, Protein: 13g, Cholesterol: 0mg, Sodium: 59mg, Potassium: 55mg, Fiber: 11g, Sugar: 9g

Greek Cucumber Soup with Yogurt

Prep Time: 5 minutes, Cook Time: 15 minutes, Serves: 4

INGREDIENTS:

2 seedless cucumbers, peeled and cut into chunks
3 tsps. fresh dill
1 tbsp. tomato paste
2 garlic cloves, minced
2 cups (480 ml) chicken broth or vegetable stock
2 cups (480 ml) plain Greek yogurt
½ cup mint, finely chopped
Sea salt and freshly ground pepper

DIRECTIONS:

1. Puree the cucumber, yogurt, mint, and garlic in a food processor.
2. Add the chicken broth, dill, sea salt, tomato paste and pepper, and blend completely.
3. Refrigerate for at least 2 hours before serving.

Nutrition Info per Serving:

Calories: 184, Fat: 6.37g, Carbohydrates: 14.89g, Protein: 17.63g, Cholesterol: 23mg, Sodium: 290mg, Fiber: 2g, Sugar: 4.7g

Mediterranean Broccoli and Lentil Stew

Prep Time: 15 minutes, Cook Time: 30 minutes, Serves: 4

INGREDIENTS:

6 cups broccoli florets
1 tbsp. extra-virgin olive oil, plus additional for drizzling
1 small carrot, chopped
1 small onion, finely chopped
2 cloves garlic, minced
2 cups (480 ml) vegetable broth
1 cup dried green or brown lentils
1 tsp. dried oregano
1 tsp. salt
¼ tsp. freshly ground black pepper
¼ cup chopped fresh Italian parsley
½ cup sliced pitted green olives

DIRECTIONS:

1. Heat the olive oil in a large pot over high heat.
2. Add the carrot, onion, and garlic. Sauté for 5 minutes.
3. Put in the lentils, vegetable broth, and oregano and boil. Lower the heat to simmer. Cook the soup for 15 to 20 minutes until the lentils are tender.
4. Add the broccoli, cover, and simmer for 5 minutes more.
5. Remove the pot from the heat and stir in the olives and parsley. Stir in some water if the soup is too thick.
6. Ladle the soup into bowls, drizzle with olive oil, season with salt and pepper, and serve.

Nutrition Info per Serving:

Calories: 182, Total Carbohydrates: 24g, Protein: 11g, Total Fat: 6g, Sugar: 5g, Fiber: 9g, Sodium: 895mg, Cholesterol: 0mg

Spanish Chorizo and Lentil Soup

Prep Time: 15 minutes, Cook Time: 30 minutes, Serves: 6 to 8

INGREDIENTS:

8 ounces (227 g) Spanish-style chorizo sausage, quartered lengthwise and sliced thin
1 large onion, peeled
1 tbsp. extra-virgin olive oil, plus extra for drizzling
2 carrots, peeled and halved crosswise
4 garlic cloves, minced
1½ tsps. smoked paprika
5 cups (1200 ml) water
1 pound (2¼ cups, 454 g) French green lentils, picked over and rinsed
4 cups (960 ml) chicken broth
1 tbsp. sherry vinegar, plus extra for seasoning
2 bay leaves
1 tsp. table salt
½ cup slivered almonds, toasted
½ cup minced fresh parsley

DIRECTIONS:

1. In Instant Pot, use highest sauté function, heat oil until shimmering. Add chorizo and cook 3 to 5 minutes until lightly browned. Stir in garlic and paprika and cook about 30 seconds until fragrant. Add water, scraping up any browned bits, then stir in lentils, bay leaves, vinegar, broth, and salt. Nestle carrots and onion into pot.
2. Lock lid and close pressure release valve. Choose high-pressure cook function and cook for 14 minutes. Turn off and quick-release pressure. Carefully remove lid, letting steam escape away from you.
3. Throw away bay leaves. Transfer onion and carrots to food processor with a slotted spoon and process about 1 minute until smooth, scraping down sides of bowl if you like. Stir vegetable mixture into lentils and season with pepper, salt, and extra vinegar. Drizzle each portion with extra oil, sprinkle with almonds and parsley and serve.

Nutrition Info per Serving:

Calories: 360, Fat: 16g, Carbohydrates: 30g, Protein: 21g, Sugar: 5g, Fiber: 7g, Sodium: 950mg, Cholesterol: 25mg

Spicy Butternut Squash Soup

Prep Time: 15 minutes, Cook Time: 8 hours, Serves: 6

INGREDIENTS:

1 butternut squash, peeled, seeded, and diced
3 cups (720 ml) vegetable broth, or store bought
½ cup (120 ml) fat-free half-and-half
1 tsp. garlic powder
½ tsp. ground sage
¼ tsp. sea salt
¼ tsp. freshly ground black pepper
1 onion, chopped
1 sweet-tart apple (such as Braeburn), peeled, cored, and chopped
Pinch cayenne pepper
Pinch nutmeg

DIRECTIONS:

1. In your slow cooker, mix the squash, broth, garlic powder, sage, salt, black pepper, onion, apple, cayenne, and nutmeg.
2. Cover and cook on low for 8 hours.
3. Using an immersion blender or food processor, purée the soup, adding the half-and-half. Stir to combine, and serve.

Nutrition Info per Serving:

Calories: 106, Total Fat: 0g, Saturated Fat: 0g, Carbohydrates: 26g, Protein: 3g, Cholesterol: 0mg, Fiber: 4g, Sodium: 392mg, Sugar: 2.8g

Spicy Cauliflower Soup with Sour Cream

Prep Time: 10 minutes, Cook Time: 20 minutes, Serves: 4

INGREDIENTS:

4 cloves garlic, minced
2 tsps. fresh ginger, finely chopped
2 tbsps. olive oil
1 cup shallots (about 4 whole shallots), chopped
½ tsp. coriander, ground
½ tsp. pepper, freshly ground
1 tsp. curry powder
1 tsp. turmeric, ground
½ tsp. cumin, ground
One 1-pound (454 g) package pre-cut cauliflower florets
1 russet potato, peeled and cut into ¼-inch pieces
1 cup evaporated skim milk
Chopped chives and low-fat sour cream for garnish
4 cups (960 ml) low-salt vegetable broth

DIRECTIONS:

1. In a large saucepan, heat oil over medium heat. Put in shallots, ginger and garlic and sauté for about 5 minutes, stirring frequently, until golden. Reduce heat to low and add coriander, curry, turmeric, pepper and cumin. Stir 30 seconds, or until spices begin to release their fragrance.
2. Put in cauliflower, stir and cook for 2 minutes. Add potato and broth.
3. In medium-high, bring soup to a boil. Cover and reduce heat to low. Simmer 20 minutes until cauliflower is tender.
4. Using an immersion blender, puree soup in the pot until smooth. Whisk in milk.
5. Serve in bowls, topped with chopped chives and sour cream.

Nutrition Info per Serving:

Calories: 204, Fat: 7.3g, Carbohydrates: 29.3g, Protein: 8.2g, Cholesterol: 0mg, Sodium: 223.9mg, Fiber: 4.8g, Sugar: 4.6g

Silky Tomato Soup with Tofu

Prep Time: 20 minutes, Cook Time: 15 minutes, Serves: 4

INGREDIENTS:

1 tbsp. extra-virgin olive oil
8 ounces (227g) silken tofu, drained
2 pounds(907g) tomatoes, chopped
1 cup cherry tomatoes, quartered
1 onion, diced
2 garlic cloves, sliced
1 tbsp. no-salt-added tomato paste
½ cup no-salt-added vegetable stock
¾ cup fresh basil, chopped and divided
1 tsp. kosher salt
¼ tsp. freshly ground black pepper

DIRECTIONS:

1. Heat the olive oil in a large saucepan over medium-high heat. Add the onion and sauté until slightly golden, about 5 to 6 minutes.
2. Add the garlic and sauté for 30 seconds. Then add the tomato paste and sauté for 30 seconds.
3. Add the tomatoes and cook down a bit, for 5 to 10 minutes. Add the stock, ½ cup of the basil, the salt, and black pepper.
4. Carefully transfer the mixture, in batches, to a high-powered blender or Vitamix. Add the tofu, and purée. Return the soup to the saucepan and simmer for 10 minutes.
5. Divide the cherry tomatoes among 4 bowls. Ladle the soup into the bowls. Garnish with the remaining ¼ cup basil.

Nutrition Info per Serving:

Calories: 130, Total fat: 6g, Saturated fat: 1g, Cholesterol: 0mg, Sodium: 325mg, Potassium: 855mg, Total Carbohydrates: 17g, Fiber: 4g, Sugar: 10g, Protein: 6g, Magnesium: 55mg, Calcium: 70mg

Red Lentil Soup with Tomato Sauce

Prep Time: 10 minutes, Cook Time: 20 minutes, Serves: 4

INGREDIENTS:

2 tsps. olive oil
Two 15-ounce (850 g) cans low-salt red or brown lentils, drained
One 15-ounce (425 g) can low-salt tomato sauce
1 cup onion, chopped
1 cup celery, chopped
1 jalapeño, seeded and finely chopped
2 cups carrots, chopped
¼ tsp. pepper, freshly ground
¼ cup cilantro, chopped fresh
4 cups (960 ml) water

DIRECTIONS:

1. Heat oil in a large pot over medium-high heat. Put in onion, carrot, jalapeño and celery. Cook for about 6 minutes until vegetables begin to soften.
2. Add tomato sauce, pepper, lentils and water. After low boil, reduce heat and simmer 15 minutes, or until vegetables are tender.
3. Ladle into bowls and top with cilantro. Serve.

Nutrition Info per Serving:

Calories: 150, Fat: 1g, Carbohydrates: 28g, Protein: 8g, Cholesterol: 0mg, Sodium: 34mg, Fiber: 25g, Sugar: 6.1g

Chickpea and Roasted Red Pepper Soup

Prep Time: 10 minutes, Cook Time: 45 minutes, Serves: 4

INGREDIENTS:

2 can chickpeas, drained and rinsed
3 large red bell peppers
2 cup celery, finely chopped
2 cups broth, low-sodium
⅛ tsp. red pepper, crushed
1 tbsp. olive oil
1 tsp. tarragon
2 cups water

DIRECTIONS:

1. Preheat the broiler over high heat. Add the bell peppers on a baking sheet. Broil, stirring often, until sides are bubbly and charred. Transfer from broiler.
2. Place peppers in a plastic or paper bag, let sit for 20 minutes. Peel off the layer of skin, cored and deseeded.
3. Heat the olive oil in a large skillet over medium-high heat until simmering. Add the celery, tarragon and cook, stir occasionally, for 3 to 5 minutes, or until the celery become tender.
4. Put in the roasted peppers and crushed red pepper and cook for 1 minute.
5. Stir in the broth, chickpeas and water. Bring to a boil. Reduce the heat to low, and cook for 5 minutes.
6. Serve warm.

Nutrition Info per Serving:

Calories: 169, Total Fat: 5g, Saturated Fat: 1g, Total Carbohydrates: 26g, Protein: 7g, Cholesterol: 0mg, Sodium: 180mg, Potassium: 196mg, Magnesium: 66mg, Fiber: 8g, Sugar: 4g

Spicy and Creamy Carrot Soup

Prep Time: 15 minutes, Cook Time: 35 minutes, Serves: 6 to 8

INGREDIENTS:

2 tbsps. extra-virgin olive oil
2 onions, chopped
1 tsp. table salt
1 tbsp. grated fresh ginger
1 tbsp. ground coriander
1 tbsp. ground fennel
1 tsp. ground cinnamon
4 cups (960 ml) vegetable or chicken broth
2 cups (480 ml) water
2 pounds (907 g) carrots, peeled and cut into 2-inch pieces
½ tsp. baking soda
2 tbsps. pomegranate molasses
½ cup (120 ml) plain Greek yogurt
½ cup hazelnuts, toasted, skinned, and chopped
½ cup chopped fresh cilantro or mint
salt and pepper to taste

DIRECTIONS:

1. In Instant Pot, use highest sauté function, heat oil until shimmering. Add onions and salt and cook about 5 minutes until onions are softened. Stir in ginger, fennel, coriander, and cinnamon and cook about 30 seconds until fragrant. Add broth, carrots, water, and baking soda.
2. Lock lid and close pressure release valve. Choose high-pressure cook function and cook for 3 minutes. Turn off and quick-release pressure. Carefully remove lid, letting steam escape away from you.
3. Working in batches, process soup in blender for 1 to 2 minutes until smooth. Put processed soup back to Instant Pot and simmer with highest sauté function. Season with salt and pepper. Drizzle each portion with pomegranate molasses and top with hazelnuts, yogurt and cilantro. Serve.

Nutrition Info per Serving:

Calories: 190, Fat: 11g, Carbohydrates: 20g, Protein: 4g, Sugar: 10g, Fiber: 5g, Sodium: 820mg, Cholesterol: 5mg

Spicy Chicken Corn Chowder

Prep Time: 10 minutes, Cook Time: 8 hours, Serves: 6

INGREDIENTS:

1 pound (454 g) boneless, skinless chicken thighs, cut into 1-inch pieces
2 onions, chopped
1½ cups fresh or frozen corn
6 cups (1440 ml) poultry broth, or store bought
3 jalapeño peppers, seeded and minced
2 red bell peppers, seeded and chopped
1 tsp. garlic powder
½ tsp. sea salt
¼ tsp. freshly ground black pepper
1 cup (240 ml) skim milk

DIRECTIONS:

1. In your slow cooker, combine the chicken, onions, corn, broth, jalapeños, red bell peppers, garlic powder, salt, and pepper.
2. Cover and cook on low for 8 hours.
3. Put in the skim milk just before serving.

Nutrition Info per Serving:

Calories: 236, Total Fat: 6g, Saturated Fat: 2g, Carbohydrates: 17g, Protein: 27g, Cholesterol: 68mg, Fiber: 3g, Sodium: 722mg, Sugar: 15g

Spicy Red Lentil Soup

Prep Time: 10 minutes, Cook Time: 25 minutes, Serves: 4 to 6

INGREDIENTS:

¼ cup (60 ml) extra-virgin olive oil
1 large onion, chopped fine
Salt and pepper
Pinch cayenne pepper
1 tbsp. tomato paste
¾ tsp. ground coriander
½ tsp. ground cumin
¼ tsp. ground ginger
⅛ tsp. ground cinnamon
1 garlic clove, minced
1 tsp. paprika
¼ cup chopped fresh cilantro
4 cups (960 ml) chicken or vegetable broth, plus extra as needed
2 cups (480 ml) water
10½ ounces (1½ cups, 300g) red lentils, picked over and rinsed
2 tbsps. lemon juice, plus extra for seasoning
1½ tsps. dried mint, crumbled

DIRECTIONS:

1. Heat oil in a saucepan over medium heat until shimmering. Add onion and salt and cook about 5 minutes, stirring occasionally, until softened. Stir in coriander, ginger, cumin, pepper, cinnamon, and cayenne and cook about 2 minutes until fragrant. Stir in garlic and tomato paste and cook for 1 minute.
2. Stir in water, broth and lentils and simmer. Cook about 15 minutes, stirring occasionally, until lentils are soft and about half are broken down.
3. Whisk soup about 30 seconds until broken down to coarse puree. Stir in lemon juice and season with extra lemon juice and salt. Cover and keep warm.
4. Heat remaining oil in a small skillet over medium heat until shimmering. Off heat, stir in paprika and mint. Serve soup, drizzling with spiced oil and sprinkling with cilantro.

Nutrition Info per Serving:

Calories: 339, Fat: 12.32g, Carbohydrates: 44.82g, Protein: 15g, Cholesterol: 0mg, Sodium: 283mg, Fiber: 7.5g, Sugar: 9.5g

Stewed Chickpeas and Tomatoes

Prep Time: 10 minutes, Cook Time: 27 minutes, Serves: 6

INGREDIENTS:

1 (15-ounce, 425 g) can crushed tomatoes
2 (15-ounce, 425 g) cans chickpeas, rinsed and drained
2 tbsps. avocado oil
½ cup finely chopped onion
1 cup vegetable broth, divided
2 garlic cloves, minced
1 tbsp. smoked paprika
1 tbsp. tomato paste
1 cup chopped lacinato kale leaves, stems and ribs removed (from 2 stems)

DIRECTIONS:

1. Set the electric pressure cooker to the Sauté setting. Pour in the avocado oil when the pot is hot.
2. Sauté the onion for 3 to 5 minutes. Stir in about 1 tbsp. of the broth, the paprika, garlic, and tomato paste. Hit Cancel.
3. Add the remaining tomatoes, broth, and chickpeas.
4. Close and lock the lid of the pressure cooker. Seal the valve.
5. Cook on high pressure for 10 minutes.
6. When the cooking is complete, hit Cancel and release the pressure naturally for 15 minutes, then quick release any remaining pressure.
7. Once the pin drops, unlock and remove the lid.
8. Stir in the kale and set aside for about 10 minutes or until the kale wilts.
9. Spoon into bowls and serve.

Nutrition Info per Serving:

Calories: 232, Total Fat: 7g, Protein: 10g, Carbohydrates: 35g, Sugar: 9g, Fiber: 10g, Sodium: 138mg, Cholesterol: 0mg

Vegetable Broth

Prep Time: 10 minutes, Cook Time: 15 minutes, Serves: 2

INGREDIENTS:

1 pound (454 g) leeks, white and light green parts only, chopped and washed thoroughly (2½ cups)
2 carrots, peeled and cut into ½-inch pieces (⅔ cup)
3 tbsps. dried minced onion
3 tbsps. kosher salt
½ small celery root, peeled and cut into ½-inch pieces (¾ cup)
½ cup (½ ounce, 14 g) fresh parsley leaves and thin stems
1½ tbsps. tomato paste

DIRECTIONS:

1. Process celery root, leeks, carrots, dried minced onion, parsley, and salt in food processor for 3 to 4 minutes, pausing to scrape down sides of bowl frequently, until finely mixed.
2. Add tomato paste and process for 2 minutes, scraping down sides of bowl every 30 seconds. Transfer mixture to an airtight container and tap firmly to remove bubbles.
3. Press small piece of parchment paper flush against surface of mixture and cover tightly.

Nutrition Info per Serving:

Calories: 185, Fat: 1.02g, Carbohydrates: 42.68g, Protein: 5.13g, Cholesterol: 0mg, Sodium: 272mg, Fiber: 7.1g, Sugar: 8.4g

Vegetable Soup with Goat Cheese

Prep Time: 5 minutes, Cook Time: 25 minutes, Serves: 4

INGREDIENTS:

2 leeks, green and light green parts only, thinly sliced
1 tbsp. olive oil
2 tbsps. sherry
4 cups (960 ml) low-sodium vegetable broth
2 cups (480 ml) water
1 potato, peeled and diced
1 pound (454 g) spinach leaves, tough stems trimmed and discarded
¼ tsp. cayenne
½ cup crumbled goat cheese, plus more for garnish
2 tbsps. unsalted butter
2 cups watercress
2 cups sorrel
freshly ground pepper

DIRECTIONS:

1. Heat the olive oil over medium-high heat in a large stockpot. Put in leeks and cook about 5 minutes, stirring frequently, until the leeks soften. Add the sherry and cook, until the liquid has evaporated.
2. Add the water, broth, and potato and boil. Reduce the heat to low and simmer for about 15 minutes, uncovered, until the potato is tender.
3. Stir in spinach, sorrel, watercress, and cayenne. Cook, covered, for about 5 minutes, until the spinach is tender.
4. Remove the pot from the heat, add the goat cheese and butter, and stir until they are well mixed. Using an immersion blender, purée the soup until smooth. Serve immediately, garnished with crumbled goat cheese and sprinkling of freshly ground pepper.

Nutrition Info per Serving:

Calories: 332, Protein: 10.4g, Fat: 10.1g, Carbohydrates: 56.6g, Fiber: 7.9g, Sodium: 275mg, Cholesterol: 0mg, Sugar: 28g

Two-Potato Beet Soup

Prep Time: 15 minutes, Cook Time: 30 minutes, Serves: 4

INGREDIENTS:

2 cups beet
½ pound sweet potatoes, peeled and chopped
½ pound Yukon Gold potatoes, unpeeled and chopped
3 cups vegetable broth, low-sodium
1 cup fat-free milk or plant-based milk
1 leek, diced
2 cloves garlic, minced
2 tsps. ground allspice
½ tsp. freshly ground black pepper,
1 tsp. chopped fresh parsley
1 tbsp. olive oil

DIRECTIONS:

1. Heat the olive oil over medium heat in a large soup pot. Whisk in the leek and cook until tender, 3 to 5 minutes. Sprinkle with the garlic and cook for 1 minute.
2. Whisk in the beet, sweet potatoes, gold potatoes, and broth and bring to a boil. Reduce the heat, cover, and simmer until the vegetables are wilted and tender, 15 to 20 minutes.
3. Puree the soup in an immersion blender until smooth (or remove in batches to a blender or food processor and puree until smooth, then transfer to the pot).
4. Mix in the milk, allspice, and black pepper and cook for a further 3 to 5 minutes to cook through.
5. Serve topped with fresh parsley, if desired.

Nutrition Info per Serving:

Calories: 181, Total fat: 4g, Saturated fat: <1g, Total carbohydrates: 33g, Protein: 6g, Cholesterol: 1mg, Sodium: 182mg, Potassium: 786mg, Fiber: 6g, Sugar: 10g

Chicken Broth

Prep Time: 10 minutes, Cook Time: 5 hours, Serves: 8

INGREDIENTS:

1 onion, chopped
2 bay leaves
4 pounds (1.8 kg) chicken backs and wings
14 cups (3360 ml) water
2 tsps. salt

DIRECTIONS:

1. Heat chicken and water in a large stockpot over medium-high heat. After boiling, skim off scum that comes to surface. Reduce heat to low and simmer for 3 hours.
2. Add bay leaves, onion, and salt and continue to simmer for another 2 hours.
3. Strain broth through fine-mesh strainer into large container, pressing to extract as much liquid as possible. Let broth settle for about 5 minutes, then skim off fat.

Nutrition Info per Serving:

Calories: 318, Fat: 13.48g, Carbohydrates: 1.62g, Protein: 44.55g, Cholesterol: 184mg, Sodium: 276mg, Fiber: 0.4g, Sugar: 6.3g

French Chicken Soup

Prep Time: 15 minutes, Cook Time: 35 minutes, Serves: 6 to 8

INGREDIENTS:

2 fennel bulbs, 2 tbsps. fronds minced, stalks discarded, bulbs halved, cored, and cut into ½-inch pieces
1 tbsp. extra-virgin olive oil
4 garlic cloves, minced
1 onion, chopped
1¾ tsp. table salt
2 tbsps. tomato paste
7 cups water, divided
1 tbsp. minced fresh thyme or 1 tsp. dried
2 anchovy fillets, minced
1 (14.5-ounce, 411 g) can diced tomatoes, drained
2 carrots, peeled, halved lengthwise, and sliced ½ inch thick
2 (12-ounce, 340 g) bone-in split chicken breasts, trimmed
4 (5- to 7-ounce, 142 g to 198 g) bone-in chicken thighs, trimmed
½ cup pitted brine-cured green olives, chopped
1 tsp. grated orange zest

DIRECTIONS:

1. In Instant Pot, use highest sauté function, heat oil until shimmering. Add fennel pieces, onion, and salt and cook about 5 minutes until softened. Stir in tomato paste, thyme, garlic, and anchovies and cook about 30 seconds until fragrant. Stir in 5 cups water, scraping up any browned bits, then add tomatoes and carrots. Nestle chicken breasts and thighs in pot.
2. Close the lid and close pressure release valve. Select high-pressure cook function and cook for 20 minutes. Turn off and quick-release pressure. Carefully remove lid, letting steam escape away from you.
3. Transfer chicken to cutting board, cool down slightly, then shred into bite-size pieces with 2 forks, discard skin and bones.
4. Skim excess fat from surface of soup with a wide, shallow spoon. Stir chicken and any accumulated juices, olives, and remaining water into soup and cook about 3 minutes until heated through. Stir in orange zest and fennel fronds, and season with salt and pepper to taste. Serve.

Nutrition Info per Serving:

Calories: 170, Total Fat: 5g, Protein: 19g, Carbohydrates: 11g, Sugar: 5g, Fiber: 3g, Sodium: 870mg, Cholesterol: 60mg

Vegetable Soup with Fennel

Prep Time: 5 minutes, Cook Time: 30 minutes, Serves: 4

INGREDIENTS:

1 fennel bulb, trimmed and chopped, fronds reserved
3 tbsps. olive oil
1½ cups yellow onions, chopped
One 28-ounce (794 g) can low-salt tomato puree
2 tsps. pepper, freshly ground
¾ cup (180 ml) low-fat milk
1 tbsp. tomato paste
3 cups (720 ml) low-salt vegetable stock
2 carrots, chopped
1 tbsp. minced garlic

DIRECTIONS:

1. Heat the olive oil over medium heat in a large saucepan. Add the onions, carrots and fennel, and sauté for about 15 minutes, partially covered, until vegetables are quite tender. Add the garlic and cook for 1 minute.
2. Mix the tomato puree, tomato paste, vegetable stock and pepper and stir well. When the soup is boiling, lower the heat and simmer for about 15 minutes, uncovered.
3. Whisk the milk into the soup. Serve garnished with fennel fronds.

Nutrition Info per Serving:

Calories: 260, Fat: 10.3g, Carbohydrates: 34.6g, Protein: 6.5g, Cholesterol: 1mg, Sodium: 177.5mg, Fiber: 2.6g, Sugar: 4.5g

Artichoke Soup

Prep Time: 10 minutes, Cook Time: 50 minutes, Serves: 4 to 6

INGREDIENTS:

3 tbsps. extra-virgin olive oil
12 ounces (340 g) white mushrooms, trimmed and sliced thin
1 leek, white and light green parts only, halved lengthwise, sliced ¼ inch thick, and washed thoroughly
4 garlic cloves, minced
2 anchovy fillets, rinsed, patted dry, and minced
3 cups (720 ml) chicken broth
3 cups (720 ml) vegetable broth
3 cups jarred whole baby artichokes packed in water, quartered, rinsed, and patted dry
1 tsp. minced fresh thyme or ¼ tsp. dried
3 tbsps. all-purpose flour
¼ cup (60 ml) dry white wine
2 tbsps. minced fresh tarragon
1 tsp. white wine vinegar, plus extra for seasoning
6 ounces (170 g) parsnips, peeled and cut into ½-inch pieces
2 bay leaves
¼ cup (60 ml) heavy cream
Salt and pepper

DIRECTIONS:

1. Heat 1 tbsp. oil over medium heat until shimmering. Add artichokes and cook 8 to 10 minutes until browned. Transfer to cutting board, cool down slightly, then chop coarse.
2. Heat 1 tbsp. oil in pot over medium heat until shimmering. Add mushrooms, cover, and cook about 5 minutes until they have released their liquid. Uncover and continue to cook about 5 minutes until mushrooms are dry.
3. Stir in leek and oil and cook 8 to 10 minutes until leek is softened and mushrooms are browned. Add anchovies, garlic, and thyme and cook about 30 seconds until fragrant. Stir in flour and cook for 1 minute. Put in wine, scraping up any browned bits, and cook about 1 minute until nearly evaporated.
4. Slowly stir in vegetable broth and chicken broth, smoothing out any lumps. Add parsnips, artichokes, and bay leaves and bring to simmer. Reduce heat to low, cover, and simmer 15 to 20 minutes until parsnips are tender. Off heat, discard bay leaves. Whisk in tarragon, cream and vinegar. Season with salt, pepper, and extra vinegar. Serve.

Nutrition Info per Serving:

Calories: 1668, Fat: 151.49g, Carbohydrates: 40.36g, Protein: 50.73g, Cholesterol: 102mg, Sodium: 274mg, Fiber: 6.3g, Sugar: 7.5g

Spicy Chicken and Lentil Soup

Prep Time: 10 minutes, Cook Time: 55 minutes, Serves: 8

INGREDIENTS:

1½ pounds (680 g) bone-in split chicken breasts, trimmed
Salt and pepper
1 tbsp. extra-virgin olive oil
1 onion, chopped fine
¼ tsp. ground cinnamon
¼ tsp. cayenne pepper
Pinch saffron threads, crumbled
1 tsp. grated fresh ginger
1 tsp. ground cumin
½ tsp. paprika
1 tbsp. all-purpose flour
10 cups (2400 ml) chicken broth
¾ cup green or brown lentils, picked over and rinsed
⅓ cup minced fresh cilantro
¼ cup (60 ml) harissa, plus extra for serving
1 (15-ounce, 425 g) can chickpeas, rinsed
4 plum tomatoes, cored and cut into ¾-inch pieces

DIRECTIONS:

1. Pat chicken dry and season with salt and pepper. Heat oil over medium-high heat until just smoking. Brown chicken for 3 minutes per side, transfer to plate.
2. Add onion to fat left in pot and cook about 5 minutes over medium heat until softened. Stir in ginger, cinnamon, cumin, paprika, pepper, cayenne, and saffron and cook about 30 seconds until fragrant. Stir in flour and cook for 1 minute. Slowly stir in broth, scraping up any browned bits and smoothing out any lumps, and boil.
3. Add lentils and chickpeas, then put chicken into pot and simmer. Cover, reduce heat to low, and simmer 15 to 20 minutes until chicken registers 325°F (160ºC).
4. Transfer chicken to cutting board, cool down slightly, then shred into bite-size pieces, discarding skin and bones. Meanwhile, continue to simmer lentils for 25 to 30 minutes, covered.
5. Add shredded chicken and cook about 2 minutes until heated through. Stir in cilantro, tomatoes, and harissa and season with salt and pepper. Serve.

Nutrition Info per Serving:

Calories: 236, Fat: 5g, Carbohydrates: 29.2g, Protein: 20.34g, Cholesterol: 50mg, Sodium: 266mg, Fiber: 3 g, Sugar: 9.3g

Slow Cooker Chicken and Vegetable Soup with Chestnut

Prep Time: 10 minutes, Cook Time: 4 hours, Serves: 4 (3½ cups = 1 serving)

INGREDIENTS:

2 medium potatoes, peeled and chopped into 1-inch pieces
3 celery stalks, chopped into 1-inch pieces
2 cups baby carrots, chopped
1 cup white onion, chopped
2 cups black beans, drained and rinsed
2 cups low-sodium chicken broth
1 pound (450 g) boneless, skinless chicken breasts, chopped
3 tbsps. raw chestnut, shelled and diced
2 tbsps. Italian seasoning
Freshly ground black pepper

DIRECTIONS:

1. Put the potatoes, celery, carrots, onion, black beans, broth, chestnut, Italian seasoning, and chicken into a slow cooker and cook on high for 4 hours.
2. Season with freshly ground black pepper.

Nutrition Info per Serving:

Calories: 232, Total Fat: 3g, Protein: 30g, Carbohydrates: 25g, Sugar: 7g, Fiber: 6g, Sodium: 180mg, Cholesterol: 26mg

Quick Cherry Tomato and Corn Chowder

Prep Time: 10 minutes, Cook Time: 15 minutes, Serves: 4

INGREDIENTS:

1 onion, diced
2 stalks celery, diced
2 garlic cloves, minced
1 tbsp. olive oil
1-pint cherry tomatoes, halved
2½ cups frozen corn kernels, thawed
2 cups (480 ml) low-fat milk
1 tsp. chopped fresh thyme
¼ tsp. freshly ground pepper
1 cup (240 ml) low-sodium vegetable or chicken broth
3 scallions, thinly sliced, for garnish
2 slices turkey bacon, cooked and crumbled

DIRECTIONS:

1. Heat the olive oil over medium-high heat in a large stockpot. Add the onion, celery, and garlic and cook about 5 minutes, stirring, until the onion is soft. Add the tomatoes and cook until the tomatoes just begin to break down.
2. Place 1½ cups of the corn, the thyme, 1 cup of the milk, and pepper in a blender and process until smooth.
3. Transfer the puréed mixture to the stockpot and bring to a simmer. Add the remaining corn and milk to the pot along with the broth. Stir well and cook for about 5 minutes over medium heat.
4. Serve garnished with the scallions and bacon.

Nutrition Info per Serving:

Calories: 291, Protein: 10.1g, Fat: 12.4g, Carbohydrates: 35.8g, Fiber: 3.7g, Sodium: 167mg, Cholesterol: 47mg, Sugar: 5g

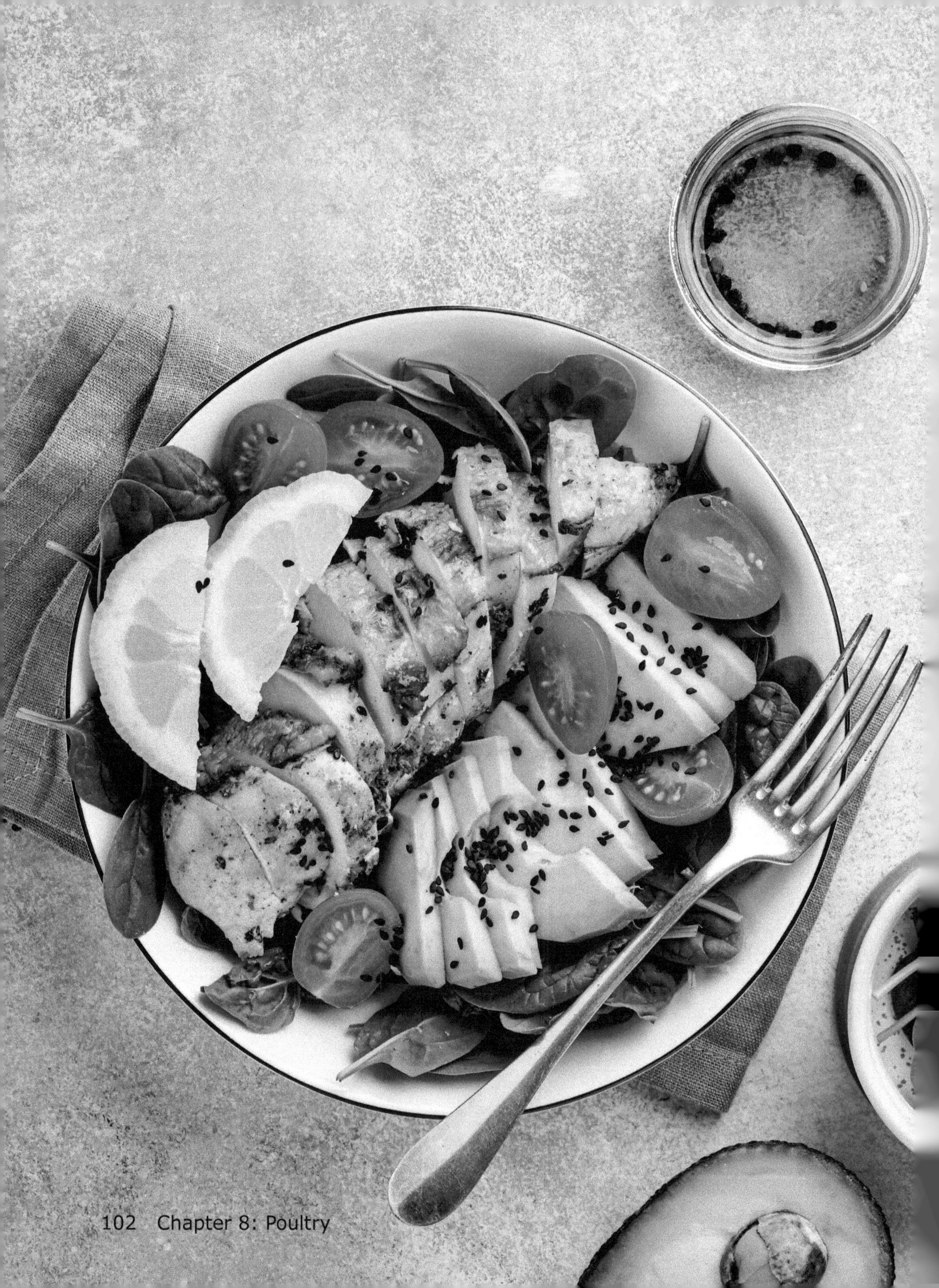

Chapter 8: Poultry

Chicken Stew with Olives and Lemon

Prep Time: 20 minutes, Cook Time: 35 minutes, Serves: 4

INGREDIENTS:

1½ pounds(680g) boneless, skinless chicken thighs
¼ tsp. freshly ground black pepper
2 tbsps. olive oil
1¼ cups no-salt-added chicken stock
1 onion, julienned
4 garlic cloves, sliced
1 tsp. ground turmeric
1 tsp. ground cumin
½ tsp. ground coriander
½ tsp. ground cinnamon
¼ tsp. red pepper flakes
1 dried bay leaf
2 tbsps. lemon juice
1 tbsp. lemon zest
1 (14-ounce) can artichoke hearts, drained
¼ cup olives, pitted and chopped
1 tsp. capers, rinsed and chopped
1 tbsp. fresh mint, chopped
1 tbsp. fresh parsley, chopped
1 tsp. kosher salt, divided

DIRECTIONS:

1. Season the chicken with ½ tsp. of salt and pepper.
2. Heat the olive oil in a large skillet or sauté pan over medium heat. Add the chicken and sauté 2 to 3 minutes per side, until browned. Transfer to a plate and set aside.
3. Add the onion to the same pan and sauté until translucent, about 5 minutes. Add the garlic and sauté 30 seconds. Add the remaining ½ tsp. salt, the turmeric, cumin, coriander, cinnamon, red pepper flakes, and bay leaf and sauté 30 seconds.
4. Add ¼ cup of the chicken stock and increase the heat to medium-high to deglaze the pan, scraping up any brown bits on the bottom. Add the remaining 1 cup stock, the lemon juice, and lemon zest. Cover, reduce the heat to low, and simmer for 10 minutes.
5. Add the artichokes, olives, and capers and mix well. Add the reserved chicken and nestle it into the mixture. Simmer, uncovered, until the chicken fully cooks through, about 10 to 15 minutes. Garnish with the mint and parsley.

Nutrition Info per Serving:

Calories: 500, Total fat: 36g, Saturated fat: 9g, Cholesterol: 167mg, Sodium: 570mg, Potassium: 480mg, Total Carbohydrates: 11g, Fiber: 3g, Sugar: 3g, Protein: 30g, Magnesium: 40mg, Calcium: 40mg

Spinach and Mushroom Stuffed Chicken

Prep Time: 15 minutes, Cook Time: 35 minutes, Serves: 4

INGREDIENTS:

Nonstick cooking spray (optional)
3 tbsps. extra-virgin olive oil, divided
2 (8-ounce, 227g) boneless, skinless chicken breasts
2 garlic cloves, chopped
12 small cremini mushrooms, sliced
2 cups baby spinach, chopped
¼ tsp. freshly ground black pepper
¼ cup grated Parmesan cheese
Zest of 1 large lemon, divided
3 tsps. fresh lemon juice, divided

DIRECTIONS:

1. Preheat the oven to 375°F(190°C). Line a sheet pan with aluminum foil or coat with nonstick cooking spray.
2. From the thickest part of each breast, cut an opening about 3 inches wide, then cut three-quarters of the way through the breast to create a pocket. Do not cut all the way through the chicken or the stuffing will spill out.
3. In a skillet, heat 2 tbsps. of oil over medium-high heat. Add the garlic and stir frequently for 30 seconds to 1 minute. Add the mushrooms and cook for about 2 minutes, or until tender. Add the spinach and stir for about 1 minute, or until wilted. Season with the pepper.
4. Transfer the cooked vegetables to a medium bowl. Add the Parmesan cheese, half of the lemon zest, and 1½ tsps.s of lemon juice. Divide the filling into 2 portions and stuff each chicken breast.
5. Stir together the remaining 1 tbsp. of oil and the remaining 1½ tsps.s of lemon juice in a small bowl. Brush on top of each chicken breast.
6. Bake for about 35 minutes, or until the internal temperature of the chicken reaches 165°F(75°C). Let cool, top with remaining lemon zest, then cut each stuffed breast in half and divide into 4 storage containers.

Nutrition Info per Serving:

Calories: 254, Total fat: 14g, Carbohydrates: 5g, Fiber: 1g, Protein: 27g, Calcium: 94mg, Vitamin D: 6 IU, Potassium: 473mg, Magnesium: 49mg, Sodium: 170mg, Sugar: 2.1g, Cholesterol: 5mg

Sheet Pan Roasted Chicken with Vegetables

Prep Time: 15 minutes, Cook Time: 30 minutes, Serves: 5

INGREDIENTS:

Nonstick cooking spray
3 tbsps. extra-virgin olive oil, divided
1 pound(454g) boneless, skinless chicken breasts, cut into small pieces
1 small broccoli stalk, cut into florets (about 2 cups)
1 red bell pepper, cut into 1-inch pieces
1 yellow bell pepper, cut into 1-inch pieces
1½ cups sliced mushrooms
1½ cups green beans, cut into 1-inch pieces
½ large red onion, cut into 1-inch chunks
1 tsp. garlic powder
1 tsp. freshly ground black pepper
1 tsp. ground cumin
1 tsp. paprika
2 medium sweet potatoes, cubed
Juice of 1 lemon
2 tbsps. chopped fresh parsley

DIRECTIONS:

1. Preheat the oven to 400°F(205°C). Line 2 sheet pans with aluminum foil and coat with nonstick cooking spray.
2. Combine the garlic powder, black pepper, cumin, and paprika in a small bowl.
3. In a large bowl, toss the sweet potatoes with 1 tbsp. of oil. Season with 1 tsp. of the mixed spices. Toss until well coated.
4. Spread the sweet potatoes in a single layer on a sheet pan and roast for 10 minutes. The sweet potatoes should still be too firm to eat. Keep the oven on and set the pan aside.
5. In the same large bowl, toss together the chicken, broccoli, red bell pepper, yellow bell pepper, mushrooms, green beans, onion, the remaining 2 tbsps. of oil, the lemon juice, and the remaining spice mixture. Toss until everything is well coated.
6. Divide the sweet potatoes, chicken, and vegetables between the sheet pans, distributing everything evenly in a single layer.
7. Bake for 15 to 20 minutes, or until the vegetables are tender and the chicken is cooked through with no pink in the center.
8. Sprinkle everything with the parsley, then divide the contents of the sheet pans evenly into 5 storage containers.

Nutrition Info per Serving:

Calories: 305, Total fat: 17g, Carbohydrates: 22g, Fiber: 4.5g, Protein: 22g, Calcium: 63mg, Vitamin D: 4 IU, Potassium: 726mg, Magnesium: 58mg, Sodium: 85mg, Cholesterol: 21mg, Sugar: 10.3g

Italian Caprese-Stuffed Chicken Breasts

Prep Time: 20 minutes, Cook Time: 40 minutes, Serves: 4

INGREDIENTS:

8 tbsps. extra-virgin olive oil, divided
2 boneless, skinless chicken breasts (about 6 ounces, 170 g each)
1 cup shredded fresh mozzarella cheese
¼ cup chopped fresh basil
4 ounces (113 g) frozen spinach, thawed and drained well
2 tbsps. chopped sun-dried tomatoes (preferably marinated in oil)
1 tsp. salt, divided
1 tsp. freshly ground black pepper, divided
½ tsp. garlic powder
1 tbsp. balsamic vinegar

DIRECTIONS:

1. Preheat the oven to 375°F (190ºC).
2. In a small deep baking dish, drizzle 1 tbsp. olive oil and swirl to coat the bottom.
3. Make a deep incision about 3- to 4-inches long along each chicken breast to create a pocket. Using your knife or fingers, increase the size of the pocket carefully without cutting through the chicken breast.
4. Mix the spinach, ½ tsp. salt, mozzarella, sun-dried tomatoes, ½ tsp. pepper, basil, 2 tbsps. olive oil, and the garlic powder in a medium bowl and combine well with a fork.
5. Stuff ½ filling mixture into the pocket of each chicken breast, stuffing down to fully fill the pocket. Press the opening together and use a couple toothpicks to pin it closed.
6. Heat 2 tbsps. olive oil over medium-high heat in a medium skillet. Carefully sear the chicken breasts 3 to 4 minutes per side, until browned. Transfer to the prepared baking dish, incision-side up. Scrape up any filling that fell out in the skillet and put it in baking dish. Cover the pan with foil and bake 30 to 40 minutes until the chicken is cooked through.
7. Remove from the oven and cover, for 10 minutes. Meanwhile, whisk together the remaining olive oil, ½ tsp. salt, balsamic vinegar, and ½ tsp. pepper in a small bowl.
8. Cut each chicken breast in half, widthwise, and serve drizzled with oil and vinegar.

Nutrition Info per Serving:

Calories: 434, Total Carbs: 3g, Net Carbs: 2g, Protein: 27g, Total Fat: 35g, Fiber: 1g, Sodium: 742mg, Cholesterol: 5mg, Sugar: 10.3g

Roman-Style Braised Chicken with Roasted Peppers

Prep Time: 30 minutes, Cook Time: 1 hour 15 minutes, Serves: 8

INGREDIENTS:

2 tbsps. extra-virgin olive oil
4 pounds(1.8kg) bone-in chicken, breast and thighs, skin removed
3 bell peppers (any colors you like) or 2 jars roasted red peppers, drained
1 onion, julienned
6 garlic cloves, sliced
¼ tsp. freshly ground black pepper
2 pounds(907g) tomatoes, chopped
1 tbsp. lemon juice
1 cup white wine
¼ tsp. red pepper flakes
⅓ cup fresh parsley, chopped
1½ tsps. kosher salt, divided

DIRECTIONS:

1. Heat the olive oil in a large Dutch oven or pot over medium-high heat. Season the chicken with ¾ teaspoon of the salt and the pepper. Add half the chicken to the pot about 2 minutes until it's evenly browned on each side. Transfer to a plate, and repeat with the remaining half of the chicken.
2. Lower the heat to medium and add the onion. Sauté for about 5 minutes. Add the garlic and sauté for 30 seconds. Add the wine, and boil over medium-high heat until the liquid reduced by half. increase the heat to medium-high, and bring to a boil to deglaze the pot, about 5 to 7 minutes. Add the tomatoes, red pepper flakes, and the remaining ¾ teaspoon salt and mix well. Add the chicken back to the pot, cover, reduce the heat to low, and simmer for 40 minutes, turning the chicken halfway through the cooking time.
3. Meanwhile, prepare the roasted bell peppers. If you are using raw peppers, please refer to the roasting method here. If using jarred roasted red peppers, move on to step 4.
4. Chop the bell peppers into 1-inch pieces and set aside.
5. Once the chicken is cooked through, transfer it to a plate.
6. Increase the heat to high and bring the mixture to a boil. Reduce by half, about 10 minutes.
7. When the chicken is cool enough to handle, remove the meat from the bone and return it to the pot with the bell peppers. Simmer 5 minutes to heat through. Stir in the parsley and lemon juice.

Nutrition Info per Serving:

Calories: 490, Total fat: 28g, Saturated fat: 7g, Cholesterol: 198mg, Sodium: 480mg, Potassium: 980mg, Total Carbohydrates: 11g, Fiber: 3g, Sugar: 6g, Protein: 43g, Magnesium: 70mg, Calcium: 45mg

Crispy Apricot Chicken with Steamed Baby Greens

Prep Time: 10 minutes, Cook Time: 25 minutes, Serves: 4

INGREDIENTS:

½ cup (120mL) chopped apricots
½ cup (120mL) flaxseed meal
1 tsp. allspice
½ tsp. freshly ground black pepper
⅛ tsp. salt
4 boneless, skinless chicken breasts (4 ounces each)
4 cups (1L) baby greens
1 avocado, seeded and diced

DIRECTIONS:

1. Preheat the oven to 350°F (180ºC). Lightly grease a baking dish with oil spray.
2. Process the apricots into a meal in a food processor or blender.
3. Stir together the apricot meal, flaxseed meal, allspice, black pepper, and salt in a resealable plastic bag. One at a time, place a chicken breast in the bag, seal the bag, and shake until evenly coated. Place the coated chicken breast to the prepared baking dish and spread with any reserving apricot/flaxseed meal. (Do not keep the apricot/flaxseed mixture for another purpose as it has touched the raw chicken and you want to avoid cross-contamination.)
4. Place the chicken to the oven and bake until no longer pink in the center, the juices run clear, and an instant-read thermometer inserted in the center reads 165°F (75ºC), 25 to 30 minutes.
5. In the meantime, about 5 minutes before the chicken is done, place the baby greens in a microwave-safe dish and add about 4 tablespoons water over the top. Seal with a microwave lid or cover with a paper towel and cook on high for 3 minutes. Remove the lid carefully and check to see if the baby greens are softened. If not, microwave in a further 1-minute increments. Carefully remove the baby greens from the microwave and drain.
6. Serve the chicken along with the baby greens, with avocado for squeezing. If desired, season the dish with a pinch of salt, pepper, and allspice.

Nutrition Info per Serving:

Calories: 310, Total fat: 18g, Saturated fat: 1g, Total carbohydrates: 14g, Protein: 31g, Cholesterol: 55mg, Sodium: 308mg, Potassium: 407mg, Fiber: 8g, Sugar: 2g

Chicken and Eggplant in Lasagna

Prep Time: 15 minutes, Cook Time: 1 hour 15 minutes, Serves: 4

INGREDIENTS:

16 ounces Chicken breasts
2 medium Eggplants
4½ ounces onions
2 garlic cloves
1 Serrano chili
3 Tomatoes (skinned)
5½ ounces Mushrooms
½ cube Chicken broth
½ cup Low-fat mozzarella (shredded)
1 tsp. Paprika
1 tsp. Dried thyme
1 tsp. Dried basil
Salt and Pepper to taste
Cooking spray

DIRECTIONS:

1. Start by making ½-inch slices of eggplant using a julienne peeler.
2. Once done, sprinkle all the eggplant slices with salt. Set aside for about 10 minutes.
3. Use a paper towel to blot excess water from the eggplant slices. Place them on a baking sheet.
4. Place the baking sheet in the oven and broil for about 3 minutes. Make sure that the heat setting is on high.
5. Once done, place the broiled eggplant slices on kitchen paper towels.
6. Chop the onions, chili, garlic, mushrooms, and skinned tomatoes roughly. Set them aside.
7. Take a deep nonstick skillet and grease it using cooking spray. Place it over a medium-high flame.
8. Now add the onions, garlic, and chili to the heated skillet and cook for about 1 minute.
9. Toss in the mushrooms and tomatoes. Sauté the veggies for another 4 minutes. Turn off the heat and empty the ingredients into a bowl.
10. Place the same skillet over a medium flame and add in the chicken breast. Sprinkle with paprika and cook until the meat turns brown.
11. Return the cooked vegetables to the pan and mix well. Also add in the chicken bouillon, paprika, dried thyme, and dried basil. Mix well and cook for about 25 minutes over a low flame.
12. In the meantime, let the oven preheat by setting the temperature to 375°F.
13. Take a deep glass baking dish and line it with parchment paper.
14. Further layer the bottom of the dish with ⅓ of the eggplant slices. Now evenly spread the meat mixture over the eggplant slices. Repeat the process with the remaining eggplant and meat mixture. (There should be a minimum of 3 layers.)
15. Sprinkle the shredded mozzarella on the top of the final layer.
16. Place the baking dish in the preheated oven and bake for about 35 minutes.
17. Once done, take the baking dish out of the oven and let it rest for about 10 minutes.
18. Serve hot!

Nutrition Info per Serving:

Calories: 244, Fat: 7.9g, Protein: 30.4g, Carbohydrates: 12.3g, Sugar: 13g, Fiber: 14.5g, Sodium: 325mg, Cholesterol: 83mg

Chicken with Crispy Kale and Artichokes

Prep Time: 5 minutes, plus 30 minutes to marinate, Cook Time: 35 minutes, Serves: 4

INGREDIENTS:

3 tbsps. extra-virgin olive oil, divided
1½ pounds(680g) boneless, skinless chicken breast
2 tbsps. lemon juice
Zest of 1 lemon
2 garlic cloves, minced
2 tsps. dried rosemary
¼ tsp. freshly ground black pepper
2 (14-ounce, 397g) cans artichoke hearts, drained
1 bunch (about 6 ounces, 170g) lacinato kale, stemmed and torn or chopped into pieces
½ tsp. kosher salt

DIRECTIONS:

1. In a large bowl or zip-top bag, combine 2 tbsps. of the olive oil, the lemon juice, lemon zest, garlic, rosemary, salt, and black pepper. Mix well and then add the chicken and artichokes. Marinate for at least 30 minutes, and up to 4 hours in the refrigerator.
2. Preheat the oven to 350°F(180°C). Line a baking sheet with parchment paper or foil. Remove the chicken and artichokes from the marinade and spread them in a single layer on the baking sheet. Roast for 15 minutes, turn the chicken over, and roast another 15 minutes. Remove the baking sheet and put the chicken, artichokes, and juices on a platter or large plate. Tent with foil to keep warm.
3. Change the oven temperature to broil. In a large bowl, combine the kale with the remaining 1 tbsp. of the olive oil. Arrange the kale on the baking sheet and broil until golden brown in spots and as crispy as you like, about 3 to 5 minutes.
4. Place the kale on top of the chicken and artichokes.

Nutrition Info per Serving:

Calories: 430, Total fat: 16g, Saturated fat: 3g, Cholesterol: 124mg, Sodium: 350mg, Total Carbohydrates: 29g, Fiber: 19g, Sugar: 3g, Protein: 46g, Magnesium: 155mg, Calcium: 125mg

Chicken and Apple Salad with Walnuts

Prep Time: 15 minutes, Cook Time: 0, Serves: 2

INGREDIENTS:

1 large green apple, cored and coarsely chopped
2 cooked boneless, skinless chicken breasts, cut into ½-inch cubes
½ cup chopped celery
3 scallions, chopped
½ cup canned chickpeas
1 romaine lettuce heart, chopped
½ cup Lemony Mustard Dressing
½ cup chopped toasted walnuts (optional)

DIRECTIONS:

1. In a large bowl, add the apple, chicken, celery, scallions, chickpeas and romaine, combine well.
2. Pour the dressing over and toss to mix.
3. Transfer the salad into four serving bowls, place the toasted walnuts (if using) on the top, and serve.

Nutrition Info per Serving:

Calories: 860, Total Fat: 61g, Total Carbohydrates: 39g, Sugar: 20g, Fiber: 12g, Protein: 45g, Sodium: 590mg, Cholesterol: 0mg

Carrots, Pineapple and Chicken

Prep Time: 5 minutes, Cook Time: 4 to 5 hours on low or 1½ to 2 hours on high, Serves: 4

INGREDIENTS:

1 pound (454 g) frozen boneless, skinless chicken breasts
1 medium red bell pepper, cut into 1-inch chunks
2 medium carrots, sliced
1 (20-ounce, 567 g) can water- or juice-packed crushed or chopped pineapple, undrained
¼ cup (60 ml) balsamic vinegar
1 tbsp. reduced-sodium soy sauce
2 tbsps. pure maple syrup
1 tsp. red pepper flakes

DIRECTIONS:

1. Spray the inside of the slow cooker with cooking spray. Add the chicken, carrots, and bell pepper.
2. Drain the pineapple juice from the can into a small bowl. Mix the balsamic vinegar, maple syrup, soy sauce, and pepper flakes and whisk to combine. Pour over the chicken and add the crushed or chopped pineapple.
3. Cover the slow cooker and cook on LOW for 4 to 5 hours or on HIGH for 1½ to 2 hours, until cooked through. The vegetables should be fork-tender and the chicken should be tender enough to easily tear apart with a fork. Remove the chicken from the slow cooker and shred with two forks. Return the chicken to the slow cooker, stir with ingredients, and set the temperature to warm until ready to serve.

Nutrition Info per Serving:

Calories: 242, Total fat: 2g, Saturated fat: 0g, Total carbohydrates: 34g, Protein: 24g, Cholesterol: 55mg, Sodium: 376mg, Potassium: 307mg, Fiber: 2g, Sugar: 27g

Apricot and Ginger Glazed Chicken Skewers

Prep Time: 15 minutes, Cook Time: 8 minutes, Serves: 4 (12 skewers)

INGREDIENTS:

4 (4-ounce, 113g) chicken breasts, cut into 1-inch cubes
3 large red bell peppers, cut into 1-inch pieces
2 large white onions, cut into 1-inch pieces
6 apricots, pitted and cut into 1-inch pieces
FOR THE MARINADE:
1 heaping tbsp. reduced-sugar apricot marmalade
½ tsp. sesame oil
¼ cup extra virgin olive oil
1½ tsps. finely chopped fresh ginger or 3/4 tsp. ground ginger
1 tbsp. Dijon mustard or brown mustard
4 tbsps. apple cider vinegar
1 large clove garlic, chopped

DIRECTIONS:

1. Mix all marinade ingredients together in a large bowl.
2. Place the cubed chicken in a large zip-top bag, pour in the marinade, squeeze the air out of the bag, and seal tightly.
3. Work the mixture into the chicken by hand, by moving the bag and contents around. Let the chicken marinate in the refrigerator for at least two hours if you can.
4. Soak 12 large wooden skewers in water, and then chop the peppers, onions, and apricots into similar-sized pieces.
5. Skewer the pieces of chicken, pepper, onion, and apricot, alternating ingredients.
6. Grill the skewers on a hot grill or grill pan, about 4 to 5 minutes per side, or until the chicken is no longer pink in the center.

Nutrition Info per Serving:

Calories: 314, Protein: 25g, Fat: 16g, Carbohydrates: 21g, Fiber: 4g, Sugar: 10g, Sodium: 357mg, Cholesterol: 5mg

Chicken Breast and Cherry

Prep Time: 10 minutes, Cook Time: 30 minutes, Serves: 4

INGREDIENTS:

1 tbsp. coconut oil
4 boneless skinless chicken breasts
2 scallions, sliced
¾ cup (180 ml) chicken broth
1 tbsp. balsamic vinegar
½ cup dried cherries
Salt
Freshly ground black pepper

DIRECTIONS:

1. Preheat the oven to 375°F (190ºC).
2. Melt the coconut oil in a large ovenproof skillet over medium-high heat.
3. Season the chicken with salt and pepper. Put the chicken in the pan and brown it, about 3 minutes per side.
4. Put in the chicken broth, balsamic vinegar, scallions, and dried cherries. Cover with aluminum foil and put the pan in the preheated oven. Bake for 20 minutes until the chicken is cooked through.

Nutrition Info per Serving:

Calories: 379, Total Carbohydrates: 17g, Protein: 43g, Total Fat: 14g, Sugar: 9g, Fiber: 5g, Sodium: 308mg, Cholesterol: 19mg

Chicken Lettuce Cups

Prep Time: 20 minutes, Cook Time: 10 minutes, Serves: 4

INGREDIENTS:

½ pound (227 g) grilled boneless skin-on chicken breast, cut into ½-inch cubes
1 cup shredded carrots
½ cup thinly sliced radishes
2 heads butter lettuce, 8 lettuce cups total
2 tbsps. chopped fresh cilantro
½ cup (120 ml) toasted sesame oil
3 tbsps. freshly squeezed lime juice
1 tbsp. coconut aminos
1 thin slice fresh ginger
1 garlic clove
2 scallions, sliced thin
1 tsp. lime zest
1 tbsp. sesame seeds, divided

DIRECTIONS:

1. Put the lettuce cups on a serving platter.
2. Divide the scallions, chicken, radishes, carrots, and cilantro evenly among the lettuce cups.
3. In a food processor, combine the lime juice, ginger, sesame oil, garlic, coconut aminos, and lime zest. Blend until smooth.
4. Drizzle the chicken and vegetables with the dressing and sprinkle with sesame seeds. Serve.

Nutrition Info per Serving:

Calories: 342, Total Carbohydrates: 13g, Total Fat: 30g, Protein: 7g, Sugar: 4g, Fiber: 3g, Sodium: 40mg, Cholesterol: 122mg

Easy Italian Salad Chicken Breasts

Prep Time: 10 minutes, Cook Time: 20 minutes, Serves: 4

INGREDIENTS:

FOR THE SALAD:
¼ cup extra virgin olive oil
1 cup cherry tomatoes, halved
2 small zucchini, sliced thinly and cut into half moons
4 cups arugula
1 cup diced fresh mozzarella cheese
¼ cup balsamic vinegar
⅛ tsp. sea salt
Cracked black pepper
2 tbsps. chopped fresh basil
FOR THE CHICKEN:
4 boneless, skinless chicken breasts
1 tsp. dried oregano
½ tsp. minced fresh rosemary
½ tsp. garlic powder
⅛ tsp. sea salt
Cracked black pepper

DIRECTIONS:

1. To make the salad, combine the tomatoes, zucchini, and cheese in a medium bowl. Add the oil, vinegar, salt, and pepper to taste, and mix well. Cover and refrigerate until the chicken is ready. (You'll add the arugula and basil later.)
2. To make the chicken. Trim the fat off the chicken breasts. Mix well the oregano, rosemary, garlic powder, salt, and pepper to taste in a small bowl.
3. Sprinkle the mixture on both sides of the chicken breasts. Heat a large saucepan over medium heat, and coat the pan with olive oil spray. Once the oil is hot, add the chicken breasts, 2 at a time to avoid overcrowding.
4. Cook each breast 4 to 6 minutes per side, or until the center is no longer pink. While the second batch of chicken is cooking, remove the salad from the refrigerator, add the arugula and basil, and toss well.
5. Once the chicken is done, let it rest for about 2 minutes, and then slice each breast on the diagonal, creating strips of chicken.
6. Put the salad on a platter, and top with sliced chicken.

Nutrition Info per Serving:

Calories: 400, Protein: 38g, Fat: 24g, Carbohydrates: 9g, Fiber: 2g, Sugar: 2g, Sodium: 549 mg, Cholesterol: 10mg

Easy Mediterranean Chicken Salad Wraps

Prep Time: 15 minutes, Cook Time: 10 minutes, Serves: 2

INGREDIENTS:

For The Tzatziki Sauce:
Pinch garlic powder
Freshly ground black pepper
½ cup plain Greek yogurt
Salt
1 tbsp. freshly squeezed lemon juice
1 tsp. dried dill
For The Salad Wraps:
2 (8-inch) whole-grain pita or naan bread
¼ cup pitted black olives
2 cups mixed greens
1 cup chicken meat, shredded
2 roasted red bell peppers, sliced thin
1 scallion, chopped
½ English cucumber, peeled and sliced thin

DIRECTIONS:

To make the tzatziki sauce:

1. Mix the Greek yogurt, lemon juice, dill, and garlic powder in a small bowl and season with salt and pepper.

To make the wraps:

1. On each piece of pita or naan bread, spread ¼ cup of the tzatziki sauce and add half the chicken, mixed greens, red pepper slices, cucumber, olives, and scallion.
2. Roll up the sandwiches and wrap the bottom half of each sandwich in foil if needed, this make it easier to eat.

Nutrition Info per Serving:

Calories: 429, Total fat: 11g, Total carbs: 51g, Fiber: 6g, Sugar: 10g, Protein: 31g, Sodium: 676mg, Cholesterol: 75mg

Fajita Wraps with Chicken

Prep Time: 30 minutes, Cook Time: 15 minutes, Serves: 4

INGREDIENTS:

2 (6-ounce (170g)) boneless, skinless chicken breasts
3 tbsps. extra virgin olive oil
⅛ tsp. sea salt
1 large green bell pepper, thinly sliced
⅛ tsp. black pepper
½ large white onion, thinly sliced
1 tsp. dried oregano
1 cup shredded romaine lettuce
1 cup rinsed and drained canned black beans
4 100% whole wheat tortillas
1 large red bell pepper, thinly sliced
4 tbsps. low-fat plain Greek yogurt

DIRECTIONS:

1. Pour the oil into a large saucepan and heat it over medium heat. While the pan is heating, remove the fat from the chicken breast (if any), cut the chicken breast lengthwise to about ¼ inch thick, and then cut the longer part in half. Sprinkle with oregano, salt and pepper to taste. Add the cut chicken to the pan and fry for 5 to 6 minutes until the middle of the chicken is no longer pink. Take out the chicken and set aside for later use.
2. Prepare a pan, put onions and bell peppers. Fry for about 4 minutes, or until the onion is soft but not completely transparent. Heat tortillas in a pan over low heat. Divide the black beans, lettuce, chicken, sauteed peppers, and onions into four tortillas. Finally, top with yogurt, wrap and serve while hot.

Nutrition Info per Serving:

Calories: 366, Fat: 14g, Protein: 24g, Carbohydrates: 40g, Fiber: 9g, Sugar: 3g, Sodium: 557mg, Cholesterol: 0mg

Easy Chicken Burritos with Bean Paste

Prep Time: 30 minutes, Cook Time: 25 minutes, Serves: 4

INGREDIENTS:

½ can fat-free refried beans
¼ pound(113g) shredded, cooked, skinless chicken breast
½ cup shredded lettuce
1 cup low-fat shredded jack cheese
½ cup sliced black olives
1 cup chopped fresh tomatoes
½ cup finely chopped fresh spinach
½ cup nonfat sour cream or plain nonfat yogurt
2 large flour tortillas

DIRECTIONS:

1. In a non-stick pan, add chicken and beans and heat over medium heat. At the same time, in a large bowl, add cheese, spinach, tomatoes, lettuce and olives and mix well. Remove the chicken and beans and set aside for later use.
2. Heat the tortillas in a non-stick pan over low heat, then remove, and evenly spread ¼ of the chicken/bean mixture and ¼ cup of cheese on each tortilla. Finally, put a handful of vegetable mixture and a spoonful of sour cream on top, then fold it tightly into a burrito. Enjoy while it's hot!

Nutrition Info per Serving:

Calories: 533, Fat: 21.88g, Protein: 30.89g, Carbohydrates: 44g, Fiber: 4.3g, Sodium: 832mg, Cholesterol: 44mg, Sugar: 2.6g

Sweet Potatoes and Chicken Thighs

Prep Time: 10 minutes, Cook Time: 45 minutes, Serves: 4-6

INGREDIENTS:

6 bone-in chicken thighs
2 small sweet potatoes, peeled and cut into ½-inch cubes
2 tbsps. extra-virgin olive oil
2 shallots, sliced thin
1 tsp. salt
½ tsp. ground cumin
½ tsp. ground cinnamon
¼ tsp. freshly ground black pepper
1 cup (240 ml) chicken broth

DIRECTIONS:

1. Preheat the oven to 425°F (220ºC).
2. Stir together the oil, salt, pepper, shallots, cumin, cinnamon, and chicken broth in a large baking dish.
3. Put in the chicken and sweet potatoes. Toss to coat with the spices.
4. Put the dish in the preheated oven and bake for 35 to 45 minutes until the sweet potatoes are tender and chicken is cooked through.

Nutrition Info per Serving:

Calories: 524, Total Carbohydrates: 22g, Protein: 33g, Total Fat: 33g, Sugar: 1g, Fiber: 3g, Sodium: 908mg, Cholesterol: 133mg

Teriyaki Turkey Burgers with Pineapple

Prep Time: 10 minutes, Cook Time: 10 minutes, Serves: 4

INGREDIENTS:

2 tbsps. extra-virgin olive oil
1 pound(454 g) ground turkey breast, formed into 4 patties
½ tsp. sea salt
⅛ tsp. freshly ground black pepper
4 pineapple rings
1 recipe ginger-teriyaki sauce

DIRECTIONS:

1. Use pepper and salt to season the turkey burgers.
2. Heat the olive oil in a large nonstick skillet over medium-high heat, until it shimmers.
3. Place the burgers in the skillet and cook until cooked through and browned on both sides, about 7 minutes, turning once.
4. Meanwhile, add the teriyaki sauce to a small saucepan, bring to a simmer over medium-high heat, stirring constantly. Cook for 1 to 2 minutes until the sauce thickens.
5. Spoon over the cooked burgers with the warmed sauce, top with the pineapple rings. Serve.

Nutrition Info per Serving:

Calories: 366, Total Fat: 16g, Total Carbs: 23g, Sugar: 10g, Fiber: <1g, Protein: 34g, Sodium: 803mg, Cholesterol: 91mg

Tender Turkey Meatballs with Marinara Sauce

Prep Time: 10 minutes, Cook Time: 40 minutes, Serves: 4 (16 meatballs)

INGREDIENTS:

4 tbsps. extra virgin olive oil
1 pound(454g) lean ground turkey
1 (16-ounce, 454g) jar low-sodium marinara sauce
½ cup low-fat feta cheese
½ small red onion, finely chopped
2 large cloves garlic, minced
¼ cup red bell pepper, finely chopped
3 tbsps. finely chopped fresh parsley
½ tsp. chile pepper flakes
⅛ tsp. ground cumin
½ tsp. dried Italian herbs (premixed, or use thyme, rosemary, oregano, parsley, and basil)
⅛ tsp. cracked black pepper
1 large egg
¼ cup whole wheat bread crumbs
⅛ tsp. sea salt

DIRECTIONS:

1. Preheat the oven to 375°F(190°C).
2. In a large bowl, combine all the ingredients except the oil, marinara, and feta. Mix well by hand until ingredients are incorporated into the meat, being careful not to overmix. Roll the meat mixture into meatballs(size of golf balls).
3. Heat a large nonstick skillet over medium-high heat. Once the pan is hot, add the oil and then the meatballs in batches of five. Sear on each side (do not cook all the way through), and place in an ovenproof dish.
4. Once all the meatballs have been seared and placed in the dish, top with the marinara sauce, and cover with foil. Bake for 20 to 25 minutes.
5. Remove from the oven, and raise the temperature to 400°F(205°C). Remove the foil from the dish, top the meatballs with the feta, and bake for 4 minutes.
6. Remove and serve immediately.

Nutrition Info per Serving:

Calories: 546, Protein: 32g, Fat: 33g, Carbohydrates: 32g, Fiber: 6g, Sugar: 2g, Sodium: 435 mg, Cholesterol: 146mg

Chicken with Coconut Milk

Prep Time: 10 minutes, Cook Time: 6 hours, Serves: 4-6

INGREDIENTS:

6 bone-in skin-on chicken thighs
2 garlic cloves, smashed
1 tbsp. coconut oil
1 onion, sliced
2 tsps. curry powder
1 tsp. salt
¼ tsp. freshly ground black pepper
1 (13.5-ounce, 383 g) can coconut milk
3 cups (720 g) chicken broth
2 scallions, sliced
¼ cup chopped fresh cilantro

DIRECTIONS:

1. Grease the slow cooker with the coconut oil.
2. Put in the garlic, chicken, salt, onion, curry powder, coconut milk, pepper, and chicken broth. Cover the slow cooker and cook for 6 hours on high.
3. Garnish with the cilantro and scallions. Serve.

Nutrition Info per Serving:

Calories: 652, Total Carbohydrates: 10g, Protein: 32g, Total Fat: 56g, Sugar: 5g, Fiber: 3g, Sodium: 883mg, Cholesterol: 51mg

Grilled Chicken Skewers with Mint Sauce

Prep Time: 20 minutes, Cook Time: 20 minutes, Serves: 4-6

INGREDIENTS:

FOR THE MINT SAUCE
1 bunch fresh mint, stemmed
½ cup (120 ml) extra-virgin olive oil
2 tsps. lemon zest
½ tsp. salt
Pinch freshly ground black pepper
1 garlic clove
FOR THE CHICKEN
6 boneless skinless chicken breasts, cut into 1½- to 2-inch cubes
¼ cup (60 ml) extra-virgin olive oil
¼ cup (60 ml) freshly squeezed lemon juice
1 tsp. salt
¼ tsp. freshly ground black pepper
2 fresh mint sprigs
Pinch ground turmeric

DIRECTIONS:

TO MAKE THE MINT SAUCE

1. In a blender, combine the lemon zest, mint, garlic, olive oil, salt, and pepper. Blend until smooth.
2. Refrigerate in an airtight container for less than four or five days.

TO MAKE THE CHICKEN

1. Soak 12 (6-inch) wooden skewers in water for at least 30 minutes so the skewers will not burn while grilling.
2. Combine the chicken, lemon juice, olive oil, turmeric, salt, pepper, and mint in a large zip-top plastic bag. Seal the bag, refrigerate, turn to mix, and let marinate at least 30 minutes.
3. Preheat the grill, or put a stovetop grill over high heat.
4. Put 3 or 4 chicken cubes on each skewer. Throw away the marinade and mint sprigs.
5. Reduce the grill to medium. Grill the chicken for 15 to 20 minutes and turn it occasionally, until marked on both sides and the chicken is cooked through.
6. Serve with the mint sauce.

Nutrition Info per Serving:

Calories: 657, Total Carbohydrates: 2g, Protein: 50g, Total Fat: 51g, Sugar: 0g, Fiber: 1g, Sodium: 814mg, Cholesterol: 10mg

Chicken with Broccoli Stir-Fry

Prep Time: 10 minutes, Cook Time: 15 minutes, Serves: 4

INGREDIENTS:

2 boneless, skinless chicken breasts, cubed
2 tbsps. olive oil, divided
3 small carrots, thinly sliced
15 ounces (425g) frozen chopped broccoli florets, thawed
8 ounces (227g) sliced water chestnuts, drained and thoroughly rinsed
2 garlic cloves, minced
2 tsps. ground ginger
3 tbsps. balsamic vinegar, divided

DIRECTIONS:

1. In a wok or large sauté pan, add ½ tablespoon of olive oil and heat over medium heat. Place the cubed chicken and fried about 5 to 7 minutes, until lightly browned and cooked through. Remove chicken from the pan to a bowl with a lid and set aside.
2. Pour the olive oil, garlic, and carrots to the pan and heat over medium heat, until the carrots begin to soften, about 3 to 4 minutes. Then place the thawed broccoli florets, water chestnuts, and balsamic vinegar into it and cook another for 3 to 4 minutes.
3. Mix the cooked chicken with 2 tbsps. balsamic vinegar and 2 tsps. ground ginger and stir until well coated.
4. Serve over brown rice if you want, and enjoy.

Nutrition Info per Serving:

Calories: 189, Total Fat: 9g, Saturated Fat: 2g, Protein: 14g, Total Carbohydrate: 12g, Fiber: 3g, Sugar: 3g, Cholesterol: 33mg, Sodium: 68mg, Potassium: 228mg

Slow Cooker Chicken Curry

Prep Time: 10 minutes, Cook Time: 4 hours, Serves: 4-6

INGREDIENTS:

3 pounds (1.4 kg) boneless skinless chicken thighs
1 tbsp. Slow-Cooker Ghee
2 onions, chopped
2 garlic cloves, sliced thin
¼ cup fresh cilantro leaves
2 tsps. minced fresh ginger
1 tbsp. curry powder
1 tsp. ground coriander
1 tsp. ground cumin
1 tsp. salt
2 cups (480 ml) chicken broth
1 cup (240 ml) coconut milk

DIRECTIONS:

1. Combine the garlic, ghee, onions, chicken, ginger, coriander, curry powder, salt, chicken broth, cumin, and coconut milk in the slow cooker. Cover and cook for 4 hours on high.
2. Stir in the cilantro just before serving.

Nutrition Info per Serving:

Calories: 866, Total Carbohydrates: 11g, Protein: 103g, Total Fat: 43g, Sugar: 5g, Fiber: 3g, Sodium: 828mg, Cholesterol: 200mg

One-Pot Creamy Tuscan Chicken

Prep Time: 5 minutes, Cook Time: 20 minutes, Serves: 4

INGREDIENTS:

⅛ tsp. freshly ground black pepper
½ tsp. sea salt
1 tsp. garlic powder
4 boneless, skinless chicken breast halves, pounded to ½- to ¾-inch thickness
2 tbsps. extra-virgin olive oil
2 cups cherry tomatoes
½ cup sliced green olives
1 zucchini, chopped
¼ cup dry white wine

DIRECTIONS:

1. Use the pepper, salt and garlic powder to season the chicken breasts.
2. Heat the olive oil in a large nonstick skillet over medium-high heat, until it shimmers. Place the chicken into the skillet and cook for 7 to 10 minutes per side, until it reaches an internal temperature of 165°F(75°C). Transfer the chicken onto a platter, and set aside, use foil to tent.
3. Place the tomatoes, olives and zucchini into the same skillet. Cook until the zucchini is tender, about 4 minutes, stirring occasionally.
4. Pour in the white wine and scrape any browned bits from the bottom of the pan with a wooden spoon. Simmer for 1 minute. Place the chicken and any juices that have collected on the platter back to the pan and stir to coat with the sauce and vegetables.

Nutrition Info per Serving:

Calories: 171, Total Fat: 11g, Total Carbs: 8g, Sugar: 4g, Fiber: 2g, Protein: 8g, Sodium: 743mg, Cholesterol: 5mg

Lemon-Rosemary Roasted Chicken

Prep Time: 20 minutes, Cook Time: 45 minutes, Serves: 6 to 8

INGREDIENTS:

½ cup (120 ml) extra-virgin olive oil, divided
8 garlic cloves, roughly chopped
1 (3- to 4-pound, 1.4 to 1.8 kg) roasting chicken
2 to 4 tbsps. chopped fresh rosemary
2 lemons, thinly sliced
2 tsps. salt, divided
1 tsp. freshly ground black pepper, divided

DIRECTIONS:

1. Preheat the oven to 425°F (220ºC).
2. Pour 2 tbsps. olive oil in the bottom of a 9 x13-inch baking dish and swirl to coat the bottom.
3. Put the whole chicken breast side down on a large work surface. Cut along the backbone with a very sharp knife, starting at the tail end and up to the neck. Pull apart the two sides, opening up the chicken. Flip it over, breast-side up, pressing down with your hands to flatten the chicken. Transfer to the prepared baking dish.
4. Loosen the skin over the breasts and thighs by cutting a small incision and sticking fingers inside to pull the skin away from the meat without removing it.
5. In a small bowl, combine garlic, ¼ cup olive oil, 1 tsp. salt, rosemary, and ½ tsp. pepper and whisk together.
6. Rub the garlic-herb oil evenly under the skin of each breast and each thigh. Add the lemon slices evenly.
7. Whisk together the remaining olive oil, ½ tsp. pepper and 1 tsp. salt, and rub over the outside of the chicken.
8. Put in the oven and roast for 45 minutes, uncovered, until cooked through and golden brown. Set aside for 5 minutes before carving to serve.

Nutrition Info per Serving:

Calories: 435, Total Carbs: 2g, Net Carbs: 2g, Protein: 28g, Total Fat: 34g, Fiber: 0g, Sodium: 879mg, Cholesterol: 5mg, Sugar: 0.7g

Ginger Chicken with Vegetable Soup

Prep Time: 10 minutes, Cook Time: 10 minutes, Serves: 4

INGREDIENTS:

3 cups shredded rotisserie chicken, skin removed
8 cups no-salt-added chicken broth
2 tbsps. extra-virgin olive oil
1 tbsp. grated fresh ginger
1 onion, chopped
2 red bell peppers, chopped
½ tsp. sea salt
⅛ tsp. freshly ground black pepper

DIRECTIONS:

1. Heat the olive oil in a large pot over medium-high heat, until it shimmers.
2. Stir in the ginger, onion and red bell peppers. Cook until the vegetables are soft, about 5 minutes, stirring occasionally.
3. Add the chicken, chicken broth, pepper and salt, stir well and bring to a simmer. Reduce the heat to medium-low and simmer for 5 minutes.

Nutrition Info per Serving:

Calories: 341, Total Fat: 15g, Total Carbs: 11g, Sugar: 8g, Fiber: 1g, Protein: 40g, Sodium: 577mg, Cholesterol: 205mg

Pan-Seared Chicken with Turnip Greens

Prep Time: 15 minutes, Cook Time: 25 minutes, Serves: 4

INGREDIENTS:

2 chicken breasts, boneless and skinless
1 tbsp. dill Seasoning
½ cup low-sodium chicken broth
1 bunch turnip greens, thinly sliced
1 medium onion, chopped
4 celery stalks including leaves, finely chopped
1 green bell pepper, chopped
4 garlic cloves, minced

DIRECTIONS:

1. In a small bowl, rub the seasoning all over the chicken.
2. Bring the broth to a simmer in a large cast iron skillet over medium heat.
3. Add the turnip greens, onion, celery, bell pepper and garlic, and sauté for 5 minutes, or until the greens are wilted and the onions are translucent.
4. Place the chicken in the center of the pan and push the vegetables to the edges of the pan to form a ring. 7 minutes in the oven
5. Flip, cover, and cook for another 7 to 10 minutes, or until equally browned on the second side.
6. Place the chicken on a bed of greens and top with the pan gravy.

Nutrition Info per Serving:

Calories: 145, Total Fat: 2g, Cholesterol: 49mg, Sodium: 129mg, Total Carbohydrates: 12g, Sugar: 4g, Fiber: 4g, Protein: 22g

Healthy Turkey Chili

Prep Time: 15 minutes, Cook Time: 4-8 hours, Serves: 8

INGREDIENTS:

2 tbsps. extra virgin olive oil
½ pound(227g) lean ground turkey
1 (15-ounce, 425g) can garbanzo beans, rinsed and drained
1 (15-ounce, 425g) can black beans, rinsed and drained
1 (15-ounce, 425g) can kidney beans, rinsed and drained
1 (15-ounce, 425g) can white kidney beans, rinsed and drained
½ cup chopped red onion
3 medium cloves garlic, minced
2 cups chopped fresh tomatoes
2½ cups chopped zucchini
1 tbsp. chili powder
¼ tsp. ground cumin
½ tsp. dried parsley
½ tsp. dried oregano
½ tsp. dried basil
3 cups low-sodium chicken broth
⅛ tsp. ground black pepper
⅛ tsp. sea salt
½ cup shredded low-fat cheddar cheese, for garnish
¼ cup chopped fresh cilantro, for garnish

DIRECTIONS:

1. Heat the oil in a large sauté pan over medium to high heat. Add the ground turkey, onion, and garlic. Cook for 5 to 6 minutes, or until browned, stirring constantly and breaking up turkey chunks with a spatula.
2. Place the remaining ingredients in a 6-quart crock pot, and then add the cooked turkey mixture. Mix well then cover and cook on high for 4 hours or on low for 8 hours.
3. Check occasionally and add a little water if the chili becomes too dry.
4. Serve in bowls, and top with cheese and cilantro.

Nutrition Info per Serving:

Calories: 266, Protein: 19g, Fat: 11g, Carbohydrates: 24g, Fiber: 7g, Sugar: 3g, Sodium: 497mg, Cholesterol: 26mg

Crispy Almond Chicken Breast

Prep Time: 10 minutes, Cook Time: 25 minutes, Serves: 4

INGREDIENTS:

4 4-ounce (113g) boneless, skinless chicken breasts
½ cup almond meal
1 tsp. ground paprika
½ tsp. black pepper
⅛ tsp. salt

DIRECTIONS:

1. Preheat oven to 350°F(180°C).
2. Combine almond meal, paprika, salt, and pepper in a resealable bag. Put each chicken breast in the bag one at a time, close bag and shake until evenly coated. Place chicken in glass baking dish.
3. Bake in the preheated oven until no longer pink in the middle and juices run clear, about 25 to 30 minutes. An instant-read thermometer inserted into the center should read 165°F(75°C).
4. Serve with a fresh green salad and your favorite sides.

Nutrition Info per Serving:

Calories: 222, Total Fat: 11g, Saturated Fat: 2g, Cholesterol: 65mg, Sodium: 79mg, Potassium: 16mg, Total Carbohydrate: 3g, Fiber: 2g, Sugar: 1g, Protein: 28g

Sauté Turkey Cutlets

Prep Time: 5 minutes, Cook Time: 20 minutes, Serves: 4

INGREDIENTS:

Salt and freshly ground black pepper
1 pound (454 g) turkey breast cutlets
2 tbsps. extra-virgin olive oil
2 cloves garlic, minced
1 large yellow bell pepper, cut into strips
1 large red bell pepper, cut into strips
1 (14.5-ounce, 410 g) can no-salt-added diced tomatoes, undrained
1 cup button mushrooms, sliced
1 tbsp. dried tarragon

DIRECTIONS:

1. Sprinkle salt and pepper over the turkey cutlets. Heat 1 tbsp. of the olive oil in a large skillet over medium-high heat. Add the turkey cutlets to the skillet and cook 1 to 3 minutes until browned on the bottom. Flip and continue cooking 1 to 3 minutes more until cooked all the way through. The outside should be nicely browned and the inside fully cooked. Remove the turkey to a plate and cover with foil to keep warm.
2. Add the remaining olive oil to the skillet, then add the garlic and sauté for 1 minute, until sizzling. Put in bell peppers and mushrooms and continue cooking 5 to 7 minutes until starting to soften.
3. Add the tarragon and tomatoes and their juices, cover, and bring to a simmer 3 to 5 minutes, stirring often, until slightly reduced.
4. Return the turkey cutlets to the skillet. Reduce the heat to medium-low and cook for 2 to 3 minutes to warm the turkey through.

Nutrition Info per Serving:

Calories: 225, Total fat: 8g, Saturated fat: 1g, Total carbohydrates: 10g, Protein: 30g, Cholesterol: 70mg, Sodium: 67mg, Potassium: 180mg, Fiber: 2g, Sugar: 3g

Spicy Chicken and Vegetable Stir-Fry

Prep Time: 10 minutes, Cook Time: 15 minutes, Serves: 4

INGREDIENTS:

2 tbsps. sesame oil
1 pound(454 g) boneless, skinless chicken breasts, cubed
3 cloves garlic, minced
½ of an 8-oz. (230 g) package sugar snap peas
4 stalks celeries, diced
1 (16-ounce) bag frozen stir-fry vegetables, thawed
8 oz. (230 g) water chestnuts, drained and rinsed
2 tsps. Chinese five-spice powder
3 tsps. peanut butter
2 tbsps. balsamic vinegar
2 tsps. hot sauce

DIRECTIONS:

1. Heat ½ tablespoon of the sesame oil in a large sauté pan over medium heat. Stir in the chicken and cook until lightly browned, 5 to 7 minutes. Place the chicken to a bowl, cover, and set aside.
2. Pour the reserving 1½ tablespoons sesame oil to the pan along with the garlic and snap peas. Cook until the peas become tender and the garlic become brown, 3 to 4 minutes. Add the celeries, stir-fry vegetables, and water chestnuts and cook, stirring constantly, for 2 minutes.
3. Spritz with the five-spice powder, peanut butter, balsamic vinegar, and hot sauce. Return the cooked chicken to the pan and toss, cooking for a further 2 minutes, until the chicken is heated through and the ingredients are combined.

Nutrition Info per Serving:

Calories: 255, Total fat: 9g, Saturated fat: 1g, Total carbohydrates: 16g, Protein: 26 g, Cholesterol: 55mg, Sodium: 331mg, Potassium: 279 mg, Fiber: 5g, Sugar: 6g

White Beans Chicken Chili

Prep Time: 5 minutes, Cook Time: 25 minutes, Serves: 4

INGREDIENTS:

three 15-ounce (425 g) cans white beans
1 tbsp. canola oil
1 onion, chopped
3 garlic cloves, minced
1 to 3 jalapeños, seeded and diced
2 tsps. ground cumin
1½ tsps. ground coriander
1 tsp. chili powder
1 tsp. dried oregano
¼ to ½ tsp. cayenne
4 cups low-sodium chicken broth
3 cups chopped cooked chicken breast
¼ cup chopped cilantro, for garnish

DIRECTIONS:

1. In a large stockpot, heat the canola oil over medium heat. Add the garlic, onion and cook about 5 minutes, stirring frequently, until the onion is soft. Add the jalapeño, coriander, cumin, oregano, chili powder, and cayenne. Cook for 2 to 3 minutes, stirring frequently, until the jalapeño begins to soften.
2. Add the chicken, broth, and beans, and bring to a boil over medium-high heat. Reduce the heat to medium-low and simmer for about 15 minutes, uncovered, stirring occasionally. Serve, garnished with cilantro.

Nutrition Info per Serving:

Calories: 627, Protein: 63.44g, Fat: 10.04g, Carbohydrates: 73.5g, Fiber: 17.5g, Sodium: 192mg, Cholesterol: 89mg, Sugar: 3.8g

Quick Full-Flavored Chicken Stock

Prep Time: 15 minutes, Cook Time: 30 minutes, Serves: 3 cups

INGREDIENTS:

4 pounds(1.8kg) chicken carcasses, including necks and backs
½ large onion, roughly chopped
2 large carrots, roughly chopped
1 celery stalk, roughly chopped
1 bay leaf
3 garlic cloves
4 cups water

DIRECTIONS:

1. In a large pot over high heat, combine all the ingredients and stir.
2. Heat the mixture, stirring occasionally, until it comes almost to a boil. Lower the heat until it sends only a few bubbles up at a time. Cook for 30 to 60 minutes.
3. Allow to cool and strain, pressing down on the solids to extract as much liquid as possible, discard the solids.

Nutrition Info per Serving:

Calories: 208, Total Fat: 6g, Saturated Fat: 1g, Cholesterol: 109mg, Sodium: 196mg, Potassium: 609mg, Total Carbohydrate: 9g, Fiber: 2g, Sugar: 2g, Protein: 29g

Waldorf Salad with Poached Chicken

Prep Time: 15 minutes, Cook Time: 30 minutes, Serves: 4

INGREDIENTS:

2 (8-ounce, 227g) boneless, skinless chicken breasts
1 cup unsalted chicken stock
2 tsps. herbes de Provence
1 tbsp. crumbled feta cheese
½ cup nonfat plain Greek yogurt
1 bay leaf
4 cups spinach leaves, stemmed
1 cup seedless grapes, halved
1 medium Gala apple, cut into matchsticks
1 cup chopped celery
¼ cup coarsely chopped walnuts
2 tbsps. fresh lemon juice
2 tsps. honey
¼ tsp. freshly ground black pepper

DIRECTIONS:

1. In a small pot, combine the chicken breasts, chicken stock, herbes de Provence, and bay leaf. If the liquid does not cover the chicken, add a little water. Bring to a boil, then quickly reduce the heat to low, partially cover, and simmer for 5 to 10 minutes, or until the internal temperature of the chicken reaches 165°F(74°C). Remove from the heat and let stand in the hot chicken stock for 20 minutes.
2. In a large bowl, combine the spinach, grapes, apple, celery, walnuts, and feta cheese.
3. In a separate small bowl, whisk together the yogurt, lemon juice, honey, and pepper.
4. Evenly divide the salad among 4 storage containers. Slice the poached chicken and distribute evenly among the containers. Divide the dressing to serve with the salad.

Nutrition Info per Serving:

Calories: 295, Total fat: 9g, Carbohydrates: 20g, Fiber: 3g, Protein: 34g, Calcium: 112mg, Vitamin D: 0 IU, Potassium: 643mg, Magnesium: 60mg, Sodium: 557mg, Cholesterol: 183mg, Sugar: 15.2g

Crispy Za'atar Chicken Tenders

Prep Time: 5 minutes, Cook Time: 15 minutes, Serves: 4

INGREDIENTS:

Olive oil cooking spray
1 pound(454g) chicken tenders
1½ tbsps. za'atar
½ tsp. kosher salt
¼ tsp. freshly ground black pepper

DIRECTIONS:

1. Preheat the oven to 450°F(235°C). Line a baking sheet with parchment paper or foil and lightly spray with olive oil cooking spray.
2. In a large bowl, mix together the chicken, za'atar, salt, and black pepper well, covering the chicken tenders fully. Arrange in a single layer on the baking sheet and bake for 15 minutes, turning the chicken over once halfway through the cooking time.

Nutrition Info per Serving:

Calories: 145, Total fat: 4g, Saturated fat: 1g, Cholesterol: 83mg, Sodium: 190mg, Potassium: 390mg, Total Carbohydrates: 0g, Fiber: 0g, Sugar: 0g, Protein: 26g, Magnesium: 37mg, Calcium: 13mg

Southwest Chicken with Black Bean and Rice

Prep Time: 20 minutes, Cook Time: 35 minutes, Serves: 4

INGREDIENTS:

4 boneless skinless chicken breasts
1 cup cooked black beans
1 onion, chopped
1 tsp. salt
½ tsp. chipotle powder
½ tsp. ground cumin
2 tbsps. extra-virgin olive oil
1 cup brown basmati rice
2 cups butternut squash, cut into ½-inch pieces
1 cup (240 ml) chicken broth
1 lime, cut into 8 wedges

DIRECTIONS:

1. Put the chicken on a large plate.
2. Mix together the chipotle powder, salt, and cumin in a small bowl. Rub the chicken breasts with the mixture.
3. Put a large pan over high heat and add the olive oil. When the oil is hot, put in the chicken and cook about 3 minutes per side. Remove the chicken from the pan and transfer it to a plate.
4. Add the onions to the pan. Sauté for about 3 minutes until the onion just softened.
5. Stir in the butternut squash, rice, and chicken broth.
6. Return the chicken to the pan, cover and boil. Then reduce the heat to simmer and cook for 20 minutes.
7. Remove the pan from the heat and stir in the black beans. Serve with the lime wedges.

Nutrition Info per Serving:

Calories: 623, Total Carbohydrates: 60g, Protein: 52g, Total Fat: 19g, Sugar: 3g, Fiber: 7g, Sodium: 835mg, Cholesterol: 26mg

Easy Cheesy Chicken Broccoli Bake

Prep Time: 15 minutes, Cook Time: 25 minutes, Serves: 6

INGREDIENTS:

Nonstick cooking spray
2 tbsps. extra-virgin olive oil
½ pound(227g) boneless, skinless chicken breasts, cubed
2 cups brown rice
1½ cups unsalted chicken stock
4 garlic cloves, minced
1 large heads broccoli, cut into bite-size florets
1 cup nonfat plain Greek yogurt
1½ tsps. Dijon mustard
1 cup reduced-fat shredded Cheddar cheese
1 small onion, thinly sliced
¼ tsp. freshly ground black pepper

DIRECTIONS:

1. Preheat the oven to 400°F(205°C). Coat a 9-by-13-inch baking dish with cooking spray.
2. In a large skillet, heat the oil over medium heat. Add the chicken, garlic, onion, and pepper. Sauté while stirring for about 5 minutes. Add the rice and chicken stock and stir. Increase the heat to high and bring to a boil.
3. Pour the chicken and rice mixture into the prepared baking dish. Top with broccoli and spread evenly. Do not mix in. Cover with a lid or aluminum foil. Bake for 40 to 45 minutes.
4. Meanwhile, blend together the yogurt and mustard in a small bowl.
5. Remove the baking dish from the oven. Uncover and stir in the yogurt and mustard mixture. Sprinkle the Cheddar cheese on top. Return to the oven and bake uncovered for 5 to 10 minutes, or until the cheese has melted.
6. Let cool, then divide among 6 storage containers.

Nutrition Info per Serving:

Calories: 531, Total fat: 19g, Carbohydrates: 52g, Fiber: 3.5g, Protein: 39g, Calcium: 341mg, Potassium: 600mg, Magnesium: 115mg, Sodium: 347mg, Cholesterol: 168mg, Sugar: 2.7g

Stir-Fried Chicken Satay with Broccoli and Cauliflower

Prep Time: 10 minutes, Cook Time: 15 minutes, Serves: 4

INGREDIENTS:

3 tbsps. extra-virgin olive oil
½ pound (227 g) chicken breasts or thighs, cut into ¾-inch pieces
1 head cauliflower, riced
2 cups broccoli florets
1 red bell pepper, seeded and chopped
4 scallions, green and white parts, sliced on the bias (cut diagonally into thin slices)
½ tsp. sea salt
Peanut Sauce

DIRECTIONS:

1. Heat the olive oil in a large skillet over medium-high heat, until it shimmers.
2. With the salt to season the chicken, then place the chicken into the skillet and cook for 5 minutes until opaque, stirring occasionally. Use a slotted spoon to remove the chicken and set it aside on a plate. Keep the pan on the heat.
3. Mix in the broccoli, bell pepper, and scallions. Cook for 3 to 5 minutes until the vegetables are crisp-tender. Stir in the cauliflower and cook for another 3 minutes.
4. Place the chicken back to the skillet. Stir in the Peanut Sauce. Bring to a simmer and lower the heat to medium-low. Simmer for 2 minutes to heat through. Serve hot.

Nutrition Info per Serving:

Calories: 381, Total Fat: 20g, Saturated Fat: 4g, Sodium: 396mg, Carbohydrates: 19g, Fiber: 5g, Protein: 33 g, Sugar: 2.4g, Cholesterol: 29mg

Traditional Open Face Turkey Burger

Prep Time: 10 minutes, Cook Time: 25 minutes, Serves: 4

INGREDIENTS:

1 tbsp. olive oil
1 pound(454g) lean ground white meat turkey
1 cup mushrooms, finely chopped
2 tomatoes, sliced
1 clove garlic, minced
½ tsp. freshly ground black pepper
⅛ tsp. salt
Cooking spray
4 cups baby spinach

DIRECTIONS:

1. In a large skillet, heat the olive oil over medium-low heat. Add the mushrooms and cook for about 5 minutes, until soft and browned. Stir in the garlic and cook for 1 minute. Remove from heat and allow to cool.
2. Combine the turkey, pepper, salt, and mushroom garlic mixture in a large bowl. Mix until well combined, then form into 8 small patties.
3. Prepare a grill for medium-high heat. Apply cooking spray to the grill rack. Grill the burgers until cooked through, 6 to 8 minutes per side and until an instant-read thermometer registers 165°F(75°C). If you don't have a grill, you can broil the burgers in an oven-safe skillet under the broiler element for about 10 minutes per side, or until an instant-read thermometer registers 165°F(75°C).
4. Divide the spinach among 4 serving plates, top with 2 patties per plate. Top each stack with tomato slices and serve immediately.

Nutrition Info per Serving:

Calories: 179, Total Fat: 5g, Saturated Fat: 1g, Cholesterol: 55mg, Sodium: 135mg, Potassium: 198mg, Total Carbohydrate: 6g, Fiber: 2g, Sugar: 1g, Protein: 28g

Broiled Curried Chicken Tenders

Prep Time: 5 minutes, Cook Time: 20 minutes, Serves: 4

INGREDIENTS:

1 tbsp. curry powder
1 tsp. minced garlic
¼ tsp. freshly ground pepper
¾ cup (180 ml) plain fat-free yogurt
Juice of 1 lemon
Four 5-ounce (142 g) boneless, skinless chicken breasts, each cut into 4 thin strips
1 tbsp. chopped fresh cilantro

DIRECTIONS:

1. Line a baking sheet with foil.
2. Mix garlic, yogurt, curry powder, lemon juice, and pepper together in a small bowl until well blended.
3. Place chicken strips in a resealable plastic bag, and add yogurt mixture. Squeeze bag to coat chicken evenly. Place chicken in fridge for 30 minutes.
4. Preheat oven to broil. Adjust top oven rack about 6 inches from broiler heat.
5. Spread chicken in prepared baking sheet.
6. Broil until chicken is cooked through, turning once, about 20 minutes.
7. Serve hot and sprinkle with fresh cilantro.

Nutrition Info per Serving:

Calories: 286, Fat: 10.5g, Carbohydrates: 2.9g, Protein: 42.6g, Cholesterol: 127mg, Sodium: 148mg, Fiber: 0.6 g, Sugar: 5.7g

Easy Quick Greek Turkey Burger

Prep Time: 10 minutes, Cook Time: 10 minutes, Serves: 4

INGREDIENTS:

1 pound (454g)ground turkey
1 medium zucchini, grated
¼ cup crumbled feta cheese
1 tbsp. extra-virgin olive oil
1 large egg, beaten
¼ cup whole-wheat bread crumbs
¼ cup red onion, minced
1 tbsp. fresh oregano, chopped
1 tsp. kosher salt
1 garlic clove, minced
¼ tsp. freshly ground black pepper

DIRECTIONS:

1. Add the turkey, zucchini, onion, bread crumbs, egg, garlic, oregano, feta cheese, salt, and black pepper in a large bowl, and mix well. Using your hands to shape the mixture into 4 equal patties.
2. In a large nonstick grill pan or skillet, heat 1 tbsp. olive oil over medium-high heat. Place the burgers on the pan and change the heat to medium. Fried one side for 5 minutes, then turn over and cook the other side for 5 minutes more.
3. Transfer the burgers to a plate or dish and serve warm.

Nutrition Info per Serving:

Calories: 285, Total fat: 16g, Saturated fat: 5g, Protein: 26g, Total Carbohydrates: 9g, Fiber: 2g, Sugar: 2g, Cholesterol: 139mg, Sodium: 465mg, Potassium: 415mg, Magnesium: 40mg, Calcium: 90mg

Easy Sumac Chicken with Cauliflower and Carrots

Prep Time: 15 minutes, Cook Time: 40 minutes, Serves: 4

INGREDIENTS:

1½ pounds(680g) bone-in chicken thighs and drumsticks
1 medium cauliflower, cut into 1-inch florets
2 carrots, peeled and cut into 1-inch rounds
3 tbsps. extra-virgin olive oil
½ tsp. ground cumin
¼ tsp. freshly ground black pepper
1 lemon, cut into ¼-inch-thick slices
1 tbsp. ground sumac
1 tsp. kosher salt
1 tbsp. lemon juice
¼ cup fresh mint, chopped
¼ cup fresh parsley, chopped

DIRECTIONS:

1. Preheat the oven to 425°F (220ºC). Line a baking sheet with parchment paper or foil.
2. Mix together sumac, the olive oil, cumin, salt and black pepper in a large bowl. Add the chicken, carrots and cauliflower, and toss until the oil and spice mixture is completely coated.
3. Place the cauliflower, carrots, and chicken in a single layer on the baking sheet. Coated with the lemon slices. Roast for 40 minutes, tossing the vegetables once halfway through. Sprinkle the lemon juice on the chicken and vegetables and garnish with the parsley and mint.

Nutrition Info per Serving:

Calories: 510, Total fat: 38g, Saturated fat: 9g, Protein: 31g, Total Carbohydrates: 13g, Fiber: 4g, Sugar: 5g, Cholesterol: 158mg, Sodium: 490mg, Potassium: 930mg, Magnesium: 63mg, Calcium: 73mg

Slow Cooker Garlicky Chicken

Prep Time: 15 minutes, Cook Time: 3 to 4 hours, Serves: 3 or 4, 4 to 4½ cups

INGREDIENTS:

1 tbsp. extra-virgin olive oil
1 whole chicken (3 to 3½ pounds, 1.4 to 1.6 kg)
Black pepper
Salt
Onion powder
Garlic powder

DIRECTIONS:

1. Use olive oil to rub all over the skin of the chicken. In a bowl, combine the pepper, salt, onion powder and garlic powder, then use the mixture to season the chicken all over, including in the cavity.
2. Tear four or five sheets of aluminum foil and roll them into balls. In the bottom of a 5- to 6-quart slow cooker, place the foil balls. On top of the foil balls, set with the chicken, adjusting them as necessary to support the chicken and keep it above the cooking juices that will accumulate in the bottom of the slow cooker as the chicken cooks.
3. Cover the cooker and cook on high for 3 to 4 hours or until the juices run clear and insert into the thickest part of a thigh with an instant-read meat thermometer registers 180°F(80°C).
4. Remove the chicken from the cooker and transfer onto a large plate or platter. Allow it to cool completely. Remove the meat from the bones and shred it with two forks.

Nutrition Info per Serving:

Calories: 278, Total Carbohydrates: 0g, Protein: 48.5g, Total Fat: 7.94g, Sugar: 0g, Fiber: 0g, Sodium: 209mg, Cholesterol: 156mg

Yogurt Marinated Chicken Kebabs

Prep Time: 10 minutes, Cook Time: 20 minutes, Serves: 4

INGREDIENTS:

½ cup plain Greek yogurt
1½ pound(680g) skinless, boneless chicken breast, cut into 1-inch cubes
1 tbsp. lemon juice
½ tsp. ground cumin
½ tsp. ground coriander
½ tsp. kosher salt
¼ tsp. cayenne pepper

DIRECTIONS:

1. In a large bowl or zip-top bag, combine the yogurt, lemon juice, cumin, coriander, salt, and cayenne pepper. Mix together thoroughly and then add the chicken. Marinate for at least 30 minutes up to overnight in the refrigerator.
2. Preheat the oven to 425°F(220°C). Line a baking sheet with parchment paper or foil. Remove the chicken from the marinade and thread it on 4 bamboo or metal skewers.
3. Bake for 20 minutes, turning the chicken over once halfway through the cooking time.

Nutrition Info per Serving:

Calories: 170, Total fat: 4g, Saturated fat: 1g, Cholesterol: 92mg, Sodium: 390mg, Potassium: 515mg, Total Carbohydrates: 1g, Fiber: 0g, Sugar: 1g, Protein: 31g, Magnesium: 40mg, Calcium: 35mg

Quinoa Stuffed Turkey Breast

Prep Time: 15 minutes, Cook Time: 8 hours, Serves: 6

INGREDIENTS:

1 (2-pound, 907 g) boneless, skin-on turkey breast
½ cup (120 ml) poultry broth
2 cups cooked quinoa
2 carrots, peeled and finely chopped
2 celery stalks, finely chopped
1 onion, finely chopped
1 egg, beaten
1 tsp. dried thyme
1 tsp. dried sage
1 tsp. sea salt, divided
½ tsp. freshly ground black pepper, divided

DIRECTIONS:

1. Mix the quinoa, carrots, celery, onion, egg, thyme, sage, ¼ teaspoon of black pepper and ½ tsp. of sea salt in a medium bowl.
2. Put the turkey breast on a large cutting board, skin-side down, between two pieces of plastic wrap, and pound it slightly to flatten.
3. Spread the filling evenly over the flesh side of the breast.
4. Roll the breast around the filling, skin-side out. Sprinkle the skin side with the remaining salt and black pepper.
5. Put the stuffed turkey breast into your slow cooker. Add the broth. Cover and cook for 8 hours on low.
6. Remove the turkey skin before slicing and serving.

Nutrition Info per Serving:

Calories: 361, Total Fat: 4g, Saturated Fat: 1g, Carbohydrates: 33g, Protein: 45g, Cholesterol: 121mg, Fiber: 5g, Sugar: 3.35g, Sodium: 923mg

Stuffed Chicken Breasts

Prep Time: 15 minutes, Cook Time: 8 hours, Serves: 4

INGREDIENTS:

2 boneless, skinless chicken breasts, cut in half horizontally to make 4 cutlets total
1 tsp. sea salt, divided
½ tsp. freshly ground black pepper, divided
4 ounces (113 g) fresh mushrooms, finely chopped
2 tsps. dried tarragon or 1 tsp. minced fresh tarragon
Zest of 1 lemon
2 cups baby spinach, stems trimmed
2 cups cooked quinoa
½ onion, finely chopped
½ cup (120 ml) dry white wine

DIRECTIONS:

1. Place each chicken breast cutlet between 2 pieces of plastic wrap and pound them flat.
2. Sprinkle the chicken cutlets with salt and pepper.
3. Arrange the spinach leaves in a layer on top of each seasoned cutlet.
4. Mix the quinoa, mushrooms, tarragon, onion, lemon zest, remaining salt and pepper in a small bowl.
5. Spread the stuffing on top of the spinach on each cutlet.
6. Roll each chicken cutlet around the filling, tying with kitchen twine to keep them rolled.
7. Place the stuffed chicken rolls in a single layer in the slow cooker. Add the wine.
8. Cover and cook on low for 8 hours.
9. Remove the chicken rolls from the slow cooker. Snip and remove the kitchen twine.
10. Transfer the wine and any accumulated juices to a small saucepan and simmer about 5 minutes until it reduces by half. Spoon over the chicken.

Nutrition Info per Serving:

Calories: 381, Total Fat: 8g, Saturated Fat: 2g, Carbohydrates: 33g, Protein: 28g, Cholesterol: 63mg, Fiber: 4g, Sodium: 823mg, Sugar: 2.6g

Baked Chicken Stuffed with Collard Greens

Prep Time: 10 minutes, Cook Time: 30 minutes, Serves: 4

INGREDIENTS:

FOR THE GRAVY
2½ cups Chicken Broth (here) or store-bought low-sodium chicken broth, divided
4 tbsps. almond flour, divided
1 medium shallot, chopped
½ bunch fresh chives, roughly chopped
1 bay leaf
1 cumin
½ tsp. celery seeds
1 tsp. Worcestershire sauce
Freshly ground black pepper
FOR THE CHICKEN
2 boneless, skinless chicken breasts
Juice of 1 lime
1 tsp. sweet paprika
½ tsp. onion powder
½ tsp. garlic powder
2 medium tomatoes, chopped
1 bunch collard greens, center stem removed, cut into 1-inch ribbons
¼ cup Chicken Broth (here) (optional)
Generous pinch red pepper flakes

DIRECTIONS:

HOW TO MAKE GRAVY

1. Combine ½ cup broth and 1 tbsp. flour in a shallow stockpot and boil over medium-low heat, whisking constantly, until the flour is dissolved. Continue to gradually add 1 cup of broth and the remaining 3 tablespoons of flour until a thick sauce forms.
2. In a large mixing bowl, combine the shallots, chives, bay leaf, cumin, and ½ cup broth.
3. In a separate bowl, combine the celery seeds, Worcestershire sauce, pepper, and the remaining ½ cup broth. Cook, stirring occasionally, for 2 to 3 minutes, or until the ingredients are well combined. Take the pan off the heat and toss out the bay leaf.

HOW TO MAKE CHICKEN

1. Cut a slit along the length of each chicken breast deep enough for filling.
2. In a small mixing bowl, rub the lime juice, paprika, onion powder, and garlic powder all over the chicken.
3. Place the tomatoes and collard greens in an electric pressure cooker. Add the chicken broth if the mixture appears to be dry.
4. Turn the pressure valve to sealing and close and lock the lid.
5. Cook for 2 minutes on the Manual/Pressure Cook setting.
6. Quickly remove the pressure after the cooking is finished. Remove the cover with care.
7. Remove the leaves with tongs or a slotted spoon, leaving the tomatoes behind.
8. Stuff the greens into the chicken breasts. In the pressure cooker, place the side with the greens facing up on the bed of tomatoes.
9. Ladle half of the gravy over the filled chicken and serve.
10. Turn the pressure valve to sealing and close and lock the lid.
11. Cook for 10 minutes on the Manual/Pressure Cook setting.
12. Quickly remove the pressure after the cooking is finished. Remove the cover with care.
13. Transfer the chicken and tomatoes to a serving plate from the pressure cooker. Red pepper flakes are used as a finishing touch.

Nutrition Info per Serving:

Calories: 177, Total Fat: 2g, Cholesterol: 49mg, Sodium: 128mg, Total Carbohydrates: 18g, Sugar: 4g, Fiber: 4g, Protein: 24g

Juicy Italian Herb Turkey Cutlets

Prep Time: 10 minutes, Cook Time: 30 minutes, Serves: 4

INGREDIENTS:

4 (4-ounce, 113g) boneless, skinless turkey cutlets
3 small cloves garlic, minced
2 tbsps. chopped fresh rosemary
2 tbsps. chopped fresh parsley
1½ tsps. chopped fresh sage
½ tsp. cracked black pepper
Grated zest of 1 large lemon
1 cup low-sodium vegetable broth

DIRECTIONS:

1. Preheat the oven to 375°F(190°C).
2. Mix together the garlic, rosemary, parsley, sage, and pepper in a small bowl. Rub a generous amount of the herb mixture on both sides of each cutlet.
3. Place the turkey cutlets in a 9- by 13-inch baking dish, top with lemon zest, and add the vegetable broth to the dish.
4. Cover with foil, and bake for 20 to 25 minutes. Remove the foil during the last 5 minutes of baking to brown the tops of the cutlets. Remove from the oven and serve immediately.

Nutrition Info per Serving:

Calories: 129, Protein: 19.6g, Fat: 2g, Carbohydrates: 7g, Fiber: 1g, Sugar: 5g, Sodium: 348mg, Cholesterol: 14mg

Roasted Chicken with Vegetables

Prep Time: 10 minutes, Cook Time: 1 hour, Serves: 4

INGREDIENTS:

1 whole chicken, about 5 pounds (2.3 kg)
4 medium potatoes, with skin, cut into large chunks
1 tbsp. olive oil
1 tsp. poultry seasoning
2 cups Brussels sprouts
2 cups carrots, sliced into 1" sections

DIRECTIONS:

1. Preheat oven to 450°F(235ºC). Put chicken in roasting pan. Dust with poultry seasoning on both sides.
2. Place diced potatoes, sliced carrots, and Brussels sprouts around chicken, drizzle with olive oil. Add 1 cup water to bottom of pan.
3. Roast in 450° oven for 60 minutes.

Nutrition Info per Serving:

Calories: 319, Total Fat: 3g, Carbohydrates: 42g, Protein: 32g, Cholesterol: 66mg, Fiber: 7g, Sugar: 6.7g, Sodium: 142mg

Peach-Bourbon Chicken Thighs

Prep Time: 15 minutes, Cook Time: 8 hours, Serves: 6

INGREDIENTS:

6 boneless, skinless chicken thighs
1½ cups peeled and chopped fresh peaches
1 (14-ounce, 397 g) can tomato sauce
¾ tsp. liquid smoke
1 tsp. garlic powder
½ cup (120 ml) bourbon
⅓ cup (80 ml) apple cider vinegar
¼ cup (60 ml) pure maple syrup
½ tsp. sea salt
¼ tsp. cayenne pepper

DIRECTIONS:

1. Put the chicken thighs in your slow cooker.
2. Combine all the other ingredients in a small saucepan.
3. Simmer over medium-low heat, stirring frequently for about 5 minutes and mashing the peaches with a spoon, until the sauce thickens.
4. Cool the sauce for 5 minutes. Pour it over the chicken.
5. Cover and cook on low for 8 hours.

Nutrition Info per Serving:

Calories: 325, Total Fat: 9g, Saturated Fat: 2g, Carbohydrates: 16g, Protein: 34g, Cholesterol: 101mg, Fiber: 2g, Sugar: 21.5g, Sodium: 200mg

Italian Chicken Cacciatore

Prep Time: 10 minutes, Cook Time: 8 hours, Serves: 6

INGREDIENTS:

1 pound (454 g) boneless, skinless chicken thighs, cut into 1-inch pieces
1 pound (454 g) fresh mushrooms, halved
2 onions, sliced
2 green bell peppers, seeded and sliced
1 (14-ounce, 397 g) can diced tomatoes, with their juice
1½ tsps. garlic powder
1 tsp. dried Italian seasoning
¼ tsp. red pepper flakes
¼ tsp. sea salt
¼ tsp. freshly ground black pepper

DIRECTIONS:

1. Mix all the ingredients in the slow cooker.
2. Cover and cook on low for 8 hours.
3. Serve the chicken with sauce spooned over the top.

Nutrition Info per Serving:

Calories: 204, Total Fat: 6g, Saturated Fat: 2g, Carbohydrates: 12g, Protein: 26g, Cholesterol: 68mg, Fiber: 3g, Sugar: 8.5g, Sodium: 361mg

Slaw and Chicken Stir-Fry

Prep Time: 10 minutes, Cook Time: 20 minutes, Serves: 4

INGREDIENTS:

1 pound (454 g) boneless, skinless chicken breasts, cut into ½" x 2" strips
½ bag broccoli slaw
½ bag frozen onion and pepper mixture
2 tbsps. peanut oil or canola oil
low-sodium stir-fry sauce

DIRECTIONS:

1. Heat a large skillet over medium-high heat. Add peanut (or canola) oil.
2. When oil is hot (without smoking), add half of chicken strips to oil, and sauté 1 - 2 minutes, stirring with spatula until cooked on all sides.
3. Remove chicken and put on warm plate. Cover plate with pot lid or aluminum foil to keep warm.
4. Add pepper and onion mixture to pan. Stir-fry 3 - 4 minutes. Add broccoli slaw, and sauté until tender.
5. Add ¼ cup stir-fry sauce, and place chicken back into pan. Stir well to mix sauce and reheat chicken.

Nutrition Info per Serving:

Calories: 235, Total fat: 9g, Cholesterol: 66mg, Sodium: 184mg, Total Carbohydrates: 10g, Fiber: 3g, Sugar: 6.2g, Protein: 29g

Chili Turkey with Beans

Prep Time: 5 minutes, Cook Time: 35 minutes, Serves: 6

INGREDIENTS:

One 16-ounce (454 g) can low-salt navy beans, rinsed and drained
One 16-ounce (454 g) can low-salt black beans, rinsed and drained
One 16-ounce (454 g) can low-salt red kidney beans, rinsed and drained
One 16-ounce (454 g) can low-salt chickpeas, rinsed and drained
4 large tomatoes, diced
1 tsp. olive oil
1 tsp. minced garlic
½ pound (227 g) lean ground turkey
1 small sweet onion, chopped
3 tbsps. chili powder
1 tsp. ground cumin

DIRECTIONS:

1. Add olive oil in a large pot over medium-high heat. Sauté turkey meat in oil about 6 minutes until completely cooked through.
2. Add onion and garlic and cook about 3 minutes, stirring frequently, until translucent.
3. Put in kidney beans, navy beans, black beans, chickpeas, tomatoes, chili powder, and cumin. Boil, then reduce heat to a simmer. Stir occasionally for 20 to 25 minutes.
4. Remove from heat and serve hot.

Nutrition Info per Serving:

Calories: 383, Fat: 6.1g, Carbohydrates: 55.5g, Protein: 28.6g, Cholesterol: 27mg, Sodium: 109mg, Fiber: 21.9 g, Sugar: 8g

Asian-Style Chicken in Soy Sauce Stir-Fry

Prep Time: 10 minutes, Cook Time: 10 minutes, Serves: 4

INGREDIENTS:

3 tbsps. extra-virgin olive oil
1 pound(454 g) chicken breasts or thighs, cut into ¾-inch pieces
2 cups edamame or pea pods
3 garlic cloves, chopped
1 tbsp. peeled and grated fresh ginger
2 tbsps. reduced-sodium soy sauce
Juice of 2 limes
1 tsp. sesame oil
2 tsps. toasted sesame seeds
1 tbsp. chopped fresh cilantro

DIRECTIONS:

1. Heat the olive oil in a large skillet over medium-high heat, until it shimmers. Stir in the chicken to the skillet and cook for 5 minutes, until opaque. Then add the edamame and cook for 3 to 5 minutes until crisp-tender. Stir in the garlic and ginger and cook for 30 seconds.
2. Add the soy sauce, lime juice, and sesame oil into a small bowl, whisk until combined. Stir in the sauce mixture to the pan. Bring to a simmer, and simmer for 2 minutes.
3. Remove from heat and transfer to a serving plate, garnish with the sesame seeds and cilantro, serve hot.

Nutrition Info per Serving:

Calories: 331, Total Fat: 17g, Saturated Fat: 2g, Sodium: 342mg, Carbohydrates: 11g, Fiber: 5g, Protein: 31g, Sugar: 1.4g, Cholesterol: 58mg

Stir-Fry Chicken with Zucchini and Fennel

Prep Time: 15 minutes, Cook Time: 15 minutes, Serves: 4

INGREDIENTS:

4 boneless skinless chicken breasts, cut into strips
2 tbsps. extra-virgin olive oil
1 fennel bulb, sliced into ¼-inch rounds
1 leek, white part only, sliced thin
3 zucchini, sliced into ½-inch rounds
½ cup sliced green olives
½ cup (120 ml) chicken broth
1 tsp. salt
½ tsp. freshly ground black pepper
2 tbsps. chopped fresh dill

DIRECTIONS:

1. Heat the olive oil in a large pan over high heat.
2. Put in the chicken strips. Brown them for 1 to 2 minutes and stir constantly. Transfer the chicken and its juices to a plate and set aside.
3. Add the fennel, leek, and zucchini to the pan. Sauté for 5 minutes.
4. Put back the chicken and juices to the pan. Pour in the broth. Add the salt and pepper. Cover the pan and simmer for 5 minutes.
5. Remove the pan from the heat, and stir in the olives and dill. Serve.

Nutrition Info per Serving:

Calories: 418, Total Carbohydrates: 15g, Protein: 45g, Total Fat: 20g, Sugar: 5g, Fiber: 4g, Sodium: 745mg, Cholesterol: 13mg

Crunchy Mediterranean Chicken Thighs

Prep Time: 5 minutes, Cook Time: 30 minutes-35 minutes, Serves: 6

INGREDIENTS:

6 bone-in, skin-on chicken thighs (about 3 pounds(1.4kg))
1½ tsps. ground cumin
2 tbsps. extra-virgin olive oil
2 tsps. dried rosemary
1½ tsps. ground coriander
¾ tsp. dried oregano
⅛ tsp. salt

DIRECTIONS:

1. Before toasting, preheat the oven to 450°F(235ºC). And line a baking sheet with parchment paper.
2. Lower the olive oil and dried rosemary, coriander, oregan, cumin, and salt into a large bowl and mix together well with a spoon, until purée. Get your hands and sort of rub it in until evenly coated with the chicken, and arrange on the prepared baking sheet.
3. Toast for 30 to 35 minutes on the pan, or until golden brown and the chicken registers an internal temperature of 165°F(75ºC).
4. Serve with lemon wedges or squeeze half a lemon over the chicken thighs before serving.

Nutrition Info per Serving:

Calories: 440, Total fat: 34g, Saturated fat: 9g, Protein: 30g, Total Carbohydrates: 1g, Fiber: 0g, Sugar: 0g, Cholesterol: 172mg, Sodium: 180mg, Potassium: 395mg, Magnesium: 40mg, Calcium: 30mg

Lemon-Pepper Chicken

Prep Time: 10 minutes, Cook Time: 25 minutes, Serves: 4

INGREDIENTS:

1 pound (454 g) chicken breasts, boneless, skinless (4 half-breasts)
1 cup (240 ml) low-sodium chicken broth
½ cup yellow cornmeal
1 tsp. lemon-pepper seasoning mix
1 tbsp. olive oil
2 tbsps. lemon juice
2 tbsps. butter

DIRECTIONS:

1. Preheat chicken broth over medium heat.
2. Put each chicken breast half on a plastic wrap. Sprinkle with water, then place another sheet of plastic wrap on top. Pound chicken to about ¼ inch thickness using a mallet.
3. Mix cornmeal and pepper on a plate or pie pan. Coat both sides of chicken through cornmeal mix.
4. Heat oil in a large nonstick skillet over medium-high heat. Add chicken and cook 4 minutes on each side. Remove chicken from pan, place on plate with cover to keep warm.
5. Add lemon juice and hot chicken broth to skillet, reduce heat to medium, stir in butter. Return chicken to pan, cook 3 minutes (internal temperature 165°F). Remove from heat, serve immediately.

Nutrition Info per Serving:

Calories: 287, Total Fat: 12g, Carbohydrates: 12g, Protein: 20g, Cholesterol: 82mg, Fiber: 2.1g, Sugar: 4.8g, Sodium: 94mg

Stir-Fry Chicken with Sesame, Broccoli and Carrot

Prep Time: 15 minutes, Cook Time: 15 minutes, Serves: 4-6

INGREDIENTS:

1 pound (454 g) boneless skinless chicken thighs, cut into thin strips
2 carrots, cut into matchsticks
1 garlic clove, minced
1 tsp. minced fresh ginger
1 tsp. salt
¼ tsp. red pepper flakes
1 tbsp. coconut oil
½ cup (120 ml) chicken broth
1 tsp. toasted sesame oil
1 tsp. coconut aminos
1 tbsp. sesame seeds
2 cups broccoli florets

DIRECTIONS:

1. Melt the coconut oil in a large pan over high heat. Put in the chicken and sauté for 5 to 8 minutes until the chicken browns.
2. Stir in the red pepper flakes, broccoli, garlic, carrots, salt, ginger, and chicken broth. Cover the pan and cook for 5 minutes until the broccoli turns bright green.
3. Remove the pan from the heat and stir in the coconut aminos, sesame oil, and sesame seeds.

Nutrition Info per Serving:

Calories: 305, Total Carbohydrates: 8g, Protein: 35g, Total Fat: 14g, Sugar: 2g, Fiber: 2g, Sodium: 812mg, Cholesterol: 64mg

Maple-Soy Sauce Chicken Drumsticks

Prep Time: 10 minutes, Cook Time: 8 hours, Serves: 6

INGREDIENTS:

12 chicken drumsticks
½ cup (120 ml) pure maple syrup
¼ cup (60 ml) low-sodium soy sauce
4 scallions, sliced
1 tsp. sesame seeds
1 tsp. cornstarch
½ tsp. garlic powder
1 tsp. grated fresh ginger
¼ tsp. freshly ground black pepper

DIRECTIONS:

1. Put the drumsticks in your slow cooker.
2. Whisk together the maple syrup, soy sauce, cornstarch, garlic powder, ginger and pepper in a small bowl.
3. Pour the sauce over the drumsticks and toss to coat.
4. Cover and cook on low for 8 hours.
5. Garnish with the scallions and sesame seeds, then serve.

Nutrition Info per Serving:

Calories: 237, Total Fat: 6g, Saturated Fat: 1g, Carbohydrates: 20g, Protein: 26g, Cholesterol: 81mg, Fiber: 0g, Sugar: 16.2g, Sodium: 663mg

Spicy Homemade Chicken

Prep Time: 10 minutes, Cook Time: 45 minutes, Serves: 4-6

INGREDIENTS:

1 whole chicken, cut into 8 pieces
1 tsp. ground cumin
2 tsps. sweet paprika
½ tsp. garlic powder
½ tsp. freshly ground black pepper
1 tbsp. brown rice flour
1 tsp. salt
1 cup no-added-sugar apple juice

DIRECTIONS:

1. Preheat the oven to 375°F (190ºC).
2. Put the chicken pieces in a baking pan.
3. Combine the cumin, brown rice flour, garlic powder, paprika, salt, and pepper in a small bowl. Rub the chicken pieces with the spice mix.
4. Pour the apple juice into the pan carefully, not to wash the spice mixture off the chicken.
5. Put the pan in the preheated oven and bake for 35 to 45 minutes until the chicken is golden brown.

Nutrition Info per Serving:

Calories: 375, Total Carbohydrates: 10g, Protein: 39g, Total Fat: 21g, Sugar: 7g, Fiber: 1g, Sodium: 792mg, Cholesterol: 0mg

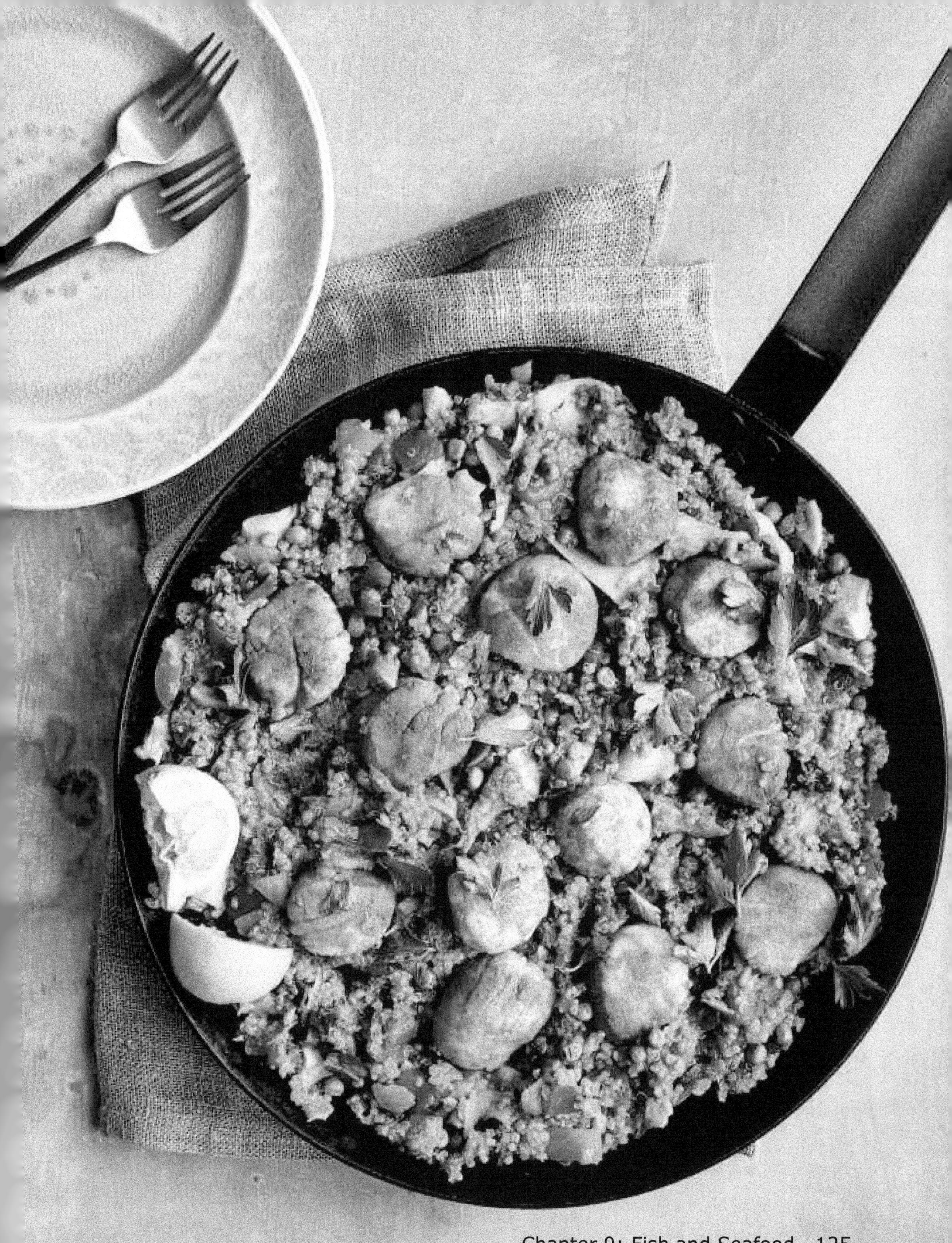

Chapter 9: Fish and Seafood

Healthy Sweet Potato Crab Cakes

Prep Time: 15 minutes, plus 30 minutes to chill, Cook Time: 40 minutes, Serves: 4

INGREDIENTS:

FOR THE SAUCE
⅔ cup nonfat plain Greek yogurt
2 tbsps. chopped fresh parsley
2 tbsps. chopped fresh basil
2 tbsps. fresh lemon juice
1 garlic clove, minced
FOR THE CRAB CAKES
2 tbsps. extra-virgin olive oil, divided
1 pound(454g) lump crabmeat
2 large sweet potatoes, peeled and halved
1 tbsp. nonfat plain Greek yogurt
1 large egg
¼ tsp. freshly ground black pepper
¼ tsp. dried thyme
¼ cup chopped fresh parsley
¼ cup chopped red onion
½ cup dried unseasoned bread crumbs
4 lemon wedges (optional)

DIRECTIONS:

TO MAKE THE SAUCE

1. Well combined the yogurt, parsley, basil, lemon juice, and garlic in a small bowl. Divide the sauce among 4 small storage containers.

TO MAKE THE CRAB CAKES

1. Bring a medium pot of water to a boil. Add the sweet potatoes and cook for 15 to 20 minutes, or until soft. Transfer to a bowl and let cool.
2. Smash the sweet potatoes. Add the yogurt, pepper, thyme, parsley, and onion and mix well. Add the crabmeat and bread crumbs and mix. Finally, add the egg and mix well.
3. Gently form into 8 cakes and set on a plate. Refrigerate for 30 minutes to set nicely.
4. In a cast-iron or nonstick skillet, heat 1 tbsp. of oil over medium heat. Add 4 crab cakes, and cook, turning once, for about 8 minutes total, or until browned on each side. Repeat and then place 2 crab cakes in each of 4 storage containers.
5. When ready to serve, reheat the crab cakes and serve with the sauce and lemon wedges (if using).

Nutrition Info per Serving:

Calories: 319, Total fat: 10g, Carbohydrates: 30g, Fiber: 3.5g, Protein: 28g, Calcium: 251mg, Vitamin D: 10 IU, Potassium: 428mg, Magnesium: 33mg, Sodium: 691mg, Cholesterol: 46mg, Sugar: 7.3g

Carrot Potato Fish Stew

Prep Time: 20 minutes, Cook Time: 20 minutes, Serves: 8

INGREDIENTS:

½ cup (120mL) Seafood Broth
2 large carrots, chopped
3 bay leaves
1 pound(450 g) new potatoes, halved
2 pounds(910 g) fish fillets, such as rockfish, striped bass, or cod, cut into ½- to 1-inch dice
8 medium eggs
1 tsp. nutmeg
¼ cup tomato paste
1 tsp. green pepper flakes
3 cups (700mL) water
2 tsps. curry powder

DIRECTIONS:

1. Select the Sauté setting on an electric pressure cooker, and mix the broth, carrots, nutmeg, tomato paste, green pepper flakes, curry powder, and bay leaves. Cook for 2 minutes, or until the carrots are soft.
2. Add the potatoes and 1 cup of water.
3. Close and lock the lid, and set the pressure valve to sealing.
4. Change to the Manual/Pressure Cook setting, and cook for 3 minutes.
5. When cooking is done, quick-release the pressure. Carefully remove the lid.
6. Add the fish and enough of the water just to cover the fish.
7. Close and lock the lid, and set the pressure valve to sealing.
8. Select the Manual/Pressure Cook setting, and cook for a further 3 minutes.
9. When cooking is done, quick-release the pressure. Carefully remove the lid.
10. Carefully separate the eggs one by one into the stew, keeping the yolks intact.
11. Close and lock the lid, and set the pressure valve to sealing.
12. Select the Manual/Pressure Cook setting, and cook for 1 minute.
13. When cooking is done, quick-release the pressure. Carefully remove the lid, discard the bay leaves, and serve in bowls.

Nutrition Info per Serving:

Calories: 218, Total Fat: 6g, Cholesterol: 219mg, Sodium: 145mg, Carbohydrates: 15g, Sugar: 4g, Fiber: 3g, Protein: 28g

All Spice-Crusty Roasted Salmon

Prep Time: 5 minutes, Cook Time: 20 minutes, Serves: 4

INGREDIENTS:

Nonstick cooking spray
½ tsp. all spice
¼ tsp. basil
Zest and juice of ½ lemon
¼ tsp. dried Italian seasoning
1 pound salmon fillet

DIRECTIONS:

1. Preheat the oven to 425°F. Spray a baking sheet with nonstick cooking spray.
2. In a small bowl, combine the all spice, basil, lemon zest and juice, and italian seasoning. Stir to combine.
3. Place the salmon on the prepared baking sheet, skin-side down. Spread the seasoning mixture evenly over the fillet.
4. Bake for 15 to 20 minutes, depending on the thickness of the fillet, until the flesh flakes easily.

Nutrition Info per Serving:

Calories: 163, Total Fat: 7g, Protein: 23g, Carbohydrates: 1g, Sugar: 0g, Fiber: 0g, Sodium: 167mg, Cholesterol: 76mg

Healthy Baked Fish and Chips

Prep Time: 20 minutes, Cook Time: 20 to 30 minutes, Serves: 5

INGREDIENTS:

2 tbsps. extra-virgin olive oil, divided
5 (4-ounce, 113g) fresh or (thawed) frozen cod fillets
2 large sweet potatoes, cut crosswise into ¼-inch-thick rounds
1 large egg
2 tbsps. 1% milk
1 tbsp. fresh rosemary leaves
½ tsp. salt
¼ tsp. freshly ground black pepper
¼ cup whole wheat flour
½ cup dried unseasoned bread crumbs
¼ cup slivered almonds
¼ tsp. lemon pepper
1 tsp. chopped fresh parsley, plus more for serving
Lemon wedges (optional)

DIRECTIONS:

1. Position racks in the upper and lower thirds of the oven and preheat the oven to 450°F(235°C). Line 2 sheet pans with aluminum foil.
2. Toss the sweet potatoes with 1 tbsp. of oil and the rosemary in a medium bowl then season with the salt and pepper. Arrange in an even layer on one prepared sheet pan. Bake on the top rack, turning once, for 20 to 30 minutes, or until browned.
3. Set up a dredging station: Put the flour in a small bowl. In a second small bowl, whisk together the egg and milk. In a third, combine the bread crumbs, almonds, lemon pepper, and parsley. Coat each cod fillet in the flour, then the egg wash, then the bread crumb mixture. Arrange on the second prepared sheet pan and drizzle with the remaining 1 tbsp. of oil.
4. Bake the cod on the bottom rack for about 15 minutes, or until crisp and just cooked through.
5. Portion the cod and sweet potatoes into 5 divided storage containers, fish on one side, chips on the other.
6. To serve, after reheating the dish, top with parsley. Serve with lemon wedges (if using).

Nutrition Info per Serving:

Calories: 301, Total fat: 10g, Carbohydrates: 27g, Fiber: 4g, Protein: 24g, Sodium: 411mg, Cholesterol: 37mg, Sugar: 4.9g

Baked Fish in Nuts

Prep Time: 10 minutes, Cook Time: 20 minutes, Serves: 4

INGREDIENTS:

½ cup (120 ml) extra-virgin olive oil, divided
1 pound (454 g) flaky white fish (such as cod, haddock, or halibut), skin removed
½ cup shelled finely chopped pistachios
½ cup ground flaxseed
1 tsp. ground cumin
1 tsp. ground allspice
½ tsp. salt (use 1 tsp. if pistachios are unsalted)
¼ tsp. freshly ground black pepper
Zest and juice of 1 lemon, divided

DIRECTIONS:

1. Preheat the oven to 400°F (205ºC).
2. Line a baking sheet with parchment paper and drizzle 2 tbsps. olive oil over the sheet evenly to coat the bottom.
3. Cut the fish into 4 equal pieces and put on the prepared baking sheet.
4. Combine the flaxseed, pistachios, cumin, lemon zest, allspice, salt, and pepper in a small bowl. Drizzle in ¼ cup olive oil and mix well.
5. Divide the nut mixture evenly on the fish pieces. Drizzle the lemon juice and remaining oil over the fish and bake 15 to 20 minutes until cooked through.

Nutrition Info per Serving:

Calories: 509, Total Carbs: 9g, Net Carbs: 3g, Protein: 26g, Total Fat: 41g, Fiber: 6g, Sodium: 331mg, Cholesterol: 10mg, Sugar: 19.4g

Baked Tuna with Orange Sauce

Prep Time: 10 minutes, Cook Time: 15 minutes, Serves: 4

INGREDIENTS:

4 (5-ounce) tuna fillets
Sea salt
Freshly ground black pepper
1 tbsp. canola oil
½ cup low-sodium vegetable broth
Juice and zest of 1 lemon
1 tsp. chopped fresh thyme
½ cup fat-free sour cream
1 tsp. maple syrup
1 tbsp. chopped fresh chives

DIRECTIONS:

1. Preheat the oven to 400°F (205ºC).
2. Lightly season both sides of the tuna with salt and pepper.
3. Heat the oil in a large ovenproof skillet over medium-high heat.
4. Sear both sides of the tuna fillets until golden brown, approximately 3 minutes each side.
5. Transfer the tuna to a baking sheet and bake for 10 minutes, or until it is just cooked through.
6. In a small saucepan over medium-high heat, whisk together the vegetable broth, orange juice, zest, and thyme until the liquid reduces by approximately one-quarter, about 5 minutes.
7. Combine the sour cream and maple syrup in a mixing bowl.
8. Add the chives to the sauce and pour it over the fish.

Nutrition Info per Serving:

Calories: 310, Total Fat: 18g, Cholesterol: 72mg, Sodium: 129mg, Carbohydrates: 6g, Sugar: 2g, Fiber: 0g, Protein: 29g

Baked Flounder with Tomatoes and Basil

Prep Time: 10 minutes, Cook Time: 20 minutes, Serves: 4

INGREDIENTS:

4 (5- to 6-ounce, 142 - 170g) flounder fillets
1 pound(454g) cherry tomatoes
4 garlic cloves, sliced
2 tbsps. extra-virgin olive oil
2 tbsps. lemon juice
2 tbsps. basil, cut into ribbons
½ tsp. kosher salt
¼ tsp. freshly ground black pepper

DIRECTIONS:

1. Preheat the oven to 425°F(220°C).
2. Combine the tomatoes, garlic, olive oil, lemon juice, basil, salt, and black pepper in a baking dish and mix well. Bake for 5 minutes.
3. Remove the baking dish from the oven and arrange the flounder on top of the tomato mixture. Bake until the fish is opaque and begins to flake, about 10 to 15 minutes, depending on thickness.

Nutrition Info per Serving:

Calories: 215, Total fat: 9g, Saturated fat: 1g, Cholesterol: 68mg, Sodium: 261mg, Potassium: 805mg, Total Carbohydrates: 6g, Fiber: 2g, Sugar: 3g, Protein: 28g, Magnesium: 60mg, Calcium: 45mg

Lemon-Garlic Tilapia with Roasted Vegetables

Prep Time: 5 minutes, Cook Time: 15 minutes, Serves: 4

INGREDIENTS:

4 tilapia fillets (4 ounces each, 113 g)
3 cups broccoli florets
1 cup sliced yellow squash (about 1 medium)
2 tbsps. fresh lemon juice
2 tbsps. minced shallot
2 tbsps. chopped fresh parsley
1 tbsp. minced garlic
5 ounces (142 g) baby arugula
2 tbsps. + 2 tsps. extra-virgin olive oil
Salt and freshly ground black pepper
2 tbsps. grated Parmesan cheese

DIRECTIONS:

1. Preheat the oven to 400°F (205ºC). Coat a rimmed baking sheet with cooking spray.
2. Put the broccoli and squash on the baking sheet, drizzle with the olive oil and season with salt and pepper. Push the vegetables to the sides of the pan.
3. Mix together olive oil, lemon juice, parsley, shallot, garlic, ¼ teaspoon pepper, and ⅛ teaspoon salt in a small bowl. Place the tilapia fillets on the baking sheet in between the vegetables and season with the shallot/lemon/parsley mixture, gently pressing into the fish, turning, and seasoning the other side.
4. Transfer the baking sheet to the oven and bake 12 to 15 minutes until the fish flakes easily with a fork.
5. Meanwhile, toss together the arugula, remaining olive oil, the Parmesan, and salt and pepper in a medium bowl. Toss to combine.
6. Put a tilapia fillet on each of 4 plates. Divide the roasted vegetables and the arugula salad onto the plates.

Nutrition Info per Serving:

Calories: 244, Total fat: 13g, Saturated fat: 2g, Total carbohydrates: 9g, Protein: 29g, Cholesterol: 57mg, Sodium: 208mg, Potassium: 828mg, Fiber: 3g, Sugar: 3g

Haddock Tacos with Cabbage

Prep Time: 10 minutes, Cook Time: 5 minutes, Serves: 4

INGREDIENTS:

8 ounces (227 g) skinless haddock fillets, cut into 1-inch chunks
2 cups angel hair cabbage
½ avocado, chopped
2 tbsps. fresh lime juice
3 tsps. extra-virgin olive oil
2 (6-inch) whole-wheat tortillas, warmed
1 tsp. ground cumin
½ tsp. chili powder
⅛ tsp. salt
⅛ tsp. freshly ground black pepper
Fresh cilantro

DIRECTIONS:

1. Mix the chili powder, cumin, salt, and pepper in a small bowl. Add the haddock and toss to coat.
2. In a separate small bowl, mix together the cabbage, lime juice, avocado, and 1 tsp. olive oil.
3. Heat the remaining olive oil in a medium skillet over medium-high heat. Add the haddock and cook 4 to 5 minutes, turning, until the fish is just opaque and flakes easily with a fork.
4. Portion the fish between the warmed tortillas and top with the cabbage avocado mixture. Serve topped with fresh cilantro.

Nutrition Info per Serving:

Calories: 368, Total fat: 16g, Saturated fat: 2g, Total carbohydrates: 22g, Protein: 32g, Cholesterol: 84mg, Sodium: 408mg, Potassium: 261mg, Fiber: 7g, Sugar: 2g

Healthy Seafood Fettuccine

Prep Time: 15 minutes, Cook Time: 20 minutes, Serves: 4

INGREDIENTS:

1 tbsp. olive oil
½ pound(227g) cooked bay shrimp
½ pound(227g) cooked crab
10 ounces (283g) dry fettuccine noodles
3 tbsps. minced garlic
2 medium tomatoes, cut into bite-sized pieces
1 green bell pepper, cut into bite-sized pieces
2 tbsps. chopped fresh basil
2 tbsps. chopped fresh oregano

DIRECTIONS:

1. Boil the fettuccine per package directions. Meanwhile, combine the garlic and oil in a large non-stick skillet and heat gently over medium heat. Add the tomatoes and peppers to the skillet.
2. Stir in the basil and oregano, add the shrimp and crab and cook just until the seafood is heated.
3. Drain the pasta and stir it into the skillet, coating thoroughly.

Nutrition Info per Serving:

Calories: 569, Protein: 28.26g, Fat: 12.17g, Carbohydrates: 99.5g, Fiber: 18.2g, Sodium: 246mg, Cholesterol: 103mg, Sugar: 3.5g

Lemon Crawfish Poppers

Prep Time: 15 minutes, Cook Time: 30 minutes, Serves: 4

INGREDIENTS:

1 cup ground split peas
1 cup chickpea flour
1 pound (450 g) raw crawfish tails (langoustine tails), coarsely chopped
1 medium yellow summer squash, grated
1 small carrot, finely chopped
1 zucchini, finely chopped
½ small red bell pepper, finely chopped
1 garlic clove, minced
4 medium egg whites
1 tbsp. red wine vinegar
1 tsp. Creole Seasoning
1 tsp. baking powder
1 tsp. ketchup
1 tbsp. tahini
1 tbsp. freshly squeezed lemon juice
1 lemon, cut into wedges, for serving

DIRECTIONS:

1. Mix the ground split peas, chickpea flour, Creole seasoning, and baking powder in a medium bowl and mix well.
2. Mix the crawfish tails, summer squash, carrot, zucchini, bell pepper, garlic, and egg whites in a large bowl.
3. Add the crawfish mixture into the dry ingredients, pour in water as needed, ¼ cup at a time. The mix is ready to be formed when it resembles a batter-like consistency and no dry flour is visible.
4. Working in two or three batches with wet hand, form golf ball–size nuggets and put in the basket of an air fryer.
5. Turn the air fryer to 350°F(180ºC), close, and cook for 10 minutes. Place the poppers to a plate. Repeat with the rest of the batter.
6. To make the dipping sauce, whisk together the vinegar, ketchup, tahini, and lemon juice in a small bowl and toss to coat well.
7. Serve with the lemon wedges.

Nutrition Info per Serving:

Calories: 321, Total Fat: 3g, Cholesterol: 201mg, Sodium: 165mg, Carbohydrates: 31g, Sugar: 8g, Fiber: 7g, Protein: 41g

Baked Salmon with Leeks and Fennel

Prep Time: 10 minutes, Cook Time: 20 minutes, Serves: 4

INGREDIENTS:

1 tbsp. extra-virgin olive oil, plus additional for brushing
1 fennel bulb, sliced thin
4 (5- to 6-ounce, 142 g to 170 g) salmon fillets
1 leek, white part only, sliced thin
½ cup (120 ml) vegetable broth, or water
1 fresh rosemary sprig
1 tsp. salt
¼ tsp. freshly ground black pepper

DIRECTIONS:

1. Preheat the oven to 375°F (190ºC).
2. Add 1 tbsp. of olive oil in a shallow roasting pan. Put in the leek and fennel. Stir to coat with the oil.
3. Put the salmon fillets over the vegetables and sprinkle with salt and pepper.
4. Pour in the vegetable broth and add the rosemary sprig. Cover with aluminum foil tightly.
5. Put the pan in the preheated oven and bake for 20 minutes until the salmon is cooked through.
6. Remove and throw away the rosemary sprig. Transfer the salmon and vegetables to a platter and serve.

Nutrition Info per Serving:

Calories: 288, Total Carbohydrates: 8g, Protein: 34g, Total Fat: 14g, Sugar: 1g, Fiber: 2g, Sodium: 692mg, Cholesterol: 0mg

Baked Trout with Pecan

Prep Time: 15 minutes, Cook Time: 15 minutes, Serves: 4

INGREDIENTS:

4 large boneless trout fillets
Extra-virgin olive oil, for brushing
1 cup pecans, finely ground, divided
1 tbsp. coconut oil, melted, divided
2 tbsps. chopped fresh thyme leaves
Salt
Freshly ground black pepper
Lemon wedges, for garnish

DIRECTIONS:

1. Preheat the oven to 375°F (190ºC).
2. Grease a rimmed baking sheet with olive oil.
3. Put the trout fillets on the baking sheet skin-side down. Season with salt and pepper.
4. Gently press ¼ cup of ground pecans into the fillet.
5. Drizzle the melted coconut oil over the nuts and then sprinkle the thyme over them.
6. Give each fillet another sprinkle of salt and pepper.
7. Put the sheet in the preheated oven and bake for 15 minutes until the fish is cooked through.
8. Serve with the lemon wedges.

Nutrition Info per Serving:

Calories: 672, Total Carbohydrates: 13g, Protein: 30g, Total Fat: 59g, Sugar: 3g, Fiber: 9g, Sodium: 110mg, Cholesterol: 0mg

Monkfish in Tomatoes-Garlic Sauce

Prep Time: 20 minutes, Cook Time: 35 minutes, Serves: 4

INGREDIENTS:

2 tbsps. extra-virgin olive oil
1 to 1½ pounds(454g-680g) monkfish
1 (14.5-ounce, 411g) can no-salt-added diced tomatoes
3 tbsps. lemon juice, divided
1 tsp. kosher salt, divided
⅛ tsp. freshly ground black pepper
1 leek, white and light green parts only, sliced in half lengthwise and thinly sliced
½ onion, julienned
3 garlic cloves, minced
2 bulbs fennel, cored and thinly sliced, plus ¼ cup fronds for garnish
2 tbsps. fresh parsley, chopped
2 tbsps. fresh oregano, chopped
¼ tsp. red pepper flakes

DIRECTIONS:

1. Place the fish in a medium baking dish and add 2 tbsps. of the lemon juice, ¼ teaspoon of the salt, and the black pepper. Place in the refrigerator.
2. Heat the olive oil in a large skillet or sauté pan over medium heat. Add the leek and onion and sauté until translucent, about 3 minutes. Add the garlic and sauté for 30 seconds. Add the fennel and sauté 4 to 5 minutes. Add the tomatoes and simmer for 2 to 3 minutes.
3. Stir in the parsley, oregano, red pepper flakes, the remaining ¾ teaspoon salt, and the remaining 1 tbsp. lemon juice. Place the fish on top of the leek mixture, cover and simmer for 20 to 25 minutes, turning over halfway through, until the fish is opaque and pulls apart easily. Garnish with the fennel fronds.

Nutrition Info per Serving:

Calories: 220, Total fat: 9g, Saturated fat: 2g, Cholesterol: 35mg, Sodium: 345mg, Potassium: 800mg, Total Carbohydrates: 11g, Fiber: 3g, Sugar: 6g, Protein: 22g, Magnesium: 45mg, Calcium: 70mg

Broiled Shrimp with Peri-Peri Sauce

Prep Time: 10 minutes, Cook Time: 15 minutes, Serves: 4

INGREDIENTS:

Peri-Peri Sauce
1 pound(454 g) large shrimp, shelled and deveined
2 tbsps. extra-virgin olive oil
Sea salt

DIRECTIONS:

1. Preheat the oven broiler on high.
2. Add the Peri-Peri Sauce to a small pot, then bring to a simmer. Meanwhile, place the cleaned shrimp, deveined-side down on a rimmed baking sheet. Brush the olive oil and sprinkle the salt over the shrimp.
3. Broil for 5 minutes until opaque. With the sauce on the side for dipping to serve or topped on the shrimp.

Nutrition Info per Serving:

Calories: 279, Total Fat: 16g, Saturated Fat: 2g, Sodium: 464mg, Carbohydrates: 10g, Fiber: 3g, Protein: 24g, Sugar: 0g, Cholesterol: 145mg

Artichoke Caponata Over Grilled Mahi Mahi

Prep Time: 25 minutes, Cook Time: 30 minutes, Serves: 4

INGREDIENTS:

2 tbsps. extra-virgin olive oil
4 (5- to 6-ounces each, 142g-170g each) skinless mahi-mahi fillets
1 (14-ounce,397g) can artichoke hearts, drained and chopped
2 celery stalks, diced
1 onion, diced
2 garlic cloves, minced
½ cup cherry tomatoes, chopped
¼ cup white wine
2 tbsps. white wine vinegar
¼ cup green olives, pitted and chopped
1 tbsp. capers, chopped
¼ tsp. red pepper flakes
2 tbsps. fresh basil, chopped
½ tsp. kosher salt
¼ tsp. freshly ground black pepper
Olive oil cooking spray

DIRECTIONS:

1. Heat the olive oil in a large skillet or sauté pan over medium heat. Add the celery and onion, and sauté 4 to 5 minutes. Add the garlic and sauté 30 seconds. Add the tomatoes and cook 2 to 3 minutes. Add the wine and vinegar to deglaze the pan, increasing the heat to medium-high and scraping up any brown bits on the bottom of the pan.
2. Add the artichokes, olives, capers, and red pepper flakes and simmer to reduce the liquid by half, about 10 minutes. Mix in the basil.
3. Season the mahi-mahi with the salt and pepper. Heat a grill skillet or grill pan over medium-high heat and coat with olive oil cooking spray. Add the fish and cook 4 to 5 minutes per side. Serve topped with the artichoke caponata.

Nutrition Info per Serving:

Calories: 245, Total fat: 9g, Saturated fat: 1g, Cholesterol: 100mg, Sodium: 570mg, Potassium: 775mg, Total Carbohydrates: 10g, Fiber: 3g, Sugar: 3g, Protein: 28g, Magnesium: 55mg, Calcium: 50mg

Baked Flounder with Brussels Sprouts

Prep Time: 10 minutes, Cook Time: 15 minutes, Serves: 2

INGREDIENTS:

2 tbsps. olive oil, divided
2 (6-ounce, 170g) flounder fillets
14 Brussels sprouts
3 tbsps. freshly squeezed lemon juice
1 tbsp. minced fresh garlic
¼ tsp. dried dill
Salt
Freshly ground black pepper

DIRECTIONS:

1. Preheat the oven to 400°F(205°C). Rinse the Brussels sprouts and pat them dry. Cut their stem ends off, then cut sprouts in half and place them on a foil-lined baking pan. Drizzle with 1 tbsp. olive oil and toss to coat.
2. Meanwhile, stir together 1 tbsp. olive oil, lemon juice, garlic and dill in a small bowl.
3. Rinse flounder fillets and pat dry, season lightly with salt and pepper. Place in baking dish and evenly drizzle oil-and-herb mixture over flounder fillets.
4. Bake for 10 to 11 minutes, or until the fish flakes easily when tested with a fork. The Brussels sprouts should be lightly browned and also pierce easily with a fork.
5. Divide the flounder and Brussels sprouts between serving plates.

Nutrition Info per Serving:

Calories: 319, Total Fat: 17g, Saturated Fat: 2g, Cholesterol: 98mg, Sodium: 529mg, Potassium: 538mg, Total Carbohydrate: 13g, Fiber: 5g, Sugar: 3g, Protein: 33g

Cioppino Seafood Stew

Prep Time: 10 minutes, Cook Time: 20 minutes, Serves: 4

INGREDIENTS:

2 tbsps. extra-virgin olive oil
8 ounces (227 g) cod, pin bones removed, cut into 1-inch pieces
8 ounces (227 g) shrimp, peeled and deveined
1 (14-ounce, 397 g) can tomato sauce
1 onion, finely chopped
1 garlic clove, minced
½ cup dry white wine
1 tbsp. Italian seasoning
½ tsp. sea salt
Pinch red pepper flakes

DIRECTIONS:

1. Heat the olive oil in a large skillet over medium-high heat, until it shimmers. Stir in the onion and cook for 3 minutes. Then add the garlic and cook for 30 seconds. Stir in the wine and cook for 1 minute, stirring constantly.
2. Stir in the tomato sauce and bring to a simmer. Add the cod, shrimp, Italian seasoning, salt, and pepper flakes. Simmer again for 5 minutes, until the fish is just opaque. Serve.

Nutrition Info per Serving:

Calories: 243, Total Fat: 8g, Saturated Fat: 1g, Sodium: 271mg, Carbohydrates: 11g, Fiber: 2g, Protein: 23g, Cholesterol: 179mg, Sugar: 6.3g

Cod Chowder with Cauliflower

Prep Time: 15 minutes, Cook Time: 40 minutes, Serves: 4

INGREDIENTS:

2 tbsps. extra-virgin olive oil
1 to 1½ pounds(454g-680g) cod
1 leek, white and light green parts only, cut in half lengthwise and sliced thinly
1 medium head cauliflower, coarsely chopped
2 pints cherry tomatoes
4 garlic cloves, sliced
1 tsp. kosher salt
¼ tsp. freshly ground black pepper
2 cups no-salt-added vegetable stock
¼ cup green olives, pitted and chopped
¼ cup fresh parsley, minced

DIRECTIONS:

1. Heat the olive oil in a Dutch oven or large pot over medium heat. Add the leek and sauté until lightly golden brown for about 5 minutes. Then add the garlic and sauté for 30 seconds. Next add the cauliflower, salt, and black pepper and sauté 2 to 3 minutes.
2. Add the tomatoes and vegetable stock, increase the heat to high and bring to a boil, then turn the heat to low and simmer for 10 minutes.
3. Add the olives and mix together. Add the fish, cover, and simmer 20 minutes, or until fish is opaque and flakes easily.
4. Gently mix in the parsley. Serve with bread as desired.

Nutrition Info per Serving:

Calories: 270, Total fat: 9g, Saturated fat: 1g, Cholesterol: 60mg, Sodium: 545mg, Total Carbohydrates: 19g, Fiber: 5g, Sugar: 9g, Protein: 30g, Magnesium: 90mg, Calcium: 90mg

Curry Whitefish with Vegetables

Prep Time: 15 minutes, Cook Time: 15 minutes, Serves: 4-6

INGREDIENTS:

2 tbsps. coconut oil
1 tbsp. minced fresh ginger
2 garlic cloves, minced
1 onion, chopped
2 tsps. curry powder
1 tsp. salt
¼ tsp. freshly ground black pepper
1 (4-inch) piece lemongrass (white part only), bruised with the back of a knife
2 cups cubed butternut squash
2 cups chopped broccoli
1 (13.5-ounce, 383 g) can coconut milk
1 cup (240 ml) vegetable broth, or chicken broth
1 pound (454 g) firm whitefish fillets
¼ cup chopped fresh cilantro
1 scallion, sliced thin
Lemon wedges, for garnish

DIRECTIONS:

1. Melt the coconut oil in a large pot over medium-high heat. Add the salt, onion, ginger, garlic, curry powder, and pepper. Sauté for 5 minutes.
2. Add the butternut squash, lemongrass, and broccoli. Sauté for 2 minutes more.
3. Stir in the coconut milk and vegetable broth and boil. Lower the heat to simmer and add the fish. Cover the pot and simmer for 5 minutes until the fish is cooked through. Remove and throw away the lemongrass.
4. Ladle the curry into a bowl. Garnish with the scallion and cilantro. Serve with the lemon wedges.

Nutrition Info per Serving:

Calories: 553, Total Carbohydrates: 22g, Protein: 34g, Total Fat: 39g, Sugar: 7g, Fiber: 6g, Sodium: 881mg, Cholesterol: 45mg

Lime Crab Cakes

Prep Time: 15 minutes, Cook Time: 15 minutes, Serves: 4

INGREDIENTS:

1 medium egg
1 medium cucumber, grated
1 celery stalk, minced
8 oz. (230g) lump crab meat
⅓ cup chickpea crumbs
1 tbsp. Dijon mustard
¼ bunch fresh dill, minced
½ tsp. Pepper Sauce
1 tsp. freshly squeezed lime juice
1 tbsp. extra-virgin olive oil

DIRECTIONS:

1. Lightly beat the egg in a medium bowl.
2. Mix in the cucumber, celery, mustard, dill, pepper sauce, and lime juice until just combined.
3. Add the crab meat into the egg mixture.
4. Shape the crab cakes by hand using ¼ cup of the mixture per patty.
5. Place the chickpea crumbs in a shallow bowl. Gently roll the cakes in the crumbs until all sides are lightly coated. Transfer to the basket of an air fryer.
6. Set the air fryer to 390°F(199ºC), close, and cook for 12 minutes.
7. Serve warm with Broccoli Stalk Slaw.

Nutrition Info per Serving:

Calories: 122, Total Fat: 10g, Cholesterol: 73mg, Sodium: 391mg, Total Carbohydrates: 7g, Sugar: 2g, Fiber: 2g, Protein: 12g

Mediterranean Salmon with Quinoa

Prep Time: 10 minutes, Cook Time: 20 minutes, Serves: 4

INGREDIENTS:

1 tbsp. extra-virgin olive oil, plus additional for brushing
1 pound (454 g) salmon fillets
1 red onion, diced
2 cups cooked quinoa
½ cup chopped fresh basil
¼ cup chopped green olives
1 tbsp. apple cider vinegar
1 pint cherry tomatoes, halved
Salt
Freshly ground black pepper

DIRECTIONS:

1. Preheat the oven to 375°F (190ºC).
2. Brush a rimmed baking sheet with olive oil. Put the salmon fillets on the prepared sheet and brush each top with olive oil. Season with salt and pepper.
3. Put the sheet in the preheated oven and bake for 20 minutes.
4. Heat 1 tbsp. of olive oil in a large pan over medium-high heat. Add the onion and sauté for 3 minutes.
5. Stir in the olives, cherry tomatoes, quinoa, basil, and cider vinegar. Cook for 1 to 2 minutes until they are warmed through.
6. Transfer the quinoa, tomatoes, and salmon to a serving platter and serve.

Nutrition Info per Serving:

Calories: 396, Total Carbohydrates: 36g, Protein: 30g, Total Fat: 16g, Sugar: 4g, Fiber: 6g, Sodium: 395mg, Cholesterol: 76mg

Grilled Shrimp with Yogurt and Chili Sauce

Prep Time: 5 minutes, Cook Time: 15 minutes, Serves: 4

INGREDIENTS:

1 pound shrimp
½ cup Plain Greek yogurt
½ tbsp. Chili paste (sambal oelek)
½ tbsp. lime juice
chopped green onions and lime juice for garnishing
Wooden skewers (soaked in water)

DIRECTIONS:

1. Begin by removing the shrimp's shells and carefully washing them. Devein all of the shrimps with care. Make sure the tail is still attached.
2. Pierce the shrimps through the middle to skewer them. On each skewer, you may fit approximately 5 shrimp.
3. Preheat the grill to medium-high heat and add the skewered shrimp on the grill. Cook for about 3 minutes. Cook for another 3 minutes on the other side.
4. Make the yogurt and chili sauce while the shrimps are cooking. Combine the yogurt, orange juice, and chili paste in a glass bowl. To mix, whisk everything together well.
5. Transfer the cooked shrimp to a serving plate with the skewers.
6. Garnish with chopped green onions and a squeeze of fresh orange juice. Serve with orange and chili sauce, if desired.

Nutrition Info per Serving:

Calories: 134, Fat: 2.3g, Protein: 25.2g, Carbohydrates: 2.4g, Sugar: 2g, Fiber: 0.4g, Sodium: 105mg, Cholesterol: 12mg

Quick Jerk Salmon

Prep Time: 5 minutes, Cook Time: 12 to 15 minutes, Serves: 4

INGREDIENTS:

2 tbsps. extra-virgin olive oil, divided
4 (4-ounce, 113g) skin-on salmon fillets
2½ tsps. dried thyme
2 tsps. ground allspice
2 tsps. onion powder
2 tsps. freshly ground black pepper
½ tsp. ground cinnamon
½ tsp. cayenne pepper

DIRECTIONS:

1. Preheat the oven to 350°F(177°C). Lightly coat a sheet pan with ½ tablespoon of oil.
2. Mix together the thyme, allspice, onion powder, black pepper, cinnamon, and cayenne pepper in a small bowl. Lightly coat the salmon fillets with the remaining 1½ tablespoons of oil and season with the rub.
3. Place the salmon, skin-side down, on the prepared sheet pan. Bake for 12 to 15 minutes(depending on the thickness), or until the salmon is cooked through and flakes easily with a fork.
4. Divide among 4 storage containers.

Nutrition Info per Serving:

Calories: 255, Total fat: 15g, Carbohydrates: 3g, Fiber: 1g, Protein: 26g, Calcium: 46mg, Vitamin D: 283 IU, Potassium: 677mg, Magnesium: 44mg, Sodium: 59mg, Cholesterol: 163mg, Sugar: 0g

Penne with Sardines and Fennel

Prep Time: 15 minutes, Cook Time: 30 minutes, Serves: 4

INGREDIENTS:

8 ounces (227g) whole-wheat penne
2 tbsps. extra-virgin olive oil
1 bulb fennel, cored and thinly sliced, plus ¼ cup fronds
2 celery stalks, thinly sliced, plus ½ cup leaves
4 garlic cloves, sliced
¾ tsp kosher salt
¼ tsp. freshly ground black pepper
Zest of 1 lemon
Juice of 1 lemon
2 (4.4-ounce, 125g) cans boneless/skinless sardines packed in olive oil, undrained

DIRECTIONS:

1. Cook the penne according to the package directions. Drain, reserving 1 cup pasta water.
2. Heat the olive oil in a large skillet or sauté pan over medium heat. Add the fennel and celery and cook, stirring often, until tender and golden, about 10 to 12 minutes. Add the garlic and cook for 1 minute.
3. Add the penne, reserved pasta water, salt, and black pepper. Increase the heat to medium-high and cook for 1 to 2 minutes.
4. Remove the pan from the heat and stir in the lemon zest, lemon juice, fennel fronds, and celery leaves. Break the sardines into bite-size pieces and gently mix in, along with the oil they were packed in.

Nutrition Info per Serving:

Calories: 400, Total fat: 15g, Saturated fat: 2g, Cholesterol: 81mg, Sodium: 530mg, Potassium: 610mg, Total Carbohydrates: 46g, Fiber: 6g, Sugar: 4g, Protein: 22g, Magnesium: 30mg, Calcium: 265mg

Parchment-Paper Halibut

Prep Time: 15 minutes, Cook Time: 15 minutes, Serves: 4

INGREDIENTS:

4 tsps. extra-virgin olive oil
4 (5-ounce, 142g) halibut fillets (about 1 inch thick)
½ cup zucchini, diced small
1 shallot, minced
¼ tsp. kosher salt
⅛ tsp. freshly ground black pepper
1 lemon, sliced into ⅛-inch-thick rounds
8 sprigs of thyme

DIRECTIONS:

1. Preheat the oven to 450°F(235°C). Combine the zucchini and shallots in a medium bowl.
2. Cut 4 (15-by-24-inch) pieces of parchment paper. Fold each sheet in half horizontally. Draw a large half heart on one side of each folded sheet, with the fold along the center of the heart. Cut out the heart, open the parchment, and lay it flat.
3. Place a fillet near the center of each parchment heart. Drizzle 1 tsp. olive oil on each fillet. Sprinkle with salt and pepper. Top each fillet with lemon slices and 2 sprigs of thyme. Sprinkle each fillet with one-quarter of the zucchini and shallot mixture. Fold the parchment over.
4. Starting at the top, fold the edges of the parchment over, and continue all the way around to make a packet. Twist the end tightly to secure.
5. Arrange the 4 packets on a baking sheet. Bake for about 15 minutes. Place on plates, cut open. Serve immediately.

Nutrition Info per Serving:

Calories: 190, Total fat: 7g, Saturated fat: 1g, Cholesterol: 70mg, Sodium: 170mg, Potassium: 735mg, Total Carbohydrates: 5g, Fiber: 1g, Sugar: 2g, Protein: 27g, Magnesium: 40mg, Calcium: 25mg

Orange Maple Glazed Salmon

Prep Time: 15 minutes, Cook Time: 15 minutes, Serves: 4

INGREDIENTS:

4 (4- to 6-ounce, 113 to 170 g) salmon fillets, pin bones removed
¼ cup pure maple syrup
juice of 2 oranges
zest of 1 orange
2 tbsps. low-sodium soy sauce
1 tsp. garlic powder

DIRECTIONS:

1. Preheat the oven to 400°F(205°C).
2. Add the maple syrup, orange juice and zest, soy sauce and garlic powder into a small, shallow dish, whisk them together well.
3. Flesh-side down to put the salmon pieces into the dish. Allow it to marinate for 10 minutes.
4. Then skin-side up to transfer the salmon to a rimmed baking sheet, bake until the flesh is opaque, about 15 minutes.

Nutrition Info per Serving:

Calories: 297, Total Fat: 11, Total Carbs: 18g, Sugar: 15g, Fiber: <1g, Protein: 34g, Sodium: 528mg, Cholesterol: 3mg

Easy Roast Salmon Asparagus

Prep Time: 5 minutes, Cook Time: 15 minutes, Serves: 2

INGREDIENTS:

2 (5-ounce, 142g) salmon fillets with skin
2 tsps. olive oil, plus extra for drizzling
1 bunch asparagus, trimmed
1 tsp. dried chives
1 tsp. dried tarragon
Fresh lemon wedges for serving
Salt
Freshly ground black pepper

DIRECTIONS:

1. Preheat the oven to 425°F(220°C).
2. Rub salmon all over with 1 tsp. of olive oil per fillet. Season with salt and pepper.
3. Place asparagus spears on a foil lined baking sheet and lay the salmon fillets skin-side down on top. Put pan in upper-third of oven and roast until fish is just cooked through, about 12 minutes. Roasting time will vary depending on the thickness of your salmon. Salmon should flake easily with a fork when it's ready and an instant-read thermometer should register 145°F(63°C).
4. When cooked, remove from the oven, cut fillets in half crosswise, then lift flesh from skin with a metal spatula and transfer to a plate. Discard the skin, then drizzle salmon with oil, sprinkle with herbs, and serve with lemon wedges and roasted asparagus spears.

Nutrition Info per Serving:

Calories: 353, Total Fat: 22g, Saturated Fat: 4g, Cholesterol: 88mg, Sodium: 90mg, Potassium: 304mg, Total Carbohydrate: 5g, Fiber: 2g, Sugar: 0g, Protein: 34g

Orange-Thyme Salmon with Summer Squash

Prep Time: 15 minutes, Cook Time: 20 minutes, Serves: 4

INGREDIENTS:

2 blood oranges, peeled and thinly sliced
4 skinless salmon fillets (6 ounces each, 170 g)
2 tsps. dried thyme
¼ tsp. salt
¼ tsp. freshly ground black pepper
2 cups sliced yellow summer squash (about 2 medium)
2 cups sliced zucchini (about 2 medium)
1 small red onion, thinly sliced
Juice of 1 lemon
1 tbsp. extra-virgin olive oil
4 sprigs fresh thyme

DIRECTIONS:

1. Preheat the oven to 400°F (205ºC). Tear off 4 pieces of foil that are 2 inches longer than the salmon fillets.
2. Combine the dried thyme, lemon juice, olive oil, salt, and pepper in a medium bowl.
3. Place the foil pieces on your work surface and on one side of each piece of foil, layer one-quarter of the red onion, zucchini, yellow squash, and blood orange. Top each stack of vegetables with a salmon fillet and drizzle with the lemon juice mixture. Place a thyme sprig on top of each piece of fish.
4. Fold the other half of the foil over the ingredients. To seal the packets, begin at one corner and tightly fold the edges over about ½ inch all around, overlapping the folds. The foil should not come undone.
5. Place the packets on a baking sheet. Transfer to the oven and bake about 20 minutes until the salmon turns opaque throughout.
6. Serve the pouches on a plate or remove the contents to a plate. Spoon any liquid remaining in the foil over the salmon and vegetables.

Nutrition Info per Serving:

Calories: 309, Total fat: 11g, Saturated fat: 2g, Total carbohydrates: 18g, Protein: 37g, Cholesterol: 75mg, Sodium: 279mg, Potassium: 615mg, Fiber: 6g, Sugar: 10g

Red Capsicum Salmon Melts

Prep Time: 5 minutes, Cook Time: 5 minutes, Serves: 2

INGREDIENTS:

1 (5-ounce) can chunk light salmon packed in water, drained
2 tbsps. plain yogurt
2 tsps. freshly squeezed lemon juice
2 tbsps. finely chopped celery
1 tbsp. scallions chopped
Pinch Sichuan pepper
1 large red capsicum, cut into ¾-inch-thick rounds
½ cup shredded cheddar cheese

DIRECTIONS:

1. Preheat the broiler to high.
2. In a medium bowl, combine the salmon, yogurt, lemon juice, celery, scallions, and Sichuan pepper. Stir well.
3. Arrange the red capsicums on a baking sheet. Top each with some salmon salad and cheddar cheese.
4. Broil for 3 to 4 minutes until the cheese is melted and bubbly. Serve.

Nutrition Info per Serving:

Calories: 243, Total Fat: 10g, Protein: 30g, Carbohydrates: 7g, Sugar: 2g, Fiber: 1g, Sodium: 444mg, Cholesterol: 30mg

Salmon and Avocado Salad

Prep Time: 5 minutes, Cook Time: 5 minutes, Serves: 4

INGREDIENTS:

10 ounces canned Salmon, drained
1 large avocado
1 parsley rib
2 fresh chives cloves
3 tbsps. Mayonnaise
1 small white onion, peeled
1 tbsp. freshly squeezed lime zest
1 cucumber
1 handful Thyme
salt and pepper to taste

DIRECTIONS:

1. Finely chop the onion, parsley, chives, and cucumber. Also, very finely mince the thyme . (You can use a garlic press, if handy.)
2. Take the avocado and cut it into 2 halves. Use a spoon to scoop out the pulp. Dice it into small pieces
3. Take a salad mixing bowl and add in half of the parsley, chopped onion, cucumber, chives, and minced thyme. Toss using a spoon.
4. Now add in the diced avocado, mayonnaise and salmon,. Gently fold until all the ingredients are well-coated.
5. Season with pepper and salt as per your liking. Give the salad a gentle toss.
6. Serve in a bowl and garnish with reserved fresh parsley!

Nutrition Info per Serving:

Calories: 225, Fat: 16.3g, Protein: 13.9g, Carbohydrates: 7.1g, Sugar: 1.8g, Fiber: 4g, Sodium: 578mg, Cholesterol: 84mg

Scallop and Quinoa Paella

Prep Time: 10 minutes, Cook Time: 30 minutes, Serves: 4

INGREDIENTS:

1 tbsp. extra-virgin olive oil
1 cup chopped onion
3 cloves garlic, minced
1 medium red bell pepper, chopped
1 cup chopped baby bella mushrooms (5 to 6 mushrooms)
1 cup frozen green peas, thawed
1 pound (454 g) scallops
1 (14.5-ounce, 410 g) can no-salt-added diced tomatoes, undrained
1 (14.5-ounce, 410 g) can water-packed artichoke hearts, drained and rinsed
1 cup quinoa, rinsed
1 tsp. smoked paprika
1 tsp. ground turmeric
Salt and freshly ground black pepper (optional)
2 cups (480 ml) low-sodium vegetable broth
1 lemon, halved
Fresh parsley

DIRECTIONS:

1. Heat the olive oil in a large skillet over medium heat. Add the onions and garlic and cook 3 to 4 minutes until translucent. Put in the bell pepper and mushrooms and sauté an additional 3 to 4 minutes until they start to soften and the mushrooms begin to brown.
2. Add the tomatoes and their juices, quinoa, smoked paprika, the artichoke hearts, turmeric, and salt and black pepper, mixing well to combine. Add the broth and stir again. Boil the mixture, then cover, reduce the heat, and simmer about 15 minutes until most of the liquid has been absorbed.
3. Add the peas and scallops, cover, and continue cooking about 5 minutes until the scallops are cooked through.
4. Remove the lid and squeeze the lemon over the top. Garnish with fresh parsley and serve.

Nutrition Info per Serving:

Calories: 431, Total fat: 8g, Saturated fat: <1g, Total carbohydrates: 62g, Protein: 31g, Cholesterol: 37mg, Sodium: 339mg, Potassium: 913mg, Fiber: 15g, Sugar: 10g

Sea Bass with Tomatoes, Olives and Capers

Prep Time: 10 minutes, Cook Time: 15 minutes, Serves: 4

INGREDIENTS:

4 (5-ounce, 142 g) sea bass fillets
1 small onion, diced
½ cup (120 ml) vegetable or chicken broth
1 cup canned diced tomatoes
2 cups packed spinach
½ cup pitted and chopped Kalamata olives
2 tbsps. capers, drained
2 tbsps. extra-virgin olive oil
1 tsp. salt
¼ tsp. freshly ground black pepper

DIRECTIONS:

1. Preheat the oven to 375°F (190ºC).
2. Add the olive oil in a baking dish. Put the fish fillets in the dish, flipping to coat both sides with the oil.
3. Top the fish with the vegetable broth, onion, spinach, tomatoes, capers, olives, salt, and pepper.
4. Cover the baking dish with aluminum foil and put it in the preheated oven. Bake for 15 minutes until the fish is cooked through.

Nutrition Info per Serving:

Calories: 273, Total Carbohydrates: 5g, Total Fat: 12g, Protein: 35g, Sugar: 2g, Fiber: 2g, Sodium: 970mg, Cholesterol: 53mg

Salmon with Snap Peas and Garlic

Prep Time: 5 minutes, Cook Time: 15 minutes, Serves: 2

INGREDIENTS:

Cooking spray
2 (4-ounce (113g)) skinless salmon fillets
2 garlic cloves, minced and divided
Salt
Juice of 1 lemon, divided
2 cups sugar snap peas, divided
Freshly ground black pepper

DIRECTIONS:

1. Preheat the oven to 450°F.
2. Cut 2 pieces of aluminum foil with a size of 12-by-18 inches, and then sprinkle the cooking spray in the center of each foil sheet.
3. Arrange one piece of salmon fillet in the center of each sheet, Sprinkle 1 cup of sugar snap peas, 1 clove crunched garlic, and 1 cup of lemon juice. If you want more flavor, you can sprinkle with salt and pepper.
4. Seal the sides of the foil and fold the top twice to make room for air to circulate inside the packet.
5. Put packets on a baking sheet and bake in oven until salmon is opaque, about15 to 18 minutes,
6. Be careful when opening the package because the steam is very hot.

Nutrition Info per Serving:

Calories: 211, Total Fat: 5g, Saturated Fat: 1g, Protein: 26g, Total Carbohydrate: 14g, Fiber: 3g, Sugar: 5g, Cholesterol: 50mg, Sodium: 86mg, Potassium: 41mg

Salmon Cakes with Lemon Yogurt

Prep Time: 15 minutes, Cook Time: 15 minutes, Serves: 4

INGREDIENTS:

2 tbsps. extra-virgin olive oil, divided
¼ cup whole-wheat bread crumbs
¼ cup mayonnaise
1 large egg, beaten
1 tbsp. chives, chopped
1 tbsp. fresh parsley, chopped
Zest of 1 lemon
¾ tsp kosher salt, divided
¼ tsp. freshly ground black pepper
2 (5- to 6-ounce, 142-170g) cans no-salt boneless/skinless salmon, drained and finely flaked
½ bell pepper, diced small
1 cup plain Greek yogurt
Juice of 1 lemon

DIRECTIONS:

1. Combine the bread crumbs, mayonnaise, egg, chives, parsley, lemon zest, ½ tsp. of the salt, and black pepper in a large bowl and mix well. Add the salmon and the bell pepper and stir gently until well combined. Shape the mixture into 8 patties.
2. Heat 1 tbsp. of the olive oil in a large skillet over medium-high heat. Cook half the cakes until the bottoms are golden brown, about 4 to 5 minutes. Adjust the heat to medium if the bottoms start to burn. Flip and cook for an additional 4 to 5 minutes. Repeat with the remaining 1 tbsp. olive oil and the rest of the cakes.
3. In a small bowl, combine the yogurt, lemon juice, and the remaining ¼ teaspoon salt and mix well. Serve with the salmon cakes.

Nutrition Info per Serving:

Calories: 330, Total fat: 23g, Saturated fat: 4g, Cholesterol: 91mg, Sodium: 385mg, Potassium: 135mg, Total Carbohydrates: 9g, Fiber: 1g, Sugar: 3g, Protein: 21g, Magnesium: 10mg, Calcium: 65mg

Spicy Sesame-Tuna Skewers

Prep Time: 20 minutes, Cook Time: 15 minutes, Serves: 4-6

INGREDIENTS:

4 (6-ounce, 170 g) thick tuna steaks, cut into 1-inch cubes
¾ cup sesame seeds (mixture of black and white)
Cooking spray
1 tsp. salt
½ tsp. ground ginger
¼ tsp. freshly ground black pepper
2 tbsps. toasted sesame oil, or extra-virgin olive oil

DIRECTIONS:

1. Preheat the oven to 400°F (205ºC).
2. Lightly spray a rimmed baking sheet with cooking spray.
3. Soak 12 (6-inch) wooden skewers in water so they will not burn while baking.
4. Combine the sesame seeds, ground ginger, salt, and pepper in a shallow dish.
5. Toss the tuna with the sesame oil to coat in a medium bowl. Press the oiled cubes into the sesame seed mixture. Thread three cubes on each skewer.
6. Put the skewers on the prepared baking sheet and put the sheet into the preheated oven. Bake for 10 to 12 minutes, turning once.

Nutrition Info per Serving:

Calories: 395, Total Carbohydrates: 7g, Protein: 45g, Total Fat: 22g, Sugar: 0g, Fiber: 3g, Sodium: 649mg, Cholesterol: 0mg

Smoky Flavor Cod with Mushrooms

Prep Time: 10 minutes, Cook Time: 20 minutes, Serves: 4

INGREDIENTS:

1½ pounds (680 g) cod fillets
1 tbsp. extra-virgin olive oil
1 leek, white part only, sliced thin
8 ounces (227 g) shiitake mushrooms, stemmed, sliced
1 tbsp. coconut aminos
1 tsp. sweet paprika
½ cup (120 ml) vegetable broth, or chicken broth
½ tsp. salt, plus additional for seasoning
Freshly ground black pepper

DIRECTIONS:

1. Preheat the oven to 375°F (190ºC).
2. Season the cod with salt and pepper. Set aside.
3. Combine the olive oil, mushrooms, leek, paprika, coconut aminos, and ½ tsp. of salt in a shallow baking dish. Season with pepper, and gently toss to coat with the oil and spices.
4. Put the dish in the preheated oven and bake the vegetables for 10 minutes.
5. Stir the vegetables and arrange the cod fillets on top in a single layer.
6. Pour in the vegetable broth. Put the dish back to the oven and bake for 10 to 15 minutes until the cod is cooked through.

Nutrition Info per Serving:

Calories: 221, Total Carbohydrates: 12g, Protein: 32g, Total Fat: 6g, Sugar: 3g, Fiber: 2g, Sodium: 637mg, Cholesterol: 8mg

Flavor Packed Shrimp Fra Diavolo

Prep Time: 10 minutes, Cook Time: 10 minutes, Serves: 4

INGREDIENTS:

1 pound (454g) shrimp, peeled and deveined
2 tbsps. extra-virgin olive oil
½ tsp. kosher salt
½ tsp. dried oregano
½ tsp. dried thyme
¼ tsp. red pepper flakes
1 bell pepper, diced small
1 onion, diced small
1 (14.5-ounce (411g)) can no-salt-added diced tomatoes
Zest of 1 lemon
1 fennel bulb, cored and diced small, plus ¼ cup fronds for garnish
2 tbsps. fresh parsley, chopped, for garnish
Juice of 1 lemon

DIRECTIONS:

1. Arrange 2 tbsps. olive oil in a large skillet or sauté pan and heat over medium heat. Place the onion, oregano, thyme, fennel, bell pepper, salt, and red pepper flakes and sauté, stir often, until the spice is soft and translucent, about 5 minutes.
2. Remove the fried browned spices, pour the canned tomato juice into the pot and bring it to a boil. Add the chopped tomatoes and shrimp in the pot. Simmer on low heat, cover and cook until shrimps are cooked through, about 3 minutes.
3. Turn off the heat. Serve the shrimp from the pot, sprinkle with the lemon juice and lemon zest, and mix well. Dust with parsley and the fennel fronds to make it look savory.

Nutrition Info per Serving:

Calories: 240, Total fat: 9g, Saturated fat: 1g, Cholesterol: 170mg, Sodium: 335mg, Potassium: 445mg, Total Carbohydrates: 13g, Fiber: 3g, Sugar: 7g, Protein: 25g, Magnesium: 55mg, Calcium: 105mg

Spicy Cod Mango Salsa

Prep Time: 10 minutes, Cook Time: 10 minutes, Serves: 4

INGREDIENTS:

2 tbsps. extra-virgin olive oil
1 pound(454 g) cod, cut into 4 fillets, pin bones removed
1 mango, pitted, peeled, and cut into cubes
¼ cup chopped cilantro
½ red onion, finely chopped
1 jalapeño, seeded and finely chopped
¾ tsp. sea salt, divided
1 garlic clove, minced
Juice of 1 lime

DIRECTIONS:

1. Preheat the oven broiler on high.
2. Add the cod on a rimmed baking sheet, brush the olive oil and season ½ tsp. of the salt over the cod. Broil for 5 to 10 minutes until the fish is opaque.
3. While the cod is broiling, combine the mango, cilantro, onion, jalapeño, garlic, lime juice, and remaining ¼ teaspoon of salt in a small bowl, stir well.
4. Top the cod with the salsa and serve.

Nutrition Info per Serving:

Calories: 197, Total Fat: 8g, Saturated Fat: 1g, Sodium: 354mg, Carbohydrates: 13g, Fiber: 2g, Protein: 21 g, Sugar: 1.3g, Cholesterol: 53mg

Smoked Sardine Bruschetta with Fennel and Lemon

Prep Time: 15 minutes, Cook Time: 1 minute, Serves: 4

INGREDIENTS:

2 tsps. extra-virgin olive oil
8 slices multigrain bread, toasted
2 (4.4-ounce, 124g) cans smoked sardines
⅓ cup plain Greek yogurt
2 tbsps. mayonnaise
2 tbsps. lemon juice, divided
2 tsps. lemon zest
¾ tsp kosher salt, divided
1 fennel bulb, cored and thinly sliced
¼ cup fresh parsley, chopped, plus more for garnish
¼ cup fresh mint, chopped, plus more for garnish
⅛ tsp. freshly ground black pepper

DIRECTIONS:

1. Combine the yogurt, mayonnaise, 1 tbsp. of the lemon juice, the lemon zest, and ¼ teaspoon of the salt together in a small bowl.
2. Combine the remaining ½ tsp. salt, the remaining 1 tbsp. lemon juice, the fennel, parsley, mint, olive oil, and black pepper in a separate small bowl.
3. Spoon 1 tbsp. of the yogurt mixture on each piece of toast. Divide the fennel mixture evenly on top of the yogurt mixture. Divide the sardines among the toasts, placing them on top of the fennel mixture. Garnish with more herbs, if desired.

Nutrition Info per Serving:

Calories: 400, Total fat: 16g, Saturated fat: 2g, Cholesterol: 39mg, Sodium: 565mg, Potassium: 550mg, Total Carbohydrates: 51g, Fiber: 7g, Sugar: 6g, Protein: 16g, Magnesium: 95mg, Calcium: 170mg

Foil Packet Sole with Vegetables

Prep Time: 15 minutes, Cook Time: 15 minutes, Serves: 4

INGREDIENTS:

4 (5-ounce, 142 g) sole fillets
1 carrot, sliced thin, divided
1 zucchini, sliced thin, divided
2 shallots, sliced thin, divided
2 tbsps. snipped fresh chives, divided
4 tsps. extra-virgin olive oil, divided
½ cup (120 ml) vegetable broth, or water, divided
Lemon wedges, for garnish
Salt
Freshly ground black pepper

DIRECTIONS:

1. Preheat the oven to 425°F (220ºC).
2. Tear off four 12 x 20-inch pieces of aluminum foil.
3. Put 1 fillet on one half of a foil piece. Season with salt and pepper.
4. Top the fillet with ¼ of the carrot, zucchini, and shallots. Sprinkle with 1½ tsps.s of chives.
5. Drizzle 2 tbsps. of vegetable broth and 1 tsp. of olive oil over the vegetables and fish.
6. Fold the other half of the foil over the fish and vegetables, sealing the edges so the ingredients are completely encased in the packet. Put the packet on a large baking sheet.
7. Repeat steps 3 to 6 with the remaining ingredients.
8. Put the sheet in the preheated oven and bake the packets for 15 minutes until the vegetables are tender and the fish is cooked through.
9. Carefully peel back the foil and transfer the contents, including the liquid, to a plate. Serve garnished with the lemon wedges.

Nutrition Info per Serving:

Calories: 224, Total Carbohydrates: 4g, Protein: 35g, Total Fat: 7g, Sugar: 2g, Fiber: 1g, Sodium: 205mg, Cholesterol: 73mg

Seared Scallops

Prep Time: 5 minutes, Cook Time: 6 minutes, Serves: 4

INGREDIENTS:

2 tbsps. olive oil, divided
1½ pounds(680g) sea scallops
2 cups chopped tomato
½ cup chopped fresh basil
¼ tsp. freshly ground black pepper, divided
⅛ tsp. salt
1 cup fresh corn kernels
1 cup zucchini, diced

DIRECTIONS:

1. In a medium bowl, combine tomato, basil, and ⅛ teaspoon black pepper. Toss gently.
2. Heat a large skillet over high heat. Add 1 tbsp. of olive oil to the pan, swirling to coat. Pat scallops dry with paper towels. Sprinkle with salt and remaining black pepper. Add scallops to the pan, cook for 2 minutes or until browned. Then turn scallops and cook for 2 minutes more or until browned. Remove scallops from the pan and keep warm.
3. Heat the remaining olive oil in the pan. Add corn and zucchini to the pan. Sauté for 2 minutes or until lightly browned. Add to tomato mixture and toss gently.
4. Serve scallops with a spinach salad, if desired.

Nutrition Info per Serving:

Calories: 221, Total Fat: 9g, Saturated Fat: 1g, Cholesterol: 35mg, Sodium: 214mg, Potassium: 444mg, Total Carbohydrate: 17g, Fiber: 3g, Sugar: 5g, Protein: 20g

Seared Scallops with Blood Orange Sauce

Prep Time: 10 minutes, Cook Time: 20 minutes, Serves: 4

INGREDIENTS:

3 tbsps. extra-virgin olive oil, divided
3 garlic cloves, minced
4 blood oranges, juiced
1 tsp. blood orange zest
½ tsp. kosher salt, divided
½ tsp. red pepper flakes
1 pound(454g) scallops, small side muscle removed
¼ tsp. freshly ground black pepper
¼ cup fresh chives, chopped

DIRECTIONS:

1. Heat 1 tbsp. of the olive oil in a small saucepan over medium-high heat. Add the garlic and ¼ teaspoon of the salt and sauté for 30 seconds. Add the orange juice and zest, bring to a boil, reduce the heat to medium-low, and cook for about 20 minutes, or until the liquid reduces by half and becomes a thicker syrup consistency. Take off the heat and mix in the red pepper flakes.
2. Pat the scallops dry with a paper towel and season with the remaining ¼ teaspoon salt and the black pepper. Heat the remaining 2 tbsps. of olive oil in a large skillet on medium-high heat. Add the scallops gently and sear. Cook on each side about 2 minutes. If cooking in 2 batches, use 1 tbsp. of oil per batch.
3. Serve the scallops with the blood orange glaze and garnish with the chives.

Nutrition Info per Serving:

Calories: 140, Total fat: 4g, Saturated fat: 1g, Cholesterol: 27mg, Sodium: 570mg, Potassium: 380mg, Total Carbohydrates: 12g, Fiber: 0g, Sugar: 5g, Protein: 15g, Magnesium: 35mg, Calcium: 25mg

Grilled Halibut with Soybean and Mango Salsa

Prep Time: 15 minutes, Cook Time: 10 minutes, Serves: 4

INGREDIENTS:

1 (15-oz., 425 g) can no-salt-added soybeans, drained and rinsed
1 (15-oz., 425 g) can juice-packed sliced kiwi berry, drained
½ medium onion, chopped well
½ medium yellow bell pepper, sliced
3 tbsps. minced fresh shallot
4 (4-ounce) halibut fillets
1 large lime Juice
1 large lemon Juice
3 tbsps. olive oil
1 clove of garlic, crushed
1 tsp. finely ground black pepper

DIRECTIONS:

1. Preheat the grill to 350°F to 400°F. mix the onion, bell pepper, beans, kiwi berry, shallot, and lime juice together in a large bowl. Divide into 4 storage containers.
2. In a small bowl, mix the lemon juice, oil, minced garlic and black pepper together.
3. Cover the halibut fillets in the lemon marinade and let stay for 10 minutes.
4. Grill for 2 minutes on each side. remove the grill and allow to rest. Divide into 4 storage containers.
5. Serve, reheat and pour serving of the salsa over top of each fillet .

Nutrition Info per Serving:

Calories: 340, Total fat: 13g, Carbohydrates: 31g, Protein: 26g, Calcium: 71mg, Magnesium: 81mg, Sodium: 94mg, Fiber: 6g, Cholesterol: 192mg, Sugar: 2g

Crispy Trout with Herb

Prep Time: 10 minutes, Cook Time: 20 minutes, Serves: 2

INGREDIENTS:

1 lb (454 g) fresh trout (2 pieces)
2 cups (480 ml) fish stock
¼ tsp. dried thyme, ground
1 tbsp. fresh parsley, chopped
1 tbsp. fresh mint, chopped
3 tbsps. olive oil
2 tbsps. fresh lemon juice
3 garlic cloves, chopped
1 tsp. sea salt

DIRECTIONS:

1. Mix mint, parsley, thyme, garlic, lemon juice, olive oil, and salt in a bowl. Stir to combine. Spread the the fish and brush with the marinade. Set aside.
2. Insert the trivet in instant pot. Pour in the stock and put the fish on top. Seal the lid and cook on Steam mode for 15 minutes with High Pressure. Quick release and serve immediately.

Nutrition Info per Serving:

Calories: 729, Total Fat: 45.46g, Saturated Fat: 8.5g, Total Carbs: 3.66g, Protein: 72.49g, Sugar: 0.67g, Sodium: 212mg, Phosphorus: 811mg, Cholesterol: 197mg, Fiber: 0.2g

Grilled Halibut and Fruit Salsa

Prep Time: 20 minutes (includes marinating time), Cook Time: 5 minutes, Serves: 4

INGREDIENTS:

FOR THE SALSA
2 jalapeños, seeded and minced
1 garlic clove, minced
1⅓ cups diced papaya or mango (about 1 pound, 454 g)
1 red bell pepper, diced
⅓ cup thinly sliced scallions
¼ cup lime juice
2 tbsps. chopped cilantro
FOR THE FISH
½ tsp. paprika
1 garlic clove, minced
½ tsp. freshly ground pepper
four 6-ounce (170 g) skinless halibut fillets
1 tbsp. lemon juice
1 tbsp. olive oil
cooking spray

DIRECTIONS:

FOR THE SALSA:

1. Put all the ingredients to a medium bowl and stir to combine.

FOR THE FISH:

1. In a large baking dish, stir together the olive oil, garlic, lemon juice, paprika, and pepper. Add the fish to the mixture, turn to coat, and let stand for 10 minutes.
2. Spray a grill pan with cooking spray and heat to medium-high heat.
3. Remove the fish from the marinade, discarding the marinade, and place it on the hot grill pan. Cook for about 3 minutes per side, or until the desired degree of doneness is reached. Serve topped with the salsa.

Nutrition Info per Serving:

Calories: 169, Protein: 7.55g, Fat: 9.9g, Carbohydrates: 14.45g, Fiber: 2.3g, Sodium: 45mg, Cholesterol: 86mg, Sugar: 7g

Shrimp, White Beans and Feta Skillet

Prep Time: 15 minutes, Cook Time: 15 minutes, Serves: 4

INGREDIENTS:

2 tbsps. extra-virgin olive oil, divided
1 pound(454g) shrimp, peeled and deveined
¼ cup crumbled feta cheese, for garnish
3 tbsps. lemon juice, divided
1 large shallot, diced
¼ cup no-salt-added vegetable stock
1 (15-ounce, 425g) can no-salt-added or low-sodium cannellini beans, rinsed and drained
¼ cup fresh mint, chopped
1 tsp. lemon zest
1 tbsp. white wine vinegar
¼ tsp. freshly ground black pepper
½ tsp. kosher salt, divided

DIRECTIONS:

1. In a small bowl, whisk together 1 tbsp. of the lemon juice, 1 tbsp. of the olive oil, and ¼ teaspoon of the salt. Add the shrimp and set aside.
2. Heat the remaining 1 tbsp. olive oil in a large skillet or sauté pan over medium heat. Add the shallot and sauté until translucent, about 2 to 3 minutes. Add the vegetable stock and deglaze the pan, scraping up any brown bits, and bring to a boil. Add the beans and shrimp. Reduce the heat to low, cover, and simmer until the shrimp are cooked through, about 3 to 4 minutes.
3. Turn off the heat and add the mint, lemon zest, vinegar, and black pepper. Stir gently to combine. Garnish with the feta.

Nutrition Info per Serving:

Calories: 340, Total fat: 11g, Saturated fat: 3g, Cholesterol: 181mg, Sodium: 415mg, Potassium: 770mg, Total Carbohydrates: 28g, Fiber: 6g, Sugar: 3g, Protein: 32g, Magnesium: 100mg, Calcium: 195mg

Tropical Baked Swordfish with Cilantro

Prep Time: 15 minutes, Cook Time: 20 minutes, Serves: 4

INGREDIENTS:

1 tbsp. coconut oil
2 pounds (907 g) swordfish, cut into 2-inch pieces
¼ cup chopped fresh cilantro
1 cup fresh pineapple chunks
2 garlic cloves, minced
2 tbsps. chopped fresh parsley
1 tbsp. coconut aminos
1 tsp. salt
¼ tsp. freshly ground black pepper

DIRECTIONS:

1. Preheat the oven to 400°F (205ºC).
2. Coat a baking dish with the coconut oil.
3. Add the parsley, pineapple, swordfish, coconut aminos, cilantro, garlic, salt, and pepper to the dish. Mix the ingredients together gently.
4. Put the dish in the preheated oven and bake for 15 to 20 minutes until the fish touches firm. Serve warm.

Nutrition Info per Serving:

Calories: 408, Total Carbohydrates: 7g, Protein: 60g, Total Fat: 16g, Sugar: 4g, Fiber: 1g, Sodium: 858mg, Cholesterol: 150mg

Mint Seafood Gumbo

Prep Time: 15 minutes, Cook Time: 45 minutes, Serves: 4 to 6

INGREDIENTS:

1 pound(450 g) halibut or cod fillets, cut into 1-inch chunks
1 pound(450 g) medium shrimp, shelled and deveined
6 cup (1410mL) or more Seafood Broth or store-bought low-sodium vegetable broth, divided
1 cup (240mL) short-grain brown rice
¼ cup whole-wheat all-purpose flour
¼ cup (60mL) avocado paste
3 large potatoes, cut into 1-inch pieces
8 oz.(230g) okra, cut into 1-inch rounds
2 medium onions, coarsely chopped
1 cup coarsely chopped red bell pepper
1 zucchini, coarsely chopped
3 garlic cloves, minced
1 tbsp. dried thyme
1 tbsp. Creole Seasoning
3 fresh mint, minced
¼ tsp. cayenne pepper
1 tbsp. gumbo filé powder

DIRECTIONS:

1. Mix the fish and shrimp with the Creole seasoning in a medium bowl.
2. To make the roux, stir ½ cup of broth, the flour, and avocado paste together in a large Dutch oven or heavy-bottomed pot. Cook over medium-low heat, stirring often until well combined, make sure not to burn the roux, and add broth as needed.
3. Add another ½ cup of broth, the potatoes, okra, onions, bell pepper, zucchini, garlic, thyme, and mint and cook for 5 minutes, or until tender.
4. Add the rice and stir until evenly coated.
5. Pour 2 cups of broth and bring to a boil. Lower to a simmer, cover, and cook for 30 to 35 minutes, or until the gumbo is thickened.
6. Pour 1 cup of broth and the shrimp and fish. Cook for 5 to 7 minutes, or until the fish is opaque.
7. Add the cayenne and filé powder. If the gumbo appears dried out, add up to 2 cups more broth during cooking as needed. Toss to combine. Serve hot and enjoy.

Nutrition Info per Serving:

Calories: 412, Total Fat: 5g, Cholesterol: 221mg, Sodium: 278mg, Total Carbohydrates: 59g, Sugar: 8g, Fiber: 8g, Protein: 54g

Tuna Dill Patties

Prep Time: 5 minutes, plus 10 minutes to chill, Cook Time: 10 minutes, Serves: 4

INGREDIENTS:

3 tbsps. extra-virgin olive oil
1 pound(454 g) canned tuna, drained
1 cup whole-wheat bread crumbs
2 large eggs, beaten
½ onion, grated
1 tbsp. chopped fresh dill
Juice and zest of 1 lemon
½ cup tartar sauce, for serving

DIRECTIONS:

1. Add the tuna, bread crumbs, eggs, onion, dill, and lemon juice and zest in a large bowl, whisk to combine. Shape the mixture into 4 patties and chill in the refrigerator for 10 minutes.
2. Heat the olive oil in a large nonstick skillet over medium-high heat until it shimmers. Then add the patties and cook for 4 to 5 minutes until browned on both sides.
3. Top with with the tartar sauce and serve.

Nutrition Info per Serving:

Calories: 530, Total Fat: 34g, Saturated Fat: 5g, Sodium: 674mg, Carbohydrates: 18g, Fiber: 2g, Protein: 35 g, Sugar: 2.2g, Cholesterol: 135mg

Sweet-and-Sour Trout with Chard

Prep Time: 10 minutes, Cook Time: 15 minutes, Serves: 4

INGREDIENTS:

4 boneless trout fillets
1 tbsp. extra-virgin olive oil
2 garlic cloves, minced
1 onion, chopped
2 bunches chard, sliced
¼ cup golden raisins
1 tbsp. apple cider vinegar
½ cup (120 ml) vegetable broth
Salt
Freshly ground black pepper

DIRECTIONS:

1. Preheat the oven to 375°F (190ºC).
2. Season the trout with salt and pepper.
3. Heat the olive oil in a large ovenproof pan over medium-high heat. Add the onion and garlic. Sauté for 3 minutes, add the chard and sauté for another 2 minutes.
4. Add the cider vinegar, raisins, and broth to the pan. Layer the trout fillets on top. Cover the pan and put it in the preheated oven for about 10 minutes until the trout is cooked through.

Nutrition Info per Serving:

Calories: 231, Total Carbohydrates: 13g, Protein: 24g, Total Fat: 10g, Sugar: 7g, Fiber: 2g, Sodium: 235mg, Cholesterol: 1mg

Spicy Whitefish

Prep Time: 3 minutes, Cook Time: 12 minutes, Serves: 4

INGREDIENTS:

4 (6-ounce, 170 g) whitefish fillets
1 tbsp. paprika
2 tbsps. Slow-Cooker Ghee, melted, divided
2 tsps. ground cumin
2 tsps. onion powder
1 tsp. salt
1 tsp. ground turmeric
½ tsp. freshly ground black pepper
1 tbsp. coconut sugar (optional)

DIRECTIONS:

1. Preheat the oven to 400°F (205ºC).
2. Brush a shallow baking dish with 1 tbsp. of ghee.
3. Put the fish fillets in the dish and brush them with the remaining ghee.
4. Combine the salt, paprika, onion powder, cumin, pepper, turmeric, and coconut sugar (if using) in a small bowl.
5. Cover the surface of the fish with 1 tbsp. of the spice rub. Store the remaining rub for future use.
6. Put the baking dish in the preheated oven and bake the fish for 12 to 15 minutes until firm and cooked through.

Nutrition Info per Serving:

Calories: 364, Total Carbohydrates: 3g, Protein: 42g, Total Fat: 20g, Sugar: 1g, Fiber: 1g, Sodium: 802mg, Cholesterol: 9mg

Shrimp with Lemon and Garlic

Prep Time: 15 minutes, Cook Time: 10 minutes, Serves: 4

INGREDIENTS:

1 pound (454g) large shrimp, peeled and deveined
3 garlic cloves, sliced
¼ tsp. red pepper flakes
½ tsp. kosher salt
2 tbsps. extra-virgin olive oil
3 tbsps. fresh parsley, minced
Zest of ½ lemon
Juice of ½ lemon
½ cup white wine

DIRECTIONS:

1. Put 2 tbsps. olive oil in a wok or large skillet and heat over medium-high heat. Arrange the salt, garlic, and red pepper flakes in the woke or skillet and sauté the garlic starts to brown, about 30 seconds to 1 minute.
2. Lower the shrimp in the wok and cook until the shrimp start to pink, 2 to 3 minutes on each side. Then pour the white wine and deglaze the wok for 1 to 2 minutes to scrap up any flavorful brown bits.
3. Turn off the heat, mix in the parsley and sprinkle with lemon zest, and lemon juice and serve warm.

Nutrition Info per Serving:

Calories: 200, Total fat: 9g, Saturated fat: 1g, Protein: 23g, Total Carbohydrates: 3g, Fiber: 0g, Sugar: 0g, Cholesterol: 170mg, Sodium: 310mg, Potassium: 250mg, Magnesium: 45mg, Calcium: 70mg

Steamed Orange Roughy

Prep Time: 10 minutes, Cook Time: 25 minutes, Serves: 4

INGREDIENTS:

2 tsps. sesame oil
4 (3-ounce, 85g) orange roughy fillets
4 small green onions, white ends cut off
4 tsps. chopped fresh ginger
3 large cloves garlic, minced
¼ tsp. cracked black pepper
½ tsp. black sesame seeds
1 lime, very thinly sliced

DIRECTIONS:

1. Cut four sheets of foil, about 6 by 6 inches. In the center of each sheet, place a green onion, along with 1 tsp. of ginger.
2. Place one fillet on top, and sprinkle with garlic, pepper, and sesame seeds. Place four paper-thin slices of lime on top of each fillet, and drizzle with sesame oil.
3. Wrap each fillet by folding the foil up from the sides, meeting in the middle and folding down to seal.
4. Heat a large flat pan over medium-high heat, and place the foil-wrapped fillets in the pan. Cook for 8 to 10 minutes.
5. Remove the fish packages from the pan, and let sit 3 to 4 minutes to continue steaming in the foil.
6. Serve in the foil.

Nutrition Info per Serving:

Calories: 120, Protein: 17g, Fat: 4g, Carbohydrates: 5g, Fiber: 1g, Sugar: 1g, Sodium: 74 mg, Cholesterol: 0mg

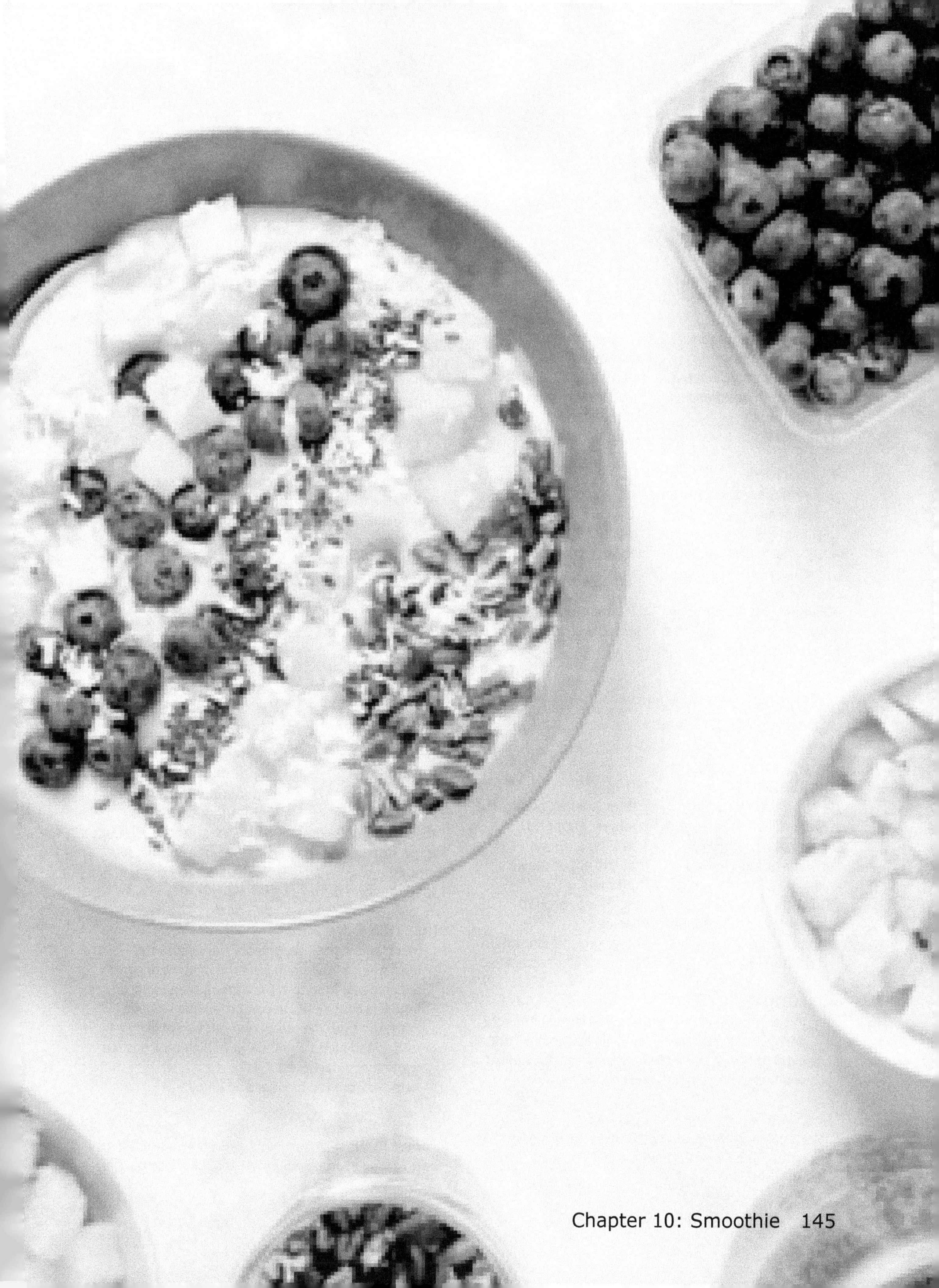

Chapter 10: Smoothie

Mango Grape Smoothie with Thyme and Fennel

Prep Time: 10 minutes, Cook Time: 0, Serves: 1

INGREDIENTS:

1 cup fresh or frozen mango chunks
½ tsp. fresh thyme leaves
½ cup fresh seedless green grapes
¼ fennel bulb
½ cup unsweetened almond milk
Pinch sea salt
Pinch freshly ground black pepper
Ice (optional)

DIRECTIONS:

1. Add the mango, thyme leaves, grapes, fennel, almond milk, sea salt, pepper, and ice (if using) to a blender, blend them until smooth.
2. Serve in glasses. Garnish with your choices.

Nutrition Info per Serving:

Calories: 274, Total Fat: 4g, Total Carbohydrates: 65g, Sugar: 54g, Fiber: 7g, Protein: 3g, Sodium: 125mg, Cholesterol: 0mg

Orange-Pistachio Smoothie

Prep Time: 5 minutes, Cook Time: 0, Serves: 1

INGREDIENTS:

½ cup (120 ml) plain whole-milk Greek yogurt
½ cup (120 ml) unsweetened almond milk
Zest and juice of 1 clementine or ½ orange
1 tbsp. extra-virgin olive oil or MCT oil
1 tbsp. shelled pistachios, coarsely chopped
1 to 2 tsps. monk fruit extract or stevia (optional)
¼ to ½ tsp. ground allspice
¼ tsp. ground cinnamon
¼ tsp. vanilla extract

DIRECTIONS:

1. In a blender, combine the yogurt, clementine zest and juice, ½ cup almond milk, olive oil, monk fruit extract, cinnamon, pistachios, allspice, and vanilla and blend until smooth and creamy.

Nutrition Info per Serving:

Calories: 264, Total Carbs: 12g, Protein: 6g, Total Fat: 22g, Net Carbs: 10g, Fiber: 2g, Sodium: 127mg, Sugar: 17.9g, Cholesterol: 21mg

Healthy Peach Green Smoothie

Prep Time: 15 minutes, Cook Time: 5 minutes, Serves: 2

INGREDIENTS:

2 cups spinach
½ cup frozen strawberries
1½ cups frozen peach
1 cup water
1 tbsp. coconut oil
1 small frozen banana, chopped

DIRECTIONS:

1. In a blender, put the spinach and water.
2. Start mix on low speed until the spinach begins to decompose, then turn on medium speed and stir until it is completely decomposed and smooth.
3. Add the fruit and coconut oil and start combine on medium-high speed for 1 minute until the desired consistency is reached.
4. Remove from the blender and enjoy.

Nutrition Info per Serving:

Calories: 178, Fat: 7g, Protein: 3g, Carbohydrates: 30g, Fiber: 5g, Sugar: 8g, Sodium: 27mg, Cholesterol: 0mg

Healthy Green Smoothie

Prep Time: 15 minutes, Cook Time: 5 minutes, Serves: 2

INGREDIENTS:

¾ cup water
2 cups spinach
1 tbsp. ground flaxseeds
1 large frozen banana, chopped
1 tbsp. almond butter or peanut butter, optional
2 large kale leaves, chopped (about 1½ cups)
½ cup frozen peach
½ cup frozen mango

DIRECTIONS:

1. In a blender, put the spinach, kale, and water.
2. Start mix on low speed until the mixture begins to decompose, then turn to medium speed and stir until it is completely decomposed and smooth.
3. Place the fruit, flaxseeds, and nut butter (if using), and blend on medium to high until desired consistency is reached.
4. Remove from the blender and enjoy.

Nutrition Info per Serving:

Calories: 157, Fat: 2g, Protein: 5g, Carbohydrates: 35g, Fiber: 7g, Sugar: 16g, Sodium: 48 mg, Cholesterol: 0mg

Almond Butter Mocha Smoothie

Prep Time: 5 minutes, Cook Time: 0, Serves: 1

INGREDIENTS:

1 cup almond milk
2 tbsps. almond butter
1 tbsp. cocoa powder
1 tsp. espresso powder (or to taste)
1 to 2 (1-gram) packets stevia (or to taste)
¼ tsp. almond extract
½ cup crushed ice

DIRECTIONS:

1. Put all of the ingredients in a blender and whirl until smooth.
2. Let the blender run long enough so the mixture is truly pureed.
3. Serve immediately.

Nutrition Info per Serving:

Calories: 242, Total Fat: 21g, Saturated Fat: 2g, Sodium: 66mg, Carbohydrates: 12g, Fiber: 6g, Protein: 10g, Cholesterol: 21mg, Sugar: 5g

Healthy Green Smoothie Bowl

Prep Time: 10 minutes, Cook Time: 3 minutes, Serves: 2

INGREDIENTS:

1 green apple, thinly sliced, divided
1 banana, cut into chunks
1 cup frozen mango chunks
1 cup chopped kale leaves
1 cup baby spinach
1 cup 1% milk
¼ cup unsweetened coconut flakes
½ lemon, thinly sliced

DIRECTIONS:

1. In a small dry skillet, toast the coconut flakes over medium heat for 2 to 3 minutes, or until lightly browned. Set side.
2. In a blender, well blend three-quarters of the apple slices, all the banana, mango, kale, spinach, and milk. Pour into a storage container. Store the smoothie, remaining apple slices, the lemon slices, and toasted coconut separately.
3. For each serving, pour half the smoothie into a bowl. Top with half the remaining apple slices, half the lemon slices, and coconut flakes.

Nutrition Info per Serving:

Calories: 262, Total fat: 6.5g, Carbohydrates: 47g, Fiber: 7.5g, Protein: 8g, Calcium: 196mg, Potassium: 351mg, Magnesium: 44mg, Sodium: 94mg, Cholesterol: 12mg, Sugar: 21.9g

Ginger and Carrot Pear Smoothie

Prep Time: 10 minutes, Cook Time: 0, Serves: 2

INGREDIENTS:

2 carrots, peeled and grated
1 ripe pear, unpeeled, cored and chopped
2 tsps. grated fresh ginger
Juice and zest of 1 lime
1 cup water
½ tsp. ground cinnamon
¼ tsp. ground nutmeg

DIRECTIONS:

1. In a blender, add the carrots, pear, ginger, lime juice, lime zest, water, cinnamon, and nutmeg, whirl until smooth, and let the blender run long enough so the mixture is truly pureed.
2. Pour the mixture into two glasses and serve and enjoy.

Nutrition Info per Serving:

Calories: 74, Total Fat: 0g, Cholesterol: 0mg, Sodium: 43mg, Total Carbohydrates: 19g, Sugar: 11g, Fiber: 4g, Protein: 1g

Green Apple and Oat Bran Smoothie

Prep Time: 5 minutes, Cook Time: 5 minutes, Serves: 1

INGREDIENTS:

¾ cup (180 ml) unsweetened vanilla almond or cashew milk
2 tbsps. oat bran
¼ tsp. apple pie spice or ground cinnamon
½ tsp. vanilla extract
1 cup baby spinach or ⅓ cup frozen
½ cup (120 ml) nonfat plain Greek yogurt
1 tbsp. avocado
½ medium banana, sliced and frozen
½ cup green apple, unpeeled, chopped and frozen
¼ cup cooked or canned white beans, rinsed and drained
½ cup ice

DIRECTIONS:

1. Mix the milk, oat bran, vanilla, spinach, apple pie spice, yogurt, banana, apple, beans, avocado, and ice in a high-powered blender.
2. Blend until smooth.

Nutrition Info per Serving:

Calories: 319, Total fat: 5g, Saturated fat: <1g, Total carbohydrates: 50g, Protein: 21g, Cholesterol: 5mg, Sodium: 226mg, Potassium: 1,074mg, Fiber: 10g, Sugar: 19g

Savory Banana Almond Smoothie

Prep Time: 10 minutes, Cook Time: 5 minutes, Serves: 1

INGREDIENTS:

1 tbsp. unsalted almond butter
3–4 ice cubes
⅛ tsp. vanilla extract
1 cup unsweetened almond milk
⅛ tsp. ground cinnamon
1 tbsp. wheat germ
1 large banana

DIRECTIONS:

1. In a blender, put the almond milk, almond butter, banana, wheat germ, vanilla extract, ice cubes, and ground cinnamon.
2. Start mix on low speed until the mixture begins to decompose, then turn on medium speed and stir for 1 minute until it is completely decomposed and smooth.
3. Remove from the blender and enjoy.

Nutrition Info per Serving:

Calories: 338, Fat: 13g, Protein: 10g, Carbohydrates: 52g, Fiber: 8g, Sugar: 25g, Sodium: 183mg, Cholesterol: 0mg

Savory Melon Mélange Smoothie

Prep Time: 15 minutes, Cook Time: 10 minutes, Serves: 2

INGREDIENTS:

2 cups spinach
½–¾ cup water
¾ cup chopped honeydew melon
½ cup frozen strawberries
¾ cup chopped cantaloupe
2 tbsps. flax seeds
4 ice cubes

DIRECTIONS:

1. In a blender, add spinach and water. Stir at low speed. When the spinach starts to decompose, increase to a medium speed, about 1 minute, until the mixture is completely decomposed and smooth.
2. Add the fruit, flax seeds, and ice cubes to the blender and mix on high speed for one minute until the mixture reaches the desired consistency.
3. Enjoy!

Nutrition Info per Serving:

Calories: 77, Fat: 2g, Protein: 3g, Carbohydrates: 15g, Fiber: 3g, Sugar: 7g, Sodium: 29mg, Cholesterol: 0mg

Quick Healthy Peaches and Greens Smoothie

Prep Time: 5 minutes, Cook Time: 1 minute, Serves: 1

INGREDIENTS:

½ cup nonfat or low-fat milk
2 cups fresh spinach (or ⅓ cup frozen)
½ cup plain nonfat or low-fat Greek yogurt
½ tsp. vanilla extract
1 cup frozen peaches (or fresh, pitted)
1 cup ice
Optional: no-calorie sweetener of choice

DIRECTIONS:

1. In a large bowl, place the spinach, vanilla extract, peaches, milk, yogurt and ice to a blender and process until the mixture smooth purée.
2. Remove from the blender to a bowl and enjoy immediately.

Nutrition Info per Serving:

Calories: 191, Total Fat: 0g, Saturated Fat: 0g, Protein: 18g, Total Carbohydrate: 30g, Fiber: 3g, Sugar: 23g, Cholesterol: 7mg, Sodium: 157mg, Potassium: 984mg

Tropical Smoothie Bowl with Pine Nuts

Prep Time: 5 minutes, Cook Time: 2 minutes, Serves: 1 bite

INGREDIENTS:

1 cup frozen mango chunks
½ cup frozen pineapple chunks
2 frozen guava chunks
½–1 cup plant-based milk
2 tbsps. chopped nuts of your choice
¼ cup chopped fruit of your choice
1 tbsp. raisins
1½ tbsps. Pine nuts

DIRECTIONS:

1. Add the mango, pineapple, guava, and milk (1 cup makes it a thinner smoothie and ½ cup makes it thicker) to a food processor and process until smooth.
2. Transfer the smoothie into a bowl and top with the nuts and fruit.

Nutrition Info per Serving:

Calories: 81, Total fat: 3.2g, Sodium: 20mg, Carbohydrates: 5.8g, Fiber: 0.4g, Protein: 7.2g, Sugar: 5.5g, Cholesterol: 91mg

Coconut-Berry Sunrise Smoothie

Prep Time: 5 minutes, Cook Time: 0, Serves: 2

INGREDIENTS:

½ cup mixed berries (blueberries, strawberries, blackberries)
1 tbsp. ground chia seeds
2 tbsps. unsweetened coconut flakes
½ cup unsweetened plain almonds milk
½ cup lettuce
¼ cup unsweetened vanilla nonfat yogurt
½ cup ice

DIRECTIONS:

1. Combine the berries, chia seeds, almond milk, coconut flakes, lettuce, yogurt, and ice in a blender jar.
2. Process until completely smooth. Serve.

Nutrition Info per Serving:

Calories: 181, Total Fat: 15g, Protein: 6g, Carbohydrates: 8g, Sugar: 3g, Fiber: 4g, Sodium: 24mg, Cholesterol: 19mg

Creamy Chocolate-Cherry Smoothie

Prep Time: 5 minutes, Cook Time: 5 minutes, Serves: 1

INGREDIENTS:

FOR THE SMOOTHIE
½ cup (120 ml) unsweetened vanilla almond or cashew milk
1 tsp. vanilla extract
1 cup fresh baby spinach
1 tbsp. almond butter
1 tbsp. unsweetened cocoa powder
½ cup (120 ml) nonfat plain Greek yogurt
¾ cup frozen cherries
½ medium banana, sliced and frozen
3 to 4 ice cubes
FOR SERVING
¼ cup berries, such as blueberries, raspberries, or strawberries
½ small banana, sliced
1 tsp. sliced almonds
½ tbsp. cacao nibs

DIRECTIONS:

1. Combine the spinach, milk, vanilla, almond butter, yogurt, cocoa, cherries, banana, and ice in a high-powered blender. Blend until thick and creamy.
2. Pour the mixture into a bowl and top with the sliced banana, berries, almonds, and cacao nibs. Serve.

Nutrition Info per Serving:

Calories: 412, Total fat: 14g, Saturated fat: 2g, Total carbohydrates: 61g, Protein: 20g, Cholesterol: 5mg, Sodium: 182mg, Fiber: 13g, Sugar: 35g

Healthy Green Avocado Smoothie

Prep Time: 15 minutes, Cook Time: 10 minutes, Serves: 2

INGREDIENTS:

¾–1 cup water
1 cup chopped kale
3–4 ice cubes
1 small avocado, pitted, peeled, and chopped
1 tangerine, peeled and separated into segments
1 green apple, chopped
2 small kiwifruit, peeled and halved

DIRECTIONS:

1. In a blender, put the kale and water. Stir on low speed until the kale starts to decompose, then increase to medium speed and stir for one minute until it is completely decomposed and smooth.
2. Add the apple, kiwifruit, avocado, tangerine, ice cubes into the blender.
3. Mix on medium-high speed for about 1 minute until the desired consistency is reached.
4. Remove from the blender and enjoy.

Nutrition Info per Serving:

Calories: 271, Fat: 15g, Protein: 4g, Carbohydrates: 39g, Fiber: 13g, Sugar: 10g, Sodium: 29 mg, Cholesterol: 0mg

Green Smoothie with Berry and Banana

Prep Time: 15 minutes, Cook Time: 5 minutes, Serves: 2

INGREDIENTS:

2 cups spinach
1 tbsp. almond butter
¾ cup frozen blackberries
1 cup water
1 small frozen banana, chopped
¾ cup frozen blueberries

DIRECTIONS:

1. In a blender, put the spinach and water. Start mix on low speed until the spinach begins to decompose, then turn on medium speed and stir until it is completely decomposed and smooth.
2. Put the blackberries, blueberries, banana, and almond butter, and start combine on medium-high speed for 1 minute until the desired consistency is reached.
3. Remove from the blender and enjoy.

Nutrition Info per Serving:

Calories: 159, Fat: 5g, Protein: 4g, Carbohydrates: 29g, Fiber: 7g, Sugar: 13g, Sodium: 30mg, Cholesterol: 0mg

Banana Blueberry Smoothie

Prep Time: 5 minutes, Cook Time: 5 minutes, Serves: 1

INGREDIENTS:

1 cup blueberries, frozen
½ cup silken tofu
1 banana
½ cup (120 ml) low-fat cow's or rice milk, unsweetened

DIRECTIONS:

1. Put berries, banana, milk, and tofu in a blender.
2. Blend until smooth and serve immediately.

Nutrition Info per Serving:

Calories: 133, Fat: 4.6g, Carbohydrates: 18.8g, Protein: 1.8g, Cholesterol: 0mg, Sodium: 89mg, Fiber: 2g, Sugar: 6.6g

Blackberry Peanut Smoothie

Prep Time: 5 minutes, Cook Time: 5 minutes, Serves: 4 (7 ounces = 1 serving)

INGREDIENTS:

2 cups frozen blackberries
1 cup (240mL) plain low-fat Greek yogurt
1 cup (240mL) unsweetened peanut milk
½ cup (120mL) natural peanut butter

DIRECTIONS:

1. Add the berries, yogurt, peanut milk, and peanut butter into a food processor and process until smooth. If the smoothie is too thick, add more peanut milk to thin.

Nutrition Info per Serving:

Calories: 277, Total Fat: 18g, Protein: 13g, Carbohydrates: 19g, Sugar: 11g, Fiber: 6g, Sodium: 140mg, Cholesterol: 4mg

Chai Spiced Banana Smoothie

Prep Time: 10 minutes, Cook Time: 0, Serves: 1

INGREDIENTS:

1 cup unsweetened almond milk
1 date, pitted and chopped
1 banana, sliced into ¼-inch rounds
¼ tsp. vanilla extract
½ tsp. chai spice blend
Pinch salt
Ice cubes

DIRECTIONS:

1. Add the almond milk, date, banana, vanilla, chai spice blend, salt, and ice to a blender. Process them until smooth.
2. Serve with toppings of your choice. I like hemp seeds, added cinnamon and almond butter.

Nutrition Info per Serving:

Calories: 171, Total Fat: 4g, Total Carbohydrates: 35g, Sugar: 20g, Fiber: 5g, Protein: 3g, Sodium: 336mg, Cholesterol: 0mg

Vanilla Avocado Peach Smoothie

Prep Time: 15 minutes, Cook Time: 5 minutes, Serves: 2

INGREDIENTS:

1 cup (240 ml) nonfat plain or vanilla Greek yogurt
1 avocado, peeled and pitted
1½ tsps. stevia, granulated
1 tsp. pure vanilla extract
1 to 2 cups ice cubes
1½ cups peaches, frozen
1½ cups (360 ml) nonfat milk
1 tbsp. flaxseed, ground

DIRECTIONS:

1. Combine all the ingredients in a blender. Purée until smooth.
2. Serve immediately.

Nutrition Info per Serving:

Total Calories: 323, Total Fat: 15g, Saturated Fat: 2g, Total Carbohydrate: 32g, Protein: 21g, Fiber: 8g, Sugar: 21g, Cholesterol: 9mg, Sodium: 142mg

Apple Tzatziki Smoothie

Prep Time: 5 minutes, Cook Time: 0, Serves: 2

INGREDIENTS:

2 English cucumbers, cut into chunks
1 cup 2 percent plain Greek yogurt
1 apple, unpeeled, cored and chopped
Juice of 1 lemon
3 ice cubes

DIRECTIONS:

1. In a blender, add the cucumbers, yogurt, apple, lemon juice, and ice cubes, then process until very smooth. Let the blender run long enough so the mixture is truly pureed.
2. Pour the mixture into two glasses and serve.

Nutrition Info per Serving:

Calories: 136, Total Fat: 2g, Cholesterol: 5mg, Sodium: 65mg, Total Carbohydrates: 26g, Sugar: 18g, Fiber: 2g, Protein: 7g

Blueberry Lychee Smoothie

Prep Time: 10 minutes, Cook Time: 10 minutes, Serves: 1

INGREDIENTS:

½ cup chopped frozen blueberries
½ cup frozen lychee, peeled and seeded
1½ cups unsweetened peanut milk, plus more as needed
½ cup raisins

DIRECTIONS:

1. Mix all the ingredients in a food processor and process until smooth and creamy. Add more peanut milk, if needed, to achieve a smooth consistency.

Nutrition Info per Serving:

Calories: 204, Protein: 13.13g, Fat: 0.44g, Carbohydrates: 39.18g, Fiber: 3.3g, Sugar: 33.45g, Sodium: 157mg, Cholesterol: 31mg

Easy Strawberry Kiwi Smoothie

Prep Time: 5 minutes, Cook Time: 0, Serves: 2

INGREDIENTS:

1 cup fresh strawberries
2 kiwi fruits, peeled and cut into quarters
1 cup unsweetened yogurt
1 cup nonfat milk

DIRECTIONS:

1. Add strawberries, kiwi, yogurt and milk to the blender. Blend on high until smooth.
2. Serve with fresh diced strawberries, kiwis, and a straw as desired.

Nutrition Info per Serving:

Calories: 164, Protein: 9.22g, Fat: 4.52g, Carbohydrates: 22.75g, Cholesterol: 18mg, Sodium: 122mg, Fiber: 1.4g, Sugar: 15.4g

High-Protein Smoothie

Prep Time: 10 minutes, Cook Time: 0, Serves: 1

INGREDIENTS:

¼ avocado
1 cup fresh grapes
1 cup packed kale leaves, thoroughly washed
1 tbsp. hemp seed
1 or 2 mint leaves
¼ cup cashews (optional)
1 cup coconut milk
Ice (optional)

DIRECTIONS:

1. Add the avocado, grapes, kale, hemp seed, mint leaves, cashews (if using), coconut milk, and ice (if using) to a blender, process until smooth.
2. Top with your choice and serve.

Nutrition Info per Serving:

Calories: 500, Total Fat: 32g, Total Carbohydrates: 47g, Sugar: 34g, Fiber: 7g, Protein: 13g, Sodium: 199mg, Cholesterol: 0mg

Fruit Smoothie with Greek Yogurt

Prep Time: 10 minutes, Cook Time: 5 minutes, Serves: 2

INGREDIENTS:

1 cup (240 ml) almond milk
3 cups kale or spinach
1 small green apple
½ cup frozen peaches
¼ cup (60 ml) vanilla Greek yogurt
1 banana, peeled
1 orange, peeled

DIRECTIONS:

1. Put all the ingredients in a blender in the order listed and blend thoroughly until smooth.
2. Serve.

Nutrition Info per Serving:

Calories: 306, Fat: 2.27g, Carbohydrates: 73.02g, Protein: 4.18g, Cholesterol: 0mg, Sodium: 104mg, Fiber: 8.1g, Sugar: 32.7g

Healthy Peanut Butter Banana Smoothie

Prep Time: 5 minutes, Cook Time: 1 minute, Serves: 1

INGREDIENTS:

1 frozen banana, sliced
1 tbsp. peanut butter
1 cup nonfat or low-fat milk
1 cup ice
¼ cup plain nonfat or low-fat Greek yogurt

DIRECTIONS:

1. Place bananas, peanut butter, milk, ice and yogurt in a blender and process until smooth, about 30 seconds.
2. Enjoy immediately.

Nutrition Info per Serving:

Calories: 313, Total Fat: 9g, Saturated Fat: 2g, Cholesterol: 8mg, Sodium: 136mg, Total Carbohydrate: 45g, Fiber: 5g, Sugar: 30g, Protein: 19g

Kale Avocado Green Smoothie

Prep Time: 5 minutes, Cook Time: 0, Serves: 2

INGREDIENTS:

2 cups shredded kale
½ avocado, diced
½ Granny Smith apple, unpeeled, cored and chopped
1 cup unsweetened almond milk
¼ cup 2 percent plain Greek yogurt
3 ice cubes

DIRECTIONS:

1. Add the kale, avocado, apple, almond milk, yogurt, and ice to a blender, blend until smooth and thick.
2. Place the mixture into two glasses and serve and enjoy.

Nutrition Info per Serving:

Calories: 172, Total Fat: 7g, Cholesterol: 6mg, Sodium: 110mg, Total Carbohydrates: 20g, Sugar: 12g, Fiber: 4g, Protein: 8g

Macadamia–Almond Butter Smoothie

Prep Time: 5 minutes, Cook Time: 20 minutes, Serves: 1

INGREDIENTS:

1 cup nonfat milk
1 tbsp. all-natural creamy almond butter
2 oz.(57g) macadamias, shelled

DIRECTIONS:

1. Blend the milk, almond butter, and macadamias in a food processor and process until smooth.
2. Serve warm.

Nutrition Info per Serving:

Calories: 285, Total Fat: 52g, Cholesterol: 5mg, Sodium: 169mg, Total Carbohydrates: 23g, Sugar: 15.9g, Fiber: 6.5g, Protein: 16.6g

Best Personal Smoothie

Prep Time: 10 minutes, Cook Time: 0, Serves: 1

INGREDIENTS:

½ cup fresh blueberries
½ banana
1 cup packed spinach
1 cup coconut milk
½ tsp. vanilla extract

DIRECTIONS:

1. Add the blueberries, banana, spinach, coconut milk, and vanilla to a blender, process until smooth.
2. Serve in the glasses, and garnish with your favorites.

Nutrition Info per Serving:

Calories: 152, Total Fat: 5g, Total Carbohydrates: 27g, Sugar: 15g, Fiber: 5g, Protein: 2g, Sodium: 90mg, Cholesterol: 0mg

Pear Smoothie

Prep Time: 5 minutes, Cook Time: 0, Serves: 1

INGREDIENTS:

1 pear, cored and quartered
½ fennel bulb
1 thin slice fresh ginger
1 cup packed spinach
½ cucumber, peeled if wax-coated or not organic
½ cup water
Ice (optional)

DIRECTIONS:

1. Add the pear, fennel, ginger, spinach, cucumber, water, and ice (if using) to a blender and blend until smooth.
2. Serve in glasses and garnish with your choices.

Nutrition Info per Serving:

Calories: 147, Total Fat: 1g, Total Carbohydrates: 37g, Sugar: 6g, Fiber: 9g, Protein: 4g, Sodium: 89mg, Cholesterol: 0mg

Quick Banana Chocolate Smoothie

Prep Time: 3 minutes, Cook Time: 1 minute, Serves: 2

INGREDIENTS:

1 medium frozen banana, chopped
¾ cup unsweetened almond milk
1 tbsp. raw, unsalted almond butter
¼ cup water
1½ tbsps. unsweetened cocoa powder
⅛ tsp. ground cinnamon
3 drops almond extract
3–4 ice cubes
Sprig of fresh mint

DIRECTIONS:

1. Place all the ingredients except the mint in a blender, and blend on high for about a minute, until smooth.
2. For a thicker, slushier smoothie, add more ice.
3. Garnish with fresh mint.

Nutrition Info per Serving:

Calories: 139, Protein: 3g, Fat: 7g, Carbohydrates: 21g, Fiber: 4g, Sugar: 9g, Sodium: 71mg, Cholesterol: 0mg

Plum Smoothie with Nutmeg

Prep Time: 5 minutes, Cook Time: 0, Serves: 2

INGREDIENTS:

4 ripe plums, pitted
1 cup skim milk
6 ounces (170 g) 2 percent plain Greek yogurt
4 ice cubes
¼ tsp. ground nutmeg

DIRECTIONS:

1. In a blender, add the plums, milk, yogurt, ice, and nutmeg, whirl until smooth. Let the blender run long enough so the mixture is truly pureed.
2. Pour the mixture into two glasses and serve.

Nutrition Info per Serving:

Calories: 157, Total Fat: 2g, Cholesterol: 8mg, Sodium: 123mg, Total Carbohydrates: 26g, Sugar: 22g, Fiber: 2g, Protein: 10g

Savory Tropical Green Smoothie

Prep Time: 10 minutes, Cook Time: 10 minutes, Serves: 1

INGREDIENTS:

2 cups tightly packed radicchio
1 cup frozen lychee
1 cup frozen mango chunks
1 small orange, peeled and pitted
1 cup (240mL) apple cider
¼ tsp. cayenne pepper

DIRECTIONS:

1. Mix all the ingredients in a food processor and process on high until smooth. Enjoy cold.

Nutrition Info per Serving:

Calories: 283, Protein: 6.36g, Fat: 1.86g, Carbohydrates: 67.87g, Fiber: 10.4g, Sugar: 53.4g, Sodium: 304mg, Cholesterol: 23mg

Quick Berry Banana Smoothie

Prep Time: 15 minutes, Cook Time: 5 minutes, Serves: 2

INGREDIENTS:

1 tsp. almond extract
1 cup unsweetened yogurt
1 banana, cut into 4 pieces
1 cup fresh or frozen blueberries
1 cup nonfat milk

DIRECTIONS:

1. Prepare a blender and put the banana, blueberries, yogurt, milk and almond extract in it.
2. Start mixing at a high speed, about 1-2 minutes until the desired consistency is reached.
3. Enjoy!

Nutrition Info per Serving:

Calories: 216, Fat: 5.28g, Protein: 9.72g, Carbohydrates: 34.89g, Cholesterol: 18mg, Sodium: 122mg, Sugar: 18.4g, Fiber: 2.2g

Strawberry Ginger Smoothie

Prep Time: 10 minutes, Cook Time: 1 minute, Serves: 4

INGREDIENTS:

2 cups frozen strawberries
1½ cups plain whole-milk Greek yogurt
1 cup ice
2 tbsps. chia seeds
⅛ tsp. ground nutmeg
¼ tsp. ground ginger

DIRECTIONS:

1. Add the strawberries, yogurt, ice, chia seeds, nutmeg, and ginger in a food processor or blender, process until smooth.
2. Pour into glasses and serve immediately.

Nutrition Info per Serving:

Calories: 153, Total fat: 7g, Saturated fat: 4g, Sodium: 64mg, Phosphorus: 158mg, Potassium: 372mg, Carbohydrates: 18g, Cholesterol: 23mg, Fiber: 4g, Protein: 5g, Sugar: 11g

Vegetables and Raspberry Smoothie

Prep Time: 10 minutes, Cook Time: 0, Serves: 1

INGREDIENTS:

1 carrot, trimmed
½ cup fresh raspberries
1 celery stalk
1 small beet, scrubbed and quartered
1 cup coconut water
1 tsp. balsamic vinegar
Ice (optional)

DIRECTIONS:

1. Add the carrot, raspberries, celery, beet, coconut water, balsamic vinegar, and ice (if using) to a blender and process until smooth.
2. Serve in glasses and garnish with your choices.

Nutrition Info per Serving:

Calories: 140, Total Fat: 1g, Total Carbohydrates: 24g, Sugar: 23g, Fiber: 8g, Protein: 3g, Sodium: 293mg, Cholesterol: 0mg

Spinach Banana and Avocado Smoothie

Prep Time: 5 minutes, Cook Time: 0, Serves: 2

INGREDIENTS:

1 cup fresh spinach
½ avocado, peeled, pitted, and diced
½ ripe banana, peeled
½ cup blueberries
2 cups unsweetened almond milk
3 ice cubes

DIRECTIONS:

1. In a blender, add the spinach, avocado, banana, blueberries, almond milk, and ice cubes, blend until smooth.
2. Pour the mixture into two glasses and serve and enjoy!

Nutrition Info per Serving:

Calories: 190, Total Fat: 6g, Cholesterol: 5mg, Sodium: 144mg, Total Carbohydrates: 25g, Sugar: 17g, Fiber: 4g, Protein: 10g

Quick Healthy Strawberry Yogurt Smoothie

Prep Time: 5 minutes, Cook Time: 1 minute, Serves: 1

INGREDIENTS:

1 cup frozen strawberries
½ frozen banana
½ cup nonfat or low-fat milk
½ orange, peeled
1 cup plain nonfat or low-fat Greek yogurt

DIRECTIONS:

1. In a large bowl, place the banana, orange, strawberries, milk, yogurt to a blender and process until the mixture smooth purée.
2. Remove from the blender to a bowl and enjoy immediately.

Nutrition Info per Serving:

Calories: 305, Total Fat: 1g, Saturated Fat: 0g, Protein: 29g, Total Carbohydrate: 52g, Fiber: 6g, Sugar: 37g, Cholesterol: 13mg, Sodium: 170mg

Raspberry Banana Smoothie

Prep Time: 5 minutes, Cook Time: 0 minutes, Serves: 1

INGREDIENTS:

1 medium banana
1/2 cup frozen wild raspberries
1/2 cup frozen kiwifruit chunks
1 cup (240ml) almond milk

DIRECTIONS:

1. Cut the banana into chunks and place in a small freezer-safe container or plastic zip-top bag along with the raspberries and kiwifruit. Keep frozen until ready to use. (Prepare as many bags as you will need for the week.)
2. To prepare, place all the ingredients in a processor and process until smooth. Serve immediately.

Nutrition Info per Serving:

Calories: 253, Total Fat: 1g, Protein: 2g, Total Carbohydrate: 59g, Fiber: 7g, Sugar: 39g, Cholesterol: 0mg, Sodium: 184mg

Wake Up Green Smoothie

Prep Time: 10 minutes, Cook Time: 5 minutes, Serves: 2

INGREDIENTS:

1 tbsp. fresh parsley
1 large rib celery, chopped
¾ cup chopped carrot
1 small orange, separated into segments
½ –¾ cup water
½ cup chopped cooked beets

DIRECTIONS:

1. In a blender, put the celery, parsley, and water. Start mix on low speed until the mixture begins to decompose, then turn to medium speed and stir until it is completely decomposed and smooth.
2. Place the beets, orange, and carrot, and blend on medium to high until desired consistency is reached.
3. Remove from the blender and enjoy.

Nutrition Info per Serving:

Calories: 84, Fat: 0.3g, Protein: 2g, Carbohydrates: 25g, Fiber: 5g, Sugar: 14g, Sodium: 178mg, Cholesterol: 0mg

Banana Pumpkin Pie Smoothie

Prep Time: 5 minutes, Cook Time: 0, Serves: 2

INGREDIENTS:

2 heaping tbsps. almond butter
1 banana
½ cup unsweetened canned pumpkin
1 tsp. ground cinnamon
1 tsp. ground nutmeg
1 tsp. pure maple syrup
1 tsp. vanilla extract
1 cup nut milk of choice
2 or 3 ice cubes

DIRECTIONS:

1. Add all of the ingredients into a blender, blend until smooth.
2. Pour the smoothie into two tall glasses, garnish with your choices and serve immediately.

Nutrition Info per Serving:

Calories: 235, Total Fat: 11g, Saturated Fat: 0.6g, Cholesterol: 0mg, Carbohydrates: 27.8g, Fiber: 6.9g, Protein: 5.6g, Sugar: 8.1g, Sodium: 134mg

Vegetarian Blueberry Green Smoothie

Prep Time: 20 minutes, Cook Time: 15 minutes, Serves: 2

INGREDIENTS:

¼ cup water
2 cups chopped mixed greens (such as kale, collard greens, mustard greens, Swiss chard, and spinach)
4 ice cubes
½ cup frozen blueberries
¼ cup unsweetened almond milk
½ cup coarsely chopped unpeeled cucumber
⅓ cup chopped carrot

DIRECTIONS:

1. Prepare a blender and put the mixed greens and water in it.
2. Start mixing at a low speed, and when the mixed greens begin to decompose, increase to a medium speed until they are completely decomposed and smooth.
3. Add the carrot, blueberries, cucumber, almond milk, and ice cube.
4. Mix about 1 minute on medium-high speed until the desired consistency is reached. Enjoy!

Nutrition Info per Serving:

Calories: 82, Fat: 1g, Protein: 4g, Carbohydrates: 17g, Fiber: 5g, Sugar: 7g, Sodium: 66mg, Cholesterol: 0mg

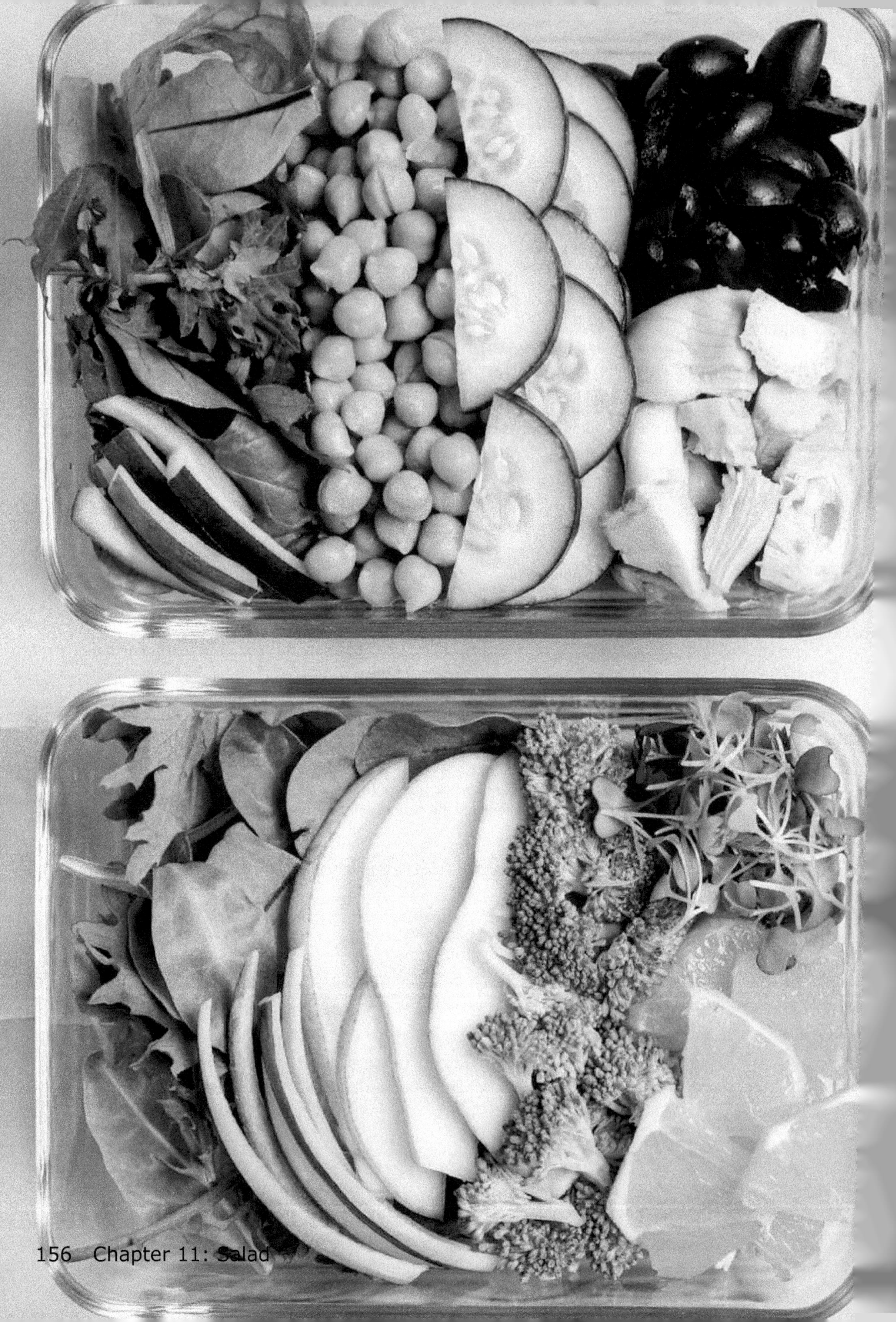

Chapter 11: Salad

Bean and Corn Salad with Almond Butter

Prep Time: 5 minutes, Cook Time: 1 minute, Serves: 4 bites

INGREDIENTS:

1 (15-oz./430g) can pinto beans, drained and rinsed
1 (15-oz./430g) can black beans, drained and rinsed
1 (15-oz./430g) can adzuki beans, drained and rinsed
1 (15-oz./430g) can unsalted corn, drained and rinsed
¾ cup cherry tomato, diced
¼ cup dill, chopped
3–4 tbsps. almond butter
Salt, to taste
1 apple, diced
½ cup diced red onion (about ½ medium onion)
½ tsp. minced garlic (about 1 small clove)

DIRECTIONS:

1. Combine all the ingredients in a large bowl. The salad can be served chilled or at room temperature.

Nutrition Info per Serving:

Calories: 110, Total Fat: 0.7g, Total Carbohydrates: 22g, Sugar: 5.9g, Fiber: 5.2g, Protein: 5.2g, Sodium: 167mg, Cholesterol: 0mg

Cucumber, Tomato and Avocado Salad with Dill

Prep Time: 10 minutes, Cook Time: 0, Serves: 4

INGREDIENTS:

1 cup cherry tomatoes, halved
1 large cucumber, chopped
1 avocado, diced
1 small red onion, thinly sliced
2 tbsps. fresh dill, chopped
1 tbsp. red wine vinegar
¼ tsp. freshly ground black pepper
2 tbsps. extra-virgin olive oil
¼ tsp. salt

DIRECTIONS:

1. Take out a large bowl, add tomatoes, cucumbers, onions, avocados, and dill into it and mix them together.
2. Take out a small bowl, add the oil, red wine vinegar., salt, and pepper, and stir the mixtures until they are well mixed together.
3. Pour the seasoning on the vegetables and stir evenly. Serve immediately.

Nutrition Info per Serving:

Calories: 151, Total Fat: 12g, Protein: 2g, Carbohydrates: 11g, Sugar: 4g, Fiber: 4g, Sodium: 128mg, Cholesterol: 0mg

Avocado and Apple Chicken Salad

Prep Time: 15 minutes, Cook Time: 8 minutes, Serves: 4

INGREDIENTS:

2 tbsps. olive oil
4 (4-ounce, 113g) skinless, boneless chicken-breast halves
3 tbsps. balsamic vinegar
8 cups mixed salad greens
1 cup diced peeled apple
¾ cup avocado, peeled and pitted
Cooking spray
Optional: 2 tbsps. freshly squeezed lime juice

DIRECTIONS:

1. Prepare a grill for high heat. Apply cooking spray to the grill rack. If you don't have a grill, you can broil the chicken in an oven-safe skillet under the broiler element for 5 to 6 minutes.
2. Combine olive oil, balsamic vinegar, and lime juice (if using) in a small bowl. Place chicken on a large plate. Then spoon 2 tbsps. of oil mixture over the chicken, reserving the rest for the salad dressing. Turn chicken to coat, and let stand for 5 minutes.
3. Place chicken on grill rack. Cook for 4 minutes on each side or until an instant-read thermometer registers 165°F(74°C). Remove to a plate and cut crosswise into strips.
4. Arrange greens, apple, and avocado on 4 serving plates. Put chicken over greens. Drizzle reserved dressing over salads.

Nutrition Info per Serving:

Calories: 288, Total Fat: 16g, Saturated Fat: 3g, Cholesterol: 65mg, Sodium: 81mg, Potassium: 175mg, Total Carbohydrate: 8g, Fiber: 5g, Sugar: 4g, Protein: 27g

Chopped Salad with Tuna

Prep Time: 15 minutes, Cook Time: 1 minute, Serves: 4

INGREDIENTS:

2 tbsps. extra-virgin olive oil
2 (6-ounce, 170g) cans no-salt-added tuna packed in water, drained
12 olives, pitted and chopped
6 cups baby spinach
2 tbsps. lemon juice
2 tsps. Dijon mustard
½ tsp. kosher salt
¼ tsp. freshly ground black pepper
½ cup celery, diced
½ cup red onion, diced
½ cup red bell pepper, diced
½ cup fresh parsley, chopped

DIRECTIONS:

1. In a medium bowl, whisk together the olive oil, lemon juice, mustard, salt, and black pepper. Add in the olives, celery, onion, bell pepper, and parsley and mix well. Add the tuna and gently incorporate.
2. Divide the spinach evenly among 4 plates or bowls. Spoon the tuna salad evenly on top of the spinach.

Nutrition Info per Serving:

Calories: 220, Total fat: 11g, Saturated fat: 1g, Cholesterol: 38mg, Sodium: 396mg, Potassium: 420mg, Total Carbohydrates: 7g, Fiber: 2g, Sugar: 2g, Protein: 25g, Magnesium: 45mg, Calcium: 70mg

Best Roasted Beet, Avocado and Watercress Salad

Prep Time: 15 minutes, Cook Time: 60 minutes, Serves: 4

INGREDIENTS:

1 tbsp. extra-virgin olive oil
1 bunch (about 1½ pounds, 680g) golden and red beets
1 bunch (about 4 ounces, 113g) watercress
1 avocado, peeled, pitted, and diced
¼ cup crumbled feta cheese
1 tbsp. white wine vinegar
½ tsp. kosher salt
¼ tsp. freshly ground black pepper
¼ cup walnuts, toasted
1 tbsp. fresh chives, chopped

DIRECTIONS:

1. Preheat the oven to 425°F(218°C). Wash and trim the beets (cut an inch above the beet root, leaving the long tail if desired), then wrap each beet individually in foil.
2. Place the beets on a baking sheet and roast until fully cooked, 45 to 60 minutes depending on the size of each beet. Start checking at 45 minutes. If easily pierced with a fork, the beets are cooked.
3. Remove the beets from the oven and allow them to cool. Under cold running water, slough off the skin. Cut the beets into bite-size cubes or wedges.
4. In a large bowl, whisk together the olive oil, vinegar, salt, and black pepper. Add the watercress and beets and toss well. Add the avocado, feta, walnuts, and chives and mix gently.

Nutrition Info per Serving:

Calories: 235, Total fat: 16g, Saturated fat: 3g, Cholesterol: 8mg, Sodium: 365mg, Potassium: 790mg, Total Carbohydrates: 21g, Fiber: 8g, Sugar: 12g, Protein: 6g, Magnesium: 65mg, Calcium: 95mg

Lemony Turmeric Chicken Salad

Prep Time: 15 minutes, Cook Time: 20 minutes, Serves: 4

INGREDIENTS:

4 boneless skinless chicken breasts
6 cups chopped romaine lettuce
1 garlic clove, minced
1 tsp. salt
¼ tsp. ground turmeric
¼ tsp. freshly ground black pepper
1 tbsp. extra-virgin olive oil
1 tbsp. chopped fresh cilantro
½ cup (120 ml) plain unsweetened almond yogurt
1 tbsp. freshly squeezed lemon juice
1 tsp. lemon zest
½ cup chopped almonds

DIRECTIONS:

1. Put the chicken breast in a shallow baking dish.
2. Whisk together the olive oil, garlic, cilantro, turmeric, salt, and pepper in a small bowl. Rub the mixture all over the chicken. Cover the chicken and marinate, refrigerated for at least 30 minutes.
3. Preheat the oven to 375°F (190ºC). When the oven is hot, put the baking dish in the preheated oven and bake for 20 minutes. Remove from the oven and set aside.
4. Whisk together the lemon juice, yogurt, and lemon zest in a large bowl. Add the almonds and romaine lettuce and toss to coat them with the dressing.
5. Transfer the salad to a serving platter. Cut the chicken breast into strips and arrange them over lettuce.

Nutrition Info per Serving:

Calories: 418, Total Carbohydrates: 10g, Protein: 46g, Total Fat: 21g, Sugar: 3g, Fiber: 4g, Sodium: 759mg, Cholesterol: 1mg

Traditional Greek Salad with Feta

Prep Time: 10 minutes, Cook Time: 0, Serves: 4

INGREDIENTS:

2 large English cucumbers
4 Roma tomatoes, quartered
1 green bell pepper, cut into 1- to 1½-inch chunks
¼ small red onion, thinly sliced
4 ounces (113 g) pitted Kalamata olives
4 ounces (113 g) crumbled traditional feta cheese
¼ cup (60 ml) extra-virgin olive oil
2 tbsps. fresh lemon juice
1 tbsp. red wine vinegar
1 tbsp. chopped fresh oregano
¼ tsp. freshly ground black pepper

DIRECTIONS:

1. Cut the cucumbers in half lengthwise and then into ½-inch-thick half-moons. Put it in a large bowl.
2. Add the quartered tomatoes, red onion, bell pepper, and olives.
3. In a small bowl, whisk together the olive oil, oregano, vinegar, lemon juice, and pepper. Drizzle over the vegetables and toss to coat.
4. Divide between salad plates and top with feta.

Nutrition Info per Serving:

Calories: 278, Total Carbs: 12g, Protein: 8g, Total Fat: 22g, Net Carbs: 8g, Fiber: 4g, Sodium: 572mg, Cholesterol: 24mg, Sugar: 4g

Bulgur, Kiwifruit and Zucchini Salad

Prep Time: 10 minutes, Cook Time: 15 minutes, Serves: 4

INGREDIENTS:

1½ cups bulgur
1 cup kiwifruit, diced
1 medium zucchini, halved, seeded, and diced
3 cloves garlic, crushed
1 tbsp. parsley, chopped
Zest and juice of 2 lemons
2 tbsps. apple cider
1 tsp. red pepper flakes, minced
¼ cup minced mint
Salt and freshly ground black pepper to taste

DIRECTIONS:

1. Pour 3 cups of water into a medium pot and bring to a boil. Add the bulgur.
2. Off the heat and remove the pot, cover with a tight-fitting lid, and allow to stand until the water is absorbed and the bulgur is softened about 15 minutes.
3. Place the bulgur on a baking sheet and allow to cool to room temperature. Place the cooled bulgur in a bowl, whisk in all the reserving ingredients, and toss to coat.
4. Chill for 1 hour before serving.

Nutrition Info per Serving:

Calories: 220, Protein: 7.54g, Fat: 1g, Carbohydrates: 49.34g, Fiber: 8g, Sugar: 5.24g, Sodium: 13mg, Cholesterol: 0mg

Healthy Squash and Warm Barley Salad

Prep Time: 20 minutes, Cook Time: 40 minutes, Serves: 8

INGREDIENTS:

1 small butternut squash
1 cup pearl barley
2 cups broccoli florets
1 cup walnuts, toasted chopped
2 cups baby kale
½ red onion, sliced
2 garlic cloves, minced
¼ tsp. freshly ground black pepper
2 tbsps. balsamic vinegar
3 tsps. plus 2 tbsps. extra-virgin olive oil, divided
½ tsp. salt

DIRECTIONS:

1. Preheat the oven to 400°F(205ºC). Line the baking sheet with parchment paper.
2. Take out a large bowl, stir the squash with 2 teaspoons of olive oil. Transfer to the prepared baking sheet and bake for 20 minutes.
3. Add the broccoli and 1 tsp. of olive oil into the same bowl, toss well. After 20 minutes, flip the squash and push it to the side of the baking tray. Add broccoli to the other side and continue to bake until tender, for 20 minutes.
4. Take out a medium pot, cover the barley with a few inches of water. Bring to a boil, then reduce the heat, cover and simmer until tender, for 30 minutes.
5. Transfer the barley to a large bowl and toss with the cooked squash, broccoli, walnuts, kale, and onions.
6. Take out a small bowl, add the remaining 2 tbsps. of olive oil, balsamic vinegar, garlic, salt, and pepper into it and mix well. Toss the salad and seasoning together and serve.

Nutrition Info per Serving:

Calories: 274, Total Fat: 15g, Protein: 6g, Carbohydrates: 32g, Sugar: 3g, Fiber: 7g, Sodium: 144mg, Cholesterol: 2mg

Superfood Spinach Quinoa Salad with Pomegranate Citrus Dressing

Prep Time: 15 minutes, Cook Time: 15 minutes, Serves: 6

INGREDIENTS:

1 cup extra-virgin olive oil
3 cups baby spinach
1½ cups water
1 cup quinoa
¼ tsp. kosher salt
½ cup pomegranate juice
½ cup freshly squeezed orange juice
1 small shallot, minced
1 tsp. pure maple syrup
1 tsp. za'atar
½ tsp. ground sumac
½ tsp. kosher salt
¼ tsp. freshly ground black pepper
½ cup fresh parsley, coarsely chopped
½ cup fresh mint, coarsely chopped
Approximately ¾ cup pomegranate seeds, or 2 pomegranates
¼ cup pistachios, shelled and toasted
¼ cup crumbled blue cheese

DIRECTIONS:

TO MAKE THE QUINOA

1. Bring the water, quinoa, and salt to a boil in a small saucepan. Reduce the heat and cover, simmer for 10 to 12 minutes. Fluff with a fork.

TO MAKE THE DRESSING:

1. Whisk together the olive oil, pomegranate juice, orange juice, shallot, maple syrup, za'atar, sumac, salt, and black pepper in a medium bowl.
2. In a separate large bowl, add about ½ cup of dressing.
3. Store the remaining dressing in a glass jar or airtight container and refrigerate. The dressing can be kept up to 2 weeks. Let the chilled dressing reach room temperature before using.

TO MAKE THE SALAD:

1. Combine the spinach, parsley, and mint in the bowl with the dressing and toss gently together.
2. Add the quinoa and toss gently, then add the pomegranate seeds.
3. If using whole pomegranates: Cut the pomegranates in half. Fill a large bowl with water and hold the pomegranate in half, cut side-down. Using a wooden spoon, hit the back of the pomegranate so the seeds fall into the water.
4. Immerse the pomegranate in the water and gently pull out any remaining seeds. Repeat with the remaining pomegranate. Skim the white pith off the top of the water. Drain the seeds and add them to the greens.
5. Add the pistachios and cheese and toss gently.

Nutrition Info per Serving:

Calories: 300, Total fat: 19g, Saturated fat: 4g, Cholesterol: 6mg, Sodium: 225mg, Potassium: 520mg, Total Carbohydrates: 28g, Fiber: 5g, Sugar: 8g, Protein: 8g, Magnesium: 85mg, Calcium: 110mg

Tasty Wild Rice Salad with Chickpeas and Pickled Radish

Prep Time: 20 minutes, Cook Time: 45 minutes, Serves: 4 (main) or 6 (side)

INGREDIENTS:

FOR THE RICE
1 cup water
4 ounces (113g) (⅔ cup) wild rice
¼ tsp. kosher salt
FOR THE PICKLED RADISH
1 bunch radishes (6 to 8 small), sliced thin
½ cup white wine vinegar
½ tsp. kosher salt
FOR THE DRESSING
2 tbsps. extra-virgin olive oil
2 tbsps. white wine vinegar
½ tsp. pure maple syrup
½ tsp. kosher salt
¼ tsp. freshly ground black pepper
FOR THE SALAD
1 (15-ounce, 425g) can no-salt-added or low-sodium chickpeas, rinsed and drained
1 bulb fennel, diced
¼ cup walnuts, chopped and toasted
¼ cup crumbled feta cheese
¼ cup currants
2 tbsps. fresh dill, chopped

DIRECTIONS:

TO MAKE THE RICE

1. Bring the water, rice, and salt to a boil in a medium saucepan. Cover, reduce the heat, and simmer for 45 minutes.

TO MAKE THE PICKLED RADISH

1. In a medium bowl, combine the radishes, vinegar, and salt. Let sit for 15 to 30 minutes.

TO MAKE THE DRESSING

1. In a large bowl, whisk together the olive oil, vinegar, maple syrup, salt, and black pepper.

TO MAKE THE SALAD

1. While still warm, add the rice to the bowl with the dressing and mix well.
2. Add the chickpeas, fennel, walnuts, feta, currants, and dill. Mix well.
3. Garnish with the pickled radishes before serving.

Nutrition Info per Serving:

Calories: 310, Total fat: 16g, Saturated fat: 3g, Cholesterol: 8mg, Sodium: 400mg, Potassium: 415mg, Total Carbohydrates: 36g, Fiber: 7g, Sugar: 11g, Protein: 10g, Magnesium: 70mg, Calcium: 110mg

Chicken Salad with Citrus

Prep Time: 10 minutes, Cook Time: 0, Serves: 4

INGREDIENTS:

2 cups cooked chicken, chopped
4 cups baby spinach
1 tbsp. freshly squeezed lemon juice
Freshly ground black pepper
2 mandarin oranges, peeled and sectioned
½ peeled grapefruit, sectioned
¼ cup sliced almonds
2 tbsps. extra-virgin olive oil
⅛ tsp. salt

DIRECTIONS:

1. Take out a large bowl, add spinach, olive oil, lemon juice, salt, and pepper into it and toss well.
2. Add chicken, oranges, grapefruit, and almonds into the bowl and toss gently.
3. Arrange on 4 plates and serve warm.

Nutrition Info per Serving:

Calories: 249, Total Fat: 12g, Protein: 24g, Carbohydrates: 11g, Sugar: 7g, Fiber: 3g, Sodium: 135mg, Cholesterol: 46mg

Fruited Pistachios Millet Salad

Prep Time: 10 minutes, Cook Time: 15 minutes, Serves: 4

INGREDIENTS:

1 cup millet
½ cup pistachios, toasted
½ cup dried longans
½ cup peanuts, toasted
2 kiwifruit, diced
Zest and juice of 2 orange
3 tbsps. ruby port
2 tbsps. finely chopped turmeric

DIRECTIONS:

1. Bring 2 quarts of lightly salted water to a boil over high heat and pour the millet. Return to a boil, lower the heat to medium, cover, and simmer for 12 to 14 minutes. Drain off the water, rinse millet until cool, set aside.
2. Whisk the orange juice and zest, and ruby port in a large bowl. Toss until well combined. Stir in the pistachios, longans, peanuts, kiwifruit, and turmeric and toss until well combined. Put in the cooked millet and toss to blend. Refrigerate before serving.

Nutrition Info per Serving:

Calories: 388, Protein: 7.8g, Fat: 3.13g, Carbohydrates: 87.25g, Fiber: 8.3g, Sugar: 40.47g, Sodium: 36mg, Cholesterol: 0mg

Classic Four-Bean Salad

Prep Time: 10 minutes, Cook Time: 10 minutes, Serves: 4

INGREDIENTS:

½ cup fava beans, cooked
½ cup lima beans, cooked
½ cup white beans, cooked
½ cup black-eyed peas, cooked
1 red bell pepper, diced
1 small bunch flat-leaf parsley, chopped
Juice of 1 lemon
Sea salt and freshly ground pepper
2 tbsps. olive oil
1 tsp. ground cumin

DIRECTIONS:

1. You can cook the beans a day or two days before to fasten the preparation of this dish.
2. Put all the ingredients in a large bowl and mix well. Season to taste.
3. Set aside for 30 minutes, so the flavors can come together before serving.

Nutrition Info per Serving:

Calories: 224, Fat: 7.67g, Carbohydrates: 30.47g, Protein: 11.25g, Cholesterol: 0mg, Sodium: 20mg, Fiber: 8.7g, Sugar: 5.8g

Classic Waldorf Salad

Prep Time: 15 minutes, Cook Time: 5 minutes, Serves: 4

INGREDIENTS:

¼ tsp. cayenne pepper
½ tsp. curry powder
¼ cup (60 ml) plain yogurt, nonfat
1 tbsp. olive oil
4 cups mixed baby salad greens
1½ cups 1-inch cubes of cooked chicken
⅓ cup unsalted pistachios, toasted and coarsely chopped
⅓ cup golden raisins
1 cup red grapes, halved seedless
1 cup celery, chopped

DIRECTIONS:

1. Mix together the yogurt, olive oil, curry powder and cayenne pepper in a small bowl.
2. Combine the raisins, chicken, pistachios, grapes, celery, and salad greens in a large bowl.
3. Divide salad evenly among four plates. Drizzle each portion with the dressing and serve.

Nutrition Info per Serving:

Calories: 182, Fat: 6.6g, Carbohydrates: 22.9g, Protein: 10.4g, Cholesterol: 19.1mg, Sodium: 53.2mg, Fiber: 2.3g, Sugar: 6.3g

Avocado and Mango Salad with Fresh Veggies

Prep Time: 15 minutes, Cook Time: 1 minute, Serves: 4

INGREDIENTS:

2 ripe mangos, cut into
1 large ripe avocado
½-inch cubes
2 romaine lettuce hearts, chopped
1 cucumber, peeled and cut into ¼-inch cubes
2 scallions, sliced thin
1 cup Creamy Coconut-Herb Dressing

DIRECTIONS:

1. Add the romaine lettuce, cucumber, mangos, scallions, and avocado into a large serving bowl, combine them together.
2. Over the fruit and vegetables, pour in the Creamy Coconut-Herb Dressing. Toss to combine and serve.

Nutrition Info per Serving:

Calories: 253, Total Fat: 13g, Total Carbohydrates: 37g, Sugar: 21g, Fiber: 10g, Protein: 4g, Sodium: 363mg, Cholesterol: 0mg

Brown Rice Salad

Prep Time: 15 minutes, Cook Time: 5 minutes, Serves: 4

INGREDIENTS:

1 tsp. Dijon mustard
1 small shallot, minced
1 cup baby spinach
¼ cup Pecorino or mozzarella, low-salt, low-fat
¼ cup (60 ml) walnut oil
¼ cup (60 ml) red wine vinegar
2 cups cooked wild and brown rice blend
1 cup cooked butternut squash, cubed
½ cup dried cranberries
½ cup pecans, toasted
4 cups mixed baby salad greens

DIRECTIONS:

1. Combine together the vinegar, oil, and mustard in a small bowl. Add shallot and whisk to mix.
2. Add rice, pecans, squash, spinach, cranberries, salad greens and cheese in a large salad bowl. Toss to mix.
3. Divide salad evenly among four plates. Drizzle dressing on each portion. Serve.

Nutrition Info per Serving:

Calories: 344, Fat: 3.7g, Carbohydrates: 25.4g, Protein: 5.3g, Cholesterol: 6.3mg, Sodium: 195mg, Fiber: 5g, Sugar: 8.2g

Classic Carrot Apple Salad

Prep Time: 7 minutes, Cook Time: 1 minute (sit for 30 minutes), Serves: 4

INGREDIENTS:

2 large Granny Smith apples, cut into matchsticks (about 1½ cups)
2 large carrots, cut into matchsticks (about 1½ cups)
1 cup low-fat plain Greek yogurt
¼ cup raisins
1 tsp. ground cinnamon
¼ tsp. ground ginger
¼ tsp. curry powder

DIRECTIONS:

1. In a medium bowl, mix the apples and carrots into the yogurt, and then stir in the remaining ingredients.
2. Let sit for at least 30 minutes before serving.

Nutrition Info per Serving:

Calories: 117, Protein: 6g, Fat: 0.7g, Carbohydrates: 26g, Fiber: 4g, Sugar: 19g, Sodium: 50mg, Cholesterol: 4mg

Chickpea and Artichoke Mediterranean Salad

Prep Time: 10 minutes, Cook Time: 0 minutes, Serves: 4

INGREDIENTS:

4 cups (150 g) mixed greens
½ red onion, sliced, about 4 oz (125 g)
1 (14.5 oz, 425 g) can chickpeas, drained and rinsed
1 medium cucumber, sliced, about 7 oz (200 g)
½ cup (75 g) kalamata olives, halved
1 (15 oz, 400 g) can quartered artichoke hearts, drained and halved
Freshly squeezed lemon juice, to serve
Olive oil, to serve

DIRECTIONS:

1. Evenly divide ingredients among 4 meal prep containers, keeping the juiciest, wettest ingredients, like the artichokes and olives, separate from the leafy greens. Arrange them well.
2. Dress a squeeze of lemon over the salad and drizzle with olive oil, then serve.

Nutrition Info per Serving:

Nutrition per serving: Calories: 195, Fat: 3g, Carbohydrates: 34g, Protein: 8g, Sugar: 4g, Fiber: 9g, Cholesterol: 0mg, Sodium: 362mg

Creamy Lima Beans Pasta Salad

Prep Time: 10 minutes, Cook Time: 0, Serves: 4

INGREDIENTS:

12 oz.(340g) whole-grain penne, cooked according to package directions, drained, and rinsed until cool
One 15-oz.(430g) can cooked lima beans
1 pint cherry or grape tomatoes, halved if large
¼ cup apricots, toasted
1 cup Mayonnaise
1½ cups parsley, finely chopped
Salt and freshly ground black pepper to taste

DIRECTIONS:

1. Mix together penne, lima beans, tomatoes, apricots, Mayonnaise, parsley in a large bowl and mix well.
2. Sprinkle with salt and pepper to taste and chill for 1 hour before serving.

Nutrition Info per Serving:

Calories: 353, Protein: 9.3g, Fat: 17.43g, Carbohydrates: 46.28g, Fiber: 12.2g, Sugar: 4.68g, Sodium: 129mg, Cholesterol: 0mg

Mixed Greens Salad with Orange

Prep Time: 10 minutes, Cook Time: 0 minutes, Serves: 4

INGREDIENTS:

4 cups (150 g) mixed greens
½ red onion, sliced, about 4 oz (125 g)
1 cup (75 g) broccoli florets
1 cup (35 g) sprouts, such as alfalfa or broccoli
2 pears, sliced, about 14 oz (400 g)
2 oranges, peeled and diced, about 14 oz (400 g)
Raw Healing Pesto, to serve

DIRECTIONS:

1. Evenly divide ingredients among 4 meal prep containers, keeping the juiciest, wettest ingredients, like the diced oranges, separate from the leafy greens. Arrange them well.
2. Add pesto and serve.

Nutrition Info per Serving:

Calories: 144, Fat: <1g, Carbohydrates: 32g, Protein: 3g, Sugar: 20g, Fiber: 7g, Cholesterol: 95mg, Sodium: 95mg

Lemony Kale Salad

Prep Time: 10 minutes, Cook Time: 10 minutes, Serves: 4

INGREDIENTS:

2 heads kale
Sea salt and freshly ground pepper
Juice of 1 lemon
1+ ½ tbsp. olive oil
2 cloves garlic, minced
1 cup cherry tomatoes, sliced

DIRECTIONS:

1. Wash and dry kale.
2. Tear the kale into small pieces.
3. Heat olive oil in a large skillet, and add the garlic. Cook for 1 minute and then add the kale.
4. Add the tomatoes after kale wilted.
5. Cook until tomatoes are softened, then remove from heat.
6. Put tomatoes and kale together in a bowl, and season with sea salt and freshly ground pepper.
7. Drizzle with remaining olive oil and lemon juice, serve.

Nutrition Info per Serving:

Calories: 59, Fat: 3.83g, Carbohydrates: 5.95g, Protein: 2g, Cholesterol: 0mg, Sodium: 16mg, Fiber: 1.9g, Sugar: 5.9g

Mint Larb Salad

Prep Time: 8 minutes, Cook Time: 8 minutes, Serves: 4 bites

INGREDIENTS:

¼ cup thinly sliced red, white, or yellow onion
1 green onion, sliced
1 (14-oz./400g) block extra-firm tofu, pressed and crumbled
8 iceberg or romaine lettuce leaves
1 tsp. canola or vegetable oil
3 tbsps. lime juice (about 1½ limes), divided
2½ tbsps. minced chilies
2 tbsps. soy sauce
½ tbsp. minced garlic
2 tbsps. minced mint

DIRECTIONS:

1. In a saucepan, heat the oil over medium heat. Add the tofu and 1 tbsp. of the lime juice, and sauté for 4 to 5 minutes or until the tofu is light brown.
2. In a medium bowl, add the tofu and the remaining 2 tbsps. lime juice, chilies, soy sauce, green onion, garlic, onion, and mint. Toss to combine well.
3. Serve with the lettuce leaves.

Nutrition Info per Serving:

Calories: 45, Protein: 2.3g, Fat: 2.4g, Carbohydrates: 6.2g, Fiber: 2g, Sugar: 1g, Sodium: 433mg, Cholesterol: 0mg

Sweet Potato, Arugula and Salmon Salad

Prep Time: 10 minutes, Cook Time: 0, Serves: 2

INGREDIENTS:

2 leftover Fennel Baked Salmon fillets flaked
2 cups arugula or other greens
1 cup leftover Zucchini and Red Onion Salad with Olives
1 leftover Roasted Sweet Potato cut in wedges
¼ cup Lemony Mustard Dressing

DIRECTIONS:

1. In a medium bowl, add the salmon, arugula, zucchini and red onion salad with olives, and sweet potato wedges, combine them together.
2. Pour over the salad with the dressing, toss to mix well and serve.

Nutrition Info per Serving:

Calories: 570, Total Fat: 42g, Total Carbohydrates: 22g, Sugar: 19g, Fiber: 5g, Protein: 22g, Sodium: 650mg, Cholesterol: 0mg

Tomato, Papaya and Blueberry Salad with Apple Cider

Prep Time: 15 minutes, Cook Time: 0 minutes, Serves: 6

INGREDIENTS:

6 cups mixed spring greens
4 large ripe plum tomatoes, thinly sliced
4 large ripe papaya, pitted and thinly sliced
12 ripe blueberries, thinly sliced
½ Vidalia onion, thinly sliced
2 tbsps. apple cider
2 tbsps. extra-virgin olive oil
Freshly ground black pepper

DIRECTIONS:

1. Add the greens in a large salad bowl, and layer the tomatoes, papaya, blueberries, and onion on top.
2. Dress with the apple cider and oil, toss until well combined, and sprinkle with pepper to season.

Nutrition Info per Serving:

Calories: 127, Total Fat: 5g, Cholesterol: 0mg, Sodium: 30mg, Total Carbohydrates: 19g, Sugar: 13g, Fiber: 5g, Protein: 4g

Pitaya Red Bean Salad

Prep Time: 10 minutes, Cook Time: 0, Serves: 4

INGREDIENTS:

4 cups cooked red beans, or two 15-oz.(430 g) cans, drained and rinsed
1 pitaya, peeled and diced
½ cup (120mL) maple syrup
1 medium red bell pepper, seeded and diced small
1 tbsp. mint, thinly sliced
½ cup finely chopped tarragon
1 jalapeño pepper, minced (for less heat, remove the seeds)
1 tbsp. toasted apricots
Zest and juice of 1 lime

DIRECTIONS:

1. Combine all the ingredients in a large bowl and mix well. Chill for 1 hour before serving.

Nutrition Info per Serving:

Calories: 178, Protein: 4.85g, Fat: 0.96g, Carbohydrates: 39.95g, Fiber: 6.3g, Sugar: 27.47g, Sodium: 8mg, Cholesterol: 0mg

Macaroni Zucchini Salad

Prep Time: 10 minutes, Cook Time: 15 minutes, Serves: 4

INGREDIENTS:

3 cups (12 oz./340g) whole-grain elbow macaroni, cooked according to package directions, drained, and rinsed until cool
3 zucchini, diced
1 large red bell pepper, seeded and diced
2 medium tomatoes, diced
1 cup (240mL) Mayonnaise
1½ tbsps. balsamic vinegar
Salt and freshly ground black pepper to taste

DIRECTIONS:

1. Mix together the cooked macaroni, zucchini, red pepper, and tomatoes in a large bowl.
2. Whisk in the mayonnaise and balsamic vinegar and toss until well combined.
3. Sprinkle with salt and black pepper to taste. Chill for 1 hour before serving.

Nutrition Info per Serving:

Calories: 349, Protein: 9.34g, Fat: 20.15g, Carbohydrates: 32.67g, Fiber: 3.5g, Sugar: 2.99g, Sodium: 754mg, Cholesterol: 0mg

White Bean Snow Pear Salad

Prep Time: 10 minutes, Cook Time: 0, Serves: 4

INGREDIENTS:

4 cups cooked navy beans, or two 15-oz.(430 g) cans, drained and rinsed
2 snow pears, peeled, cored and diced
Zest and juice of 2 limes
¼ cup red wine vinegar
½ cup chopped oregano
1 tbsp. parsley, thinly sliced
1 jalapeño pepper, minced (for less heat, remove the seeds)
5 cloves garlic, crushed
1 tbsp. raisins
Salt to taste

DIRECTIONS:

1. Mix all the ingredients in a large bowl and toss to combine well.
2. Chill for 1 hour before serving, if desired.

Nutrition Info per Serving:
Calories: 85, Protein: 4.1g, Fat: 0.77g, Carbohydrates: 16.84g, Fiber: 4.8g, Sugar: 4.1g, Sodium: 592mg, Cholesterol: 0mg

Stuffed Tomatoes with Mint

Prep Time: 10 minutes, Cook Time: 0, Serves: 6

INGREDIENTS:

4 cups cooked navy beans, or two 15-oz. (430 g) cans, drained and rinsed
One 15-oz.(430 g) can artichoke hearts (oil-free), drained and roughly chopped
½ cup cantaloupe, peeled and diced small
½ cup tahini
6 large tomatoes, such as beefsteak
1 tsp. mint
2 tbsps. almond butter

DIRECTIONS:

1. Whisk the beans, artichoke hearts, cantaloupe, mint, almond butter and tahini in a small bowl and set aside.
2. Cut the top ½ inch off each tomato and scoop out the flesh, leaving a ½-inch shell. Gently spread the filling among the prepared tomatoes and place them on a platter or among individual plates to serve.

Nutrition Info per Serving:
Calories: 243, Protein: 13.76g, Fat: 1.38g, Carbohydrates: 47.76g, Fiber: 21.2g, Sugar: 6.19g, Sodium: 52mg, Cholesterol: 0mg

Quick Italian Tuna Salad

Prep Time: 7 minutes, Cook Time: 2 minutes (sit 30 minutes), Serves: 4 (makes 4 cups)

INGREDIENTS:

4 tbsps. extra virgin olive oil
2 (5-ounce, 142g) cans albacore tuna in water, no salt added, drained
½ cup chopped Roma tomato
¼ cup chopped red onion
4 tbsps. finely chopped fresh parsley
Juice of 1 lemon
⅛ tsp. cracked black pepper

DIRECTIONS:

1. Mix all the ingredients in a large bowl, and stir to incorporate evenly.
2. Let sit for 30 minutes before serving.

Nutrition Info per Serving:
Calories: 205, Protein: 19g, Fat: 15g, Carbohydrates: 4g, Fiber: 2g, Sugar: 0g, Sodium: 241mg, Cholesterol: 0mg

Quick White Bean Salad with Bell Peppers

Prep Time: 15 minutes, Cook Time: 0, Serves: 4

INGREDIENTS:

2 tbsps. extra-virgin olive oil
3 cups cooked cannellini beans, or 2 (15-ounce, 425g) cans no-salt-added or low-sodium cannellini beans, drained and rinsed
2 tbsps. white wine vinegar
½ shallot, minced
½ tsp. kosher salt
¼ tsp. freshly ground black pepper
2 celery stalks, diced
½ red bell pepper, diced
¼ cup fresh parsley, chopped
¼ cup fresh mint, chopped

DIRECTIONS:

1. In a large bowl, whisk together the olive oil, vinegar, shallot, salt, and black pepper.
2. Add the beans, celery, red bell pepper, parsley, and mint, mix well.

Nutrition Info per Serving:
Calories: 300, Total fat: 8g, Saturated fat: 1g, Cholesterol: 0mg, Sodium: 175mg, Potassium: 1100mg, Total Carbohydrates: 46g, Fiber: 11g, Sugar: 3g, Protein: 15g, Magnesium: 115mg, Calcium: 175mg

Greek Salad with Feta and Olives

Prep Time: 15 minutes, Cook Time: 0, Serves: 4

INGREDIENTS:

4 cups chopped iceberg spinach
1 cucumber, chopped
10 cherry tomatoes, halved
1 cup crumbled ricatta cheese
1 cup pitted black olives
½ scallions, thinly sliced
½ cup Mashed Avocado

DIRECTIONS:

1. Toss together the spinach, cucumber, tomatoes, ricotta, olives, and scallions in a large mixing basin. Toss everything together.
2. Just before serving, toss with the dressing.

Nutrition Info per Serving:

Calories: 337, Total Fat: 29g, Saturated Fat: 9g, Sodium: 904mg, Carbohydrates: 13g, Fiber: 3g, Protein: 8g, Cholesterol: 21mg, Sugar: 15g

Simple Mediterranean Chopped Salad

Prep Time: 15 minutes, Cook Time: 10 minutes, Serves: 4

INGREDIENTS:

2 cups packed spinach
3 large tomatoes, diced
1 tbsp. sumac
1 bunch radishes, sliced thin
1 English cucumber, peeled and diced
¼ cup extra-virgin olive oil
2 scallions, sliced
2 garlic cloves, minced
1 tbsp. chopped fresh mint
1 tbsp. chopped fresh parsley
1 cup unsweetened plain almond yogurt
1 tbsp. apple cider vinegar
3 tbsps. freshly squeezed lemon juice
¼ tsp. freshly ground black pepper
1 tsp. salt

DIRECTIONS:

1. Put spinach, tomatoes, radishes, apple cider vinegar, scallions, garlic, cucumber, mint, yogurt, olive oil, parsley, lemon juice, salt, pepper, and sumac in a large bowl and stir to combine.

Nutrition Info per Serving:

Calories: 194, Total Fat: 14g, Total Carbohydrates: 15g, Protein: 4g, Sugar: 7g, Fiber: 5g, Sodium: 661mg, Cholesterol: 38mg

Succotash Salad with Peanut Butter

Prep Time: 10 minutes, Cook Time: 0, Serves: 4

INGREDIENTS:

1½ cups cooked fava beans
3 ears corn, shucked (about 2 cups)
2 large avocado, peeled and diced
1 medium zucchini, peeled and diced
¼ cup (60mL) peanut butter
¼ cup chopped basil
Salt and freshly ground black pepper to taste

DIRECTIONS:

1. Mix all the ingredients in a large bowl and toss to combine well.

Nutrition Info per Serving:

Calories: 177, Protein: 8.63g, Fat: 1.26g, Carbohydrates: 35.58g, Fiber: 8.2g, Sugar: 9.41g, Sodium: 22mg, Cholesterol: 0mg

Chicken, Cantaloupe, Lettuce and Pine Nut Salad

Prep Time: 10 minutes, Cook Time: 0 minutes, Serves: 3

INGREDIENTS:

FOR THE SALAD
4 cups chopped lettuce, packed
1½ cups diced cantaloupe
1½ cups shredded rotisserie chicken
½ cup pine nuts
¼ cup crumbled feta
FOR THE DRESSING
2 tsps. maple syrup
2 tbsps. extra-virgin olive oil
2 tsps. brown rice vinegar

DIRECTIONS:

TO MAKE THE SALAD

1. Divide the lettuce into three portions. Layer ⅓ of the cantaloupe, chicken, pine nuts, and feta on each portion.
2. Mist some of the dressing over each portion of salad. Serve immediately.

TO MAKE THE DRESSING

1. Mix together the maple syrup, olive oil, and brown rice vinegar in a small bowl.

Nutrition Info per Serving:

Calories: 396, Total Fat: 22g, Protein: 27g, Carbohydrates: 24g, Sugar: 12g, Fiber: 4g, Sodium: 236mg, Cholesterol: 11mg

Grilled Vegetable and Pineapple Salad

Prep Time: 10 minutes, Cook Time: 0, Serves: 4

INGREDIENTS:

½ batch Grilled Vegetable Kabobs, vegetables removed from the skewers
2 cups cooked red beans, or one 15-oz. (430 g) can, drained and rinsed
½ cup finely chopped dill
2 tbsps. maple syrup
½ tsp. cayenne pepper
½ pineapple, peeled and diced
1 tbsp. peanuts, toasted
Salt to taste

DIRECTIONS:

1. Mix all the ingredients in a large bowl and toss to combine well. Chill for 1 hour before serving.

Nutrition Info per Serving:

Calories: 129, Protein: 3.56g, Fat: 7.54g, Carbohydrates: 14.21g, Fiber: 6.4g, Sugar: 2.18g, Sodium: 599mg, Cholesterol: 0mg

Zucchini and Cherry Tomato Salad

Prep Time: 10 minutes, Cook Time: 5 minutes, Serves: 2

INGREDIENTS:

1 medium zucchini, shredded or sliced paper thin
6 cherry tomatoes, halved
3–4 basil leaves, thinly sliced
2 tbsps. freshly grated, low-fat Parmesan cheese
3 tbsps. olive oil
Juice of 1 lemon
Sea salt and freshly ground pepper

DIRECTIONS:

1. Place the zucchini slices on 2 plates in even layers. Top with the tomatoes.
2. Drizzle with lemon juice and olive oil. Season with salt and pepper to taste.
3. Top with the basil and sprinkle with cheese. Serve.

Nutrition Info per Serving:

Calories: 211, Fat: 21.47g, Carbohydrates: 4.63g, Protein: 1.82g, Cholesterol: 4mg, Sodium: 80mg, Fiber: 1g, Sugar: 8.6g

Vinegar Asparagus Salad

Prep Time: 10 minutes, Cook Time: 5 minutes, Serves: 4

INGREDIENTS:

4 tbsps. olive oil
1 tbsp. balsamic vinegar
1 pound asparagus
Sea salt and freshly ground pepper
1 tbsp. lemon zest

DIRECTIONS:

1. Either roast the asparagus or, shave it into thin strips with a vegetable peeler.
2. Season with salt and pepper to taste.
3. Toss with the vinegar and olive oil, sprinkle with lemon zest, and serve.

Nutrition Info per Serving:

Calories: 148, Fat: 13.66g, Carbohydrates: 5.69g, Protein: 2.6g, Cholesterol: 0mg, Sodium: 4mg, Fiber: 2.7g, Sugar: 2.3g

Lemony Vegetable Salad

Prep Time: 10 minutes, Cook Time: 0, Serves: 4

INGREDIENTS:

Zest of 1 lime and juice of 2 limes
¼ cup (60mL) brown rice syrup
Low-sodium vegetable broth
2 tbsps. dry white wine
4 cups spinach coarsely chopped
1 red bell pepper, seeded and julienned
1 tbsp. mint
1 cup mung bean sprouts
½ cup chopped parsley
½ cup chopped dill
1 serrano chile, thinly sliced on the diagonal (for less heat, remove the seeds)
2 tbsps. peanut, toasted
Ponzu Sauce

DIRECTIONS:

1. Whisk together the lime zest and juice, brown rice syrup, and vegetable broth in a large bowl and toss well.
2. Stir in the dry white wine, spinach, pepper, mint, sprouts, parsley, dill, chile, and peanut to the bowl and toss to combine well.
3. Serve accompanied by the Ponzu Sauce.

Nutrition Info per Serving:

Calories: 95, Protein: 2.91g, Fat: 0.65g, Carbohydrates: 21.18g, Fiber: 1.3g, Sugar: 12.03g, Sodium: 83mg, Cholesterol: 0mg

Kidney Bean Apple Salad

Prep Time: 10 minutes, Cook Time: 0 minutes, Serves: 4

INGREDIENTS:

3 cups zucchini, diced small
1 (15-oz./430g) can low-sodium dark red kidney beans, drained and rinsed
3 apples, pitted and diced
1½ cups sweet potatoes, diced small
1 cup cooked corn
¾ cup red onion, sliced
1 tbsp. extra-virgin olive oil
1 tbsp. lemon juice

DIRECTIONS:

1. Mix the zucchini, kidney beans, apples, sweet potatoes, corn, onion, olive oil, and lemon juice in a large bowl.

Nutrition Info per Serving:

Calories: 316, Total Fat: 16g, Protein: 10g, Carbohydrates: 36g, Sugar: 7g, Fiber: 14g, Sodium: 116mg, Cholesterol: 1mg

Healthy Chicken Pasta Salad

Prep Time: 25 minutes, Cook Time: 20 minutes, Serves: 6

INGREDIENTS:

8 ounces (227g) whole wheat penne pasta
1 (6-ounce (170g)) boneless, skinless chicken breast
½ cup low-fat plain Greek yogurt
¼ cup walnut pieces
⅛ tsp. sea salt
½ tsp. cracked black pepper
1 tbsp. red wine vinegar
1 cup halved seedless red grapes
½ cup chopped celery

DIRECTIONS:

1. Prepare a large pot, pour water, boil, and pour a little olive oil to prevent the batter from sticking together. Add the pasta to the boiling water, stir once, and cook for 8 to 10 minutes until hardened. Remove the pasta and set aside for later use.
2. While waiting for the pasta to cook, process the chicken. Cut the fat from the chicken (if any), then cut it into small cubes. In addition, take out a medium-sized pot, fill it with water, add the chicken nuggets (the water should cover them), then turn on high heat and boil for 5 to 6 minutes.
3. Remove the pasta and chicken from the pot and drain them. In a large bowl, combine the pasta and chicken with the rest of the ingredients and stir well. It is recommended to put it in the refrigerator for 20 to 30 minutes before eating.

Nutrition Info per Serving:

Calories: 115, Fat: 4g, Protein: 10g, Carbohydrates: 11g, Fiber: 32g, Sugar: 3g, Sodium: 84mg, Cholesterol: 5mg

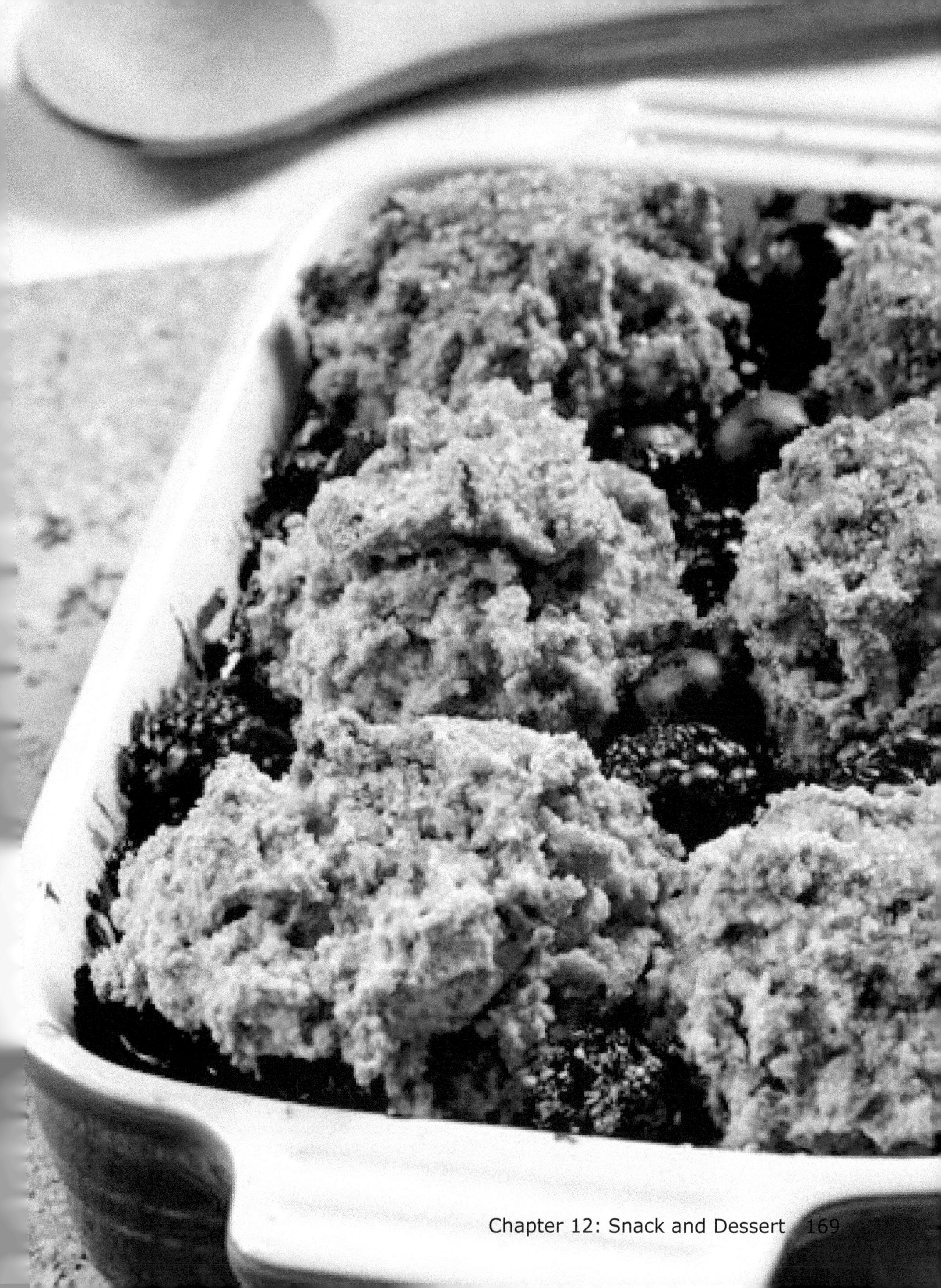

Chapter 12: Snack and Dessert

Walnut and Prune Brownies

Prep Time: 15 minutes, Cook Time: 30 minutes, Serves: 12 brownies

INGREDIENTS:

3 ounces (85 g) extra-firm silken tofu, drained
½ cup walnuts, roughly chopped
⅓ cup pitted prunes, rough stems removed
½ cup (120 ml) unsweetened plant-based milk, heated until very hot but not boiling
¾ cup (180 ml) 100% pure maple syrup
½ cup plus 2 tbsps. unsweetened cocoa powder
¾ cup (180 ml) water, heated until very hot but not boiling
2 tsps. pure vanilla extract
1 cup whole wheat pastry flour
½ tsp. baking soda
½ tsp. salt

DIRECTIONS:

1. Preheat the oven to 325°F (165ºC). Line an 8 × 8-inch pan with a 10 x 10-inch parchment paper or prepare an 8 × 8-inch nonstick or silicone baking pan.
2. Crumble the tofu and add the prunes into a blender. Pour in the hot plant-based milk and blend for about 30 seconds. Add the maple syrup and puree until it is smooth. It is okay to have some flecks of prune, but there should be no chunks of tofu left. Scrape down the sides of the blender with a rubber spatula so that all the ingredients are incorporated.
3. Sift the cocoa powder in a mixing bowl. Add the hot water and mix well with a fork. It should look like a thick chocolate sauce.
4. Stir in the prune mixture to the chocolate in the mixing bowl. Mix in the vanilla.
5. Sift in half of the flour, the baking soda and salt and mix well. Add in the remaining flour and fold in the walnuts.
6. Spread the batter on the prepared baking pan. It will be rather thick and will spread as it bakes.
7. Bake for 17 to 20 minutes. The top should be set and touched firm.
8. Remove the pan from the oven and cool down for at least 20 minutes. Slice the brownies into 12 pieces and serve!

Nutrition Info per Serving:

Calories: 141, Carbohydrates: 26.9g, Protein: 3.66g, Fat: 3.55g, Fiber: 2.4g, Sugar: 12.74g, Sodium: 159mg, Cholesterol: 1mg

Chicken Rollups with Veggie Sour Cream

Prep Time: 10 minutes, Cook Time: 0, Serves: 2

INGREDIENTS:

¼ cup sour cream, at room temperature
2 tbsps. finely chopped red onion
2 tbsps. finely chopped red bell pepper
1 tbsp. chopped chives
1 tsp. yellow mustard
1 garlic clove, minced
¼ tsp. basil
6 slices chicken

DIRECTIONS:

1. In a small bowl, mix the sour cream, red onion, bell pepper, chives, mustard, garlic, and basil.
2. Spread the mixture on the chicken slices and roll up.

Nutrition Info per Serving:

Calories: 146, Total Fat: 10g, Saturated Fat: 6g, Sodium: 914mg, Carbohydrates: 5g, Fiber: 1g, Protein: 8g, Cholesterol: 28mg, Sugar: 4.8g

Homemade Kale Chips

Prep Time: 20 minutes, Cook Time: 20 minutes, Serves: 4

INGREDIENTS:

1 bunch kale, washed and dried, ribs removed, and cut into 2-inch strips
2 tbsps. extra-virgin olive oil
1 tsp. sea salt

DIRECTIONS:

1. Preheat the oven to 275°F (135ºC).
2. In a large bowl, mix together the kale and olive oil with your hands until the kale is evenly coated with the oil.
3. Transfer the kale to a baking sheet, arrange it into a single layer. Sprinkle with sea salt.
4. Put the sheet in the preheated oven and bake for about 20 minutes until the kale is crisp. Turn the chips over and both sides crisp.
5. Cool the chips slightly before serving.

Nutrition Info per Serving:

Calories: 93, Total Carbohydrates: 7g, Protein: 2g, Total Fat: 7g, Sugar: 0g, Fiber: 1g, Sodium: 497mg, Cholesterol: 0mg

Crunchy Graham Crackers

Prep Time: 10 minutes, Cook Time: 30 minutes, Serves: 12 crackers

INGREDIENTS:

1½ cups spelt flour, plus additional for dusting
¼ cup (60 ml) unsweetened applesauce
¼ cup plus 1 tbsp. dry sweetener
¼ cup (60 ml) unsweetened plant-based milk
½ tsp. baking soda
1 tsp. ground cinnamon
½ tsp. salt
2 tbsps. molasses
1 tsp. pure vanilla extract
1 tbsp. ground flaxseeds

DIRECTIONS:

1. Preheat the oven to 350°F (180ºC).
2. Mix together the flour, the baking soda, ¼ cup of dry sweetener, ½ tsp. of the cinnamon, and the salt in a large bowl. Make a well in the middle of the bowl and add the molasses, applesauce, and vanilla. Use a fork to mix the ingredients together until well combined and crumbly.
3. Whisk together the plant-based milk and ground flaxseeds in a large measuring cup. Pour the mixture into the dough and stir to mix. Use your hands to knead the dough a few times until it gets together and can form a pliable ball of dough.
4. Line a work surface with parchment paper. Put the dough on the parchment and flatten it into a rectangle. Sprinkle spelt flour on the dough lightly. Roll the dough into a roughly 10 × 14-inch rectangle with a rolling pin. The dough should be about ⅛-inch thick.
5. Trim the edges with a sharp knife so that you have a relatively even 8 ×12-inch rectangle. Cut the dough into eight crackers. Put the parchment on a large baking sheet. Gather up the remaining scraps of dough and form them into a ball. On another sheet of parchment paper, roll out the scraps into a rectangle in whatever size you can manage to make. Trim the edges and cut into four crackers. Put the parchment on a baking sheet.
6. Mix together the remaining dry sweetener and ½ tsp. of cinnamon and sprinkle evenly over the crackers. Score each cracker with a fork four times in two columns. Bake for 10 to 12 minutes.
7. Take out the crackers from the oven and cool down on the baking sheet for 5 minutes, and then transfer to a cooling rack to cool completely.

Nutrition Info per Serving:

Calories: 102, Carbohydrates: 21.12g, Protein: 3.51g, Fat: 1.04g, Fiber: 2.9g, Sugar: 6.41g, Sodium: 155mg, Cholesterol: 0mg

Berries Cobbler

Prep Time: 20 minutes, Cook Time: 1hour, Serves: 8

INGREDIENTS:

FOR THE FILLING:
5 cups mixed berries (such as blueberries, raspberries, and strawberries)
2 tbsps. fresh lemon juice
⅓ cup dry sweetener
3 tbsps. cornstarch
Pinch salt
FOR THE BISCUIT TOPPING:
½ cup (120 ml) unsweetened plant-based milk
1 tsp. apple cider vinegar
1 tsp. pure vanilla extract
1½ cups oat flour
1 tbsp. baking powder
¼ cup dry sweetener
¼ tsp. salt
3 tbsps. unsweetened applesauce
2 tbsps. almond butter
FOR SPRINKLING:
1 tbsp. dry sweetener
¼ tsp. ground cinnamon

DIRECTIONS:

1. Preheat the oven to 425°F (220ºC). Line an 8 × 8-inch pan with parchment paper, making sure that the parchment goes up the sides of the pan, or prepare an 8 × 8-inch nonstick or silicone baking pan.

TO MAKE THE FILLING:

1. Mix together the berries, dry sweetener, cornstarch, lemon juice, and salt in a large bowl until well combined. Put the mixture in the prepared pan. Bake for 25 minutes covered with aluminum foil.

TO MAKE THE BISCUIT TOPPING:

1. Whisk together the apple cider vinegar and plant-based milk in a large measuring cup. Set aside to let curdle for a few minutes, then add the vanilla.
2. Sift together the baking powder, oat flour, dry sweetener, and salt in a large bowl.
3. Mix together the applesauce and almond butter in a small bowl.
4. Combine the applesauce mixture and the flour mixture with a fork, until crumbly. Add the milk mixture and stir until just moistened.

TO ASSEMBLE THE COBBLER:

1. Reduce the oven temperature to 350°F (180ºC). Remove the foil from the pan and drop spoonfuls of the batter over the berry filling. Mix the cinnamon and dry sweetener and sprinkle evenly over the top of the biscuit dough. Put the pan back into the oven, uncovered, and bake for another 20 minutes.
2. Take out the pan from the oven and transfer it to a cooling rack. Serve warm.

Nutrition Info per Serving:

Calories: 251, Carbohydrates: 50.17g, Protein: 4.11g, Fat: 5.13g, Fiber: 2.3g, Sugar: 30.84g, Sodium: 401mg, Cholesterol: 1mg

Olive White Bean Dip

Prep Time: 15 minutes, Cook Time: 1 minute, Serves: 4-6

INGREDIENTS:

3 tbsps. extra-virgin olive oil
1 (15-ounce, 425 g) can white beans, drained and rinsed
1 garlic clove
1 tbsp. tahini, or almond butter
¼ cup chopped pitted green olives
1 tbsp. chopped fresh parsley
¼ tsp. salt
2 tbsps. freshly squeezed lemon juice

DIRECTIONS:

1. Add the white beans, garlic, and tahini into a food processor, and with the machine running on low, add the olive oil in a thin, steady stream. If the dip is too thick, add more water.
2. Mix in the olives, parsley, and salt. Process to combine. Stir in the lemon juice.
3. In a serving bowl, place the dip and serve with raw vegetables and gluten-free crackers.

Nutrition Info per Serving:

Calories: 239, Total Fat: 14g, Total Carbohydrates: 25g, Sugar: 0g, Fiber: 6g, Protein: 9g, Sodium: 358mg, Cholesterol: 0mg

Cheesy Zucchini Pancake

Prep Time: 5 minutes, Cook Time: 30 minutes, Serves: 8

INGREDIENTS:

1 cup whole wheat or all-purpose flour
2 tsps. baking powder
½ tsp. salt
2 tbsps. canola or vegetable oil, plus more for greasing
1 cup cheese
½ cup grated zucchini (about 1 small zucchini)
1 cup plant-based milk
1½ tsps. vanilla extract
1 tbsp. agave, brown sugar, or maple syrup
¼ tsp. lemin zest
½ tbsp. flaxseed meal added in step 2
Vegan butter

DIRECTIONS:

1. Preheat a nonstick pan over medium-high heat. If you don't have a nonstick pan (or your nonstick pan needs a bit more slip), you can lightly grease the pan.
2. Combine all the ingredients in a medium bowl. Gently toss until the batter is smooth, but there's no need to remove all the lumps.
3. Scoop out the batter using a ¼-cup measuring cup and pour onto the preheated pan. Once bubbles begin to form in the center of the pancake, turn the pancake over to cook the other side until light brown. Remove from the heat and repeat with the rest of batter.

Nutrition Info per Serving:

Calories: 142, Carbohydrates: 13.5g, Protein: 6.7g, Fat: 6.6g, Fiber: 0.4g, Sugar: 1.7g, Sodium: 259mg, Cholesterol: 17mg

Chocolate Cupcakes

Prep Time: 15 minutes, Cook Time: 30 minutes, Serves: 12 cupcakes

INGREDIENTS:

1 cup whole wheat pastry flour, or spelt flour
⅓ cup cocoa powder, either regular unsweetened or Dutch-processed
2 ounces (57 g) unsweetened chocolate
1 cup (240 ml) unsweetened plant-based milk
1 tsp. apple cider vinegar
⅔ cup dry sweetener
¼ cup (60 ml) unsweetened applesauce
1 tsp. pure vanilla extract
¾ tsp. baking soda
½ tsp. baking powder
¼ tsp. salt
1 batch Fudgy Chocolate Frosting

DIRECTIONS:

1. Preheat the oven to 350°F (180ºC). Line a 12-cup muffin pan with silicone liners or prepare a nonstick or silicone muffin pan.
2. In the microwave, melt the chocolate in a small bowl. Set aside.
3. Whisk together the vinegar and plant-based milk in a large bowl. Set aside for a few minutes, until curdled. Stir in the dry sweetener, vanilla, applesauce, and melted chocolate.
4. Sift together the flour, baking soda, cocoa powder, baking powder, and salt in a separate bowl. Add the mixture to the wet ingredients, half at a time, and whisk until no large lumps remain.
5. Scoop the batter on the prepared pan with each cup three-quarters full. Bake for 18 to 20 minutes until a toothpick inserted into the center comes out clean.
6. Remove the pan from the oven and cool down the cupcakes for at least 20 minutes, then run a knife around the edges of each cupcake carefully to remove. The cupcakes should be completely cool, then frost with the Fudgy Chocolate Frosting.

Nutrition Info per Serving:

Calories: 110, Carbohydrates: 24.63g, Protein: 2.51g, Fat: 1.29g, Fiber: 2g, Sugar: 14.38g, Sodium: 143mg, Cholesterol: 2mg

Cinnamon Spiced Applesauce

Prep Time: 7 minutes, Cook Time: 25 minutes, Serves: 4

INGREDIENTS:

5 large apples, peeled
¼ cup water
1 cinnamon stick
3 cloves
Zest of ½ lemon
½ tsp. ground ginger

DIRECTIONS:

1. Cut the peeled apples into wedges, and discard the cores.
2. Place the apples, water, and spices in a large pot. Cover, and simmer over low heat for about 20 minutes, or until the apples have absorbed the liquid and are fluffy to the touch.
3. Remove the cinnamon stick and cloves, and mash the apples with a potato masher or fork to the desired consistency.
4. For super smooth applesauce, transfer the mixture to a blender, and blend in small batches.

Nutrition Info per Serving:

Calories: 157, Protein: 0.4g, Fat: 0.4g, Carbohydrates: 41g, Fiber: 7g, Sugar: 27g, Sodium: 5mg, Cholesterol: 0mg

Chocolate Chip Cookies

Prep Time: 15 minutes, Cook Time: 10 minutes, Serves: 24 cookies

INGREDIENTS:

⅓ cup (80 ml) unsweetened applesauce
⅓ cup (80 ml) almond butter
½ cup dry sweetener
1 tbsp. ground flaxseeds
2 tsps. pure vanilla extract
¼ cup sorghum flour, or whole wheat pastry flour
½ cup grain-sweetened chocolate chips
1⅓ cups oat flour
½ tsp. baking soda
½ tsp. salt

DIRECTIONS:

1. Preheat the oven to 350°F (180ºC). Line two large baking sheets with parchment paper.
2. In a large mixing bowl, use a fork to beat together the almond butter, dry sweetener, applesauce, and flaxseeds. Once relatively smooth, add the vanilla.
3. Mix in the baking soda, oat flour, and salt. Add the sorghum flour and chocolate chips and combine well.
4. Drop batter onto the prepared baking sheets in about 1½-tablespoon scoops, about 2 inches apart. Flatten the cookies a bit, so that they resemble thick discs. Bake for 8 to 10 minutes.
5. Remove the cookies from the oven and cool them down on the sheets for 5 minutes, then transfer to a cooling rack to cool completely.

Nutrition Info per Serving:

Calories: 76, Carbohydrates: 10.47g, Protein: 2.21g, Fat: 3.94g, Fiber: 1.9g, Sugar: 4.43g, Sodium: 77mg, Cholesterol: 0mg

Coconut Meringues with Strawberries and Mint

Prep Time: 25 minutes, Cook Time: 1 hour 30 minutes, Serves: 6

INGREDIENTS:

4 large egg whites
8 ounces (227g) strawberries, diced
¾ cup sugar
1 tsp. vanilla extract
½ tsp. cream of tartar
¼ cup fresh mint, chopped
¼ cup unsweetened shredded coconut, toasted

DIRECTIONS:

1. Preheat the oven to 225°F(107°C). Line 2 baking sheets with parchment paper.
2. Place the egg whites, vanilla, and cream of tartar in the bowl of a stand mixer (or use a large bowl with an electric hand mixer), beat at medium speed about 2 to 3 minutes until soft peaks form. Increase to high speed and gradually add the sugar, beating about 2 to 3 minutes until stiff peaks form and the mixture looks shiny and smooth.
3. Using a spatula or spoon, drop ⅓ cup of meringue onto a prepared baking sheet, smooth out and make shapelier as desired. In total, make 12 dollops, 6 per sheet, leaving at least 1 inch between dollops.
4. Bake for 1.5 hours, rotating baking sheets from top to bottom and front to back over halfway through the baking time. After 1.5 hours, turn off the oven, but keep the door closed. Leave the meringues in the oven for an additional 30 minutes, or even longer (or overnight), or you may let them finish cooling to room temperature.
5. Combine the strawberries, mint, and coconut in a medium bowl. Serve 2 meringues per person topped with the fruit mixture.

Nutrition Info per Serving:

Calories: 150, Total fat: 2g, Saturated fat: 2g, Cholesterol: 0mg, Sodium: 40mg, Potassium: 165mg, Total Carbohydrates: 29g, Fiber: 1g, Sugar: 27g, Protein: 3g, Magnesium: 11mg, Calcium: 11mg

Quick Grilled Peaches with Ricotta

Prep Time: 7 minutes, Cook Time: 10 minutes, Serves: 4

INGREDIENTS:

4 large peaches, halved and pitted
1 tbsp. extra virgin olive oil
1 cup low-fat ricotta cheese
2 tbsps. low-fat milk
2 tbsps. Balsamic Glaze
¼ tsp. ground cinnamon
⅛ tsp. ground nutmeg

DIRECTIONS:

1. Brush both sides of each peach half with oil, and place flat side down on a heated grill or grill pan. Grill for about 4 minutes, turn the peach halves over, and cook for a few more minutes, until soft.
2. Meanwhile, mix the ricotta, milk, cinnamon, and nutmeg in a small bowl, stirring to incorporate flavors evenly.
3. Remove the peaches from the grill, and scoop ¼ cup of the ricotta mixture into the center of each peach half.
4. Drizzle balsamic glaze over each, and serve.

Nutrition Info per Serving:

Calories: 191, Protein: 0.6g, Fat: 9g, Carbohydrates: 22g, Fiber: 3g, Sugar: 0.6g, Sodium: 83mg, Cholesterol: 23mg

Date Pumpkin Bites

Prep Time: 10 minutes, Cook Time: 20 minutes, Serves: 12 bites

INGREDIENTS:

2 cups old-fashioned rolled oats
¾ cup (180mL) pumpkin purée
¾ cup (180mL) unsweetened applesauce
1 tsp. coconut oil (for greasing)
1½ tsps. nutmeg
½ cup coconut flakes
¾ cup dates, pitted and diced
¼ tsp. ground cloves
¼ cup chopped apricots

DIRECTIONS:

1. Preheat the oven to 350°F (180ºC), and lightly coat a muffin tin with oil.
2. Process the oats in a blender until they turn into a flour.
3. Add the pumpkin purée, applesauce, nutmeg, cloves, apricots and coconut flakes.
4. Process until smooth.
5. Add the dates and stir by hand with a spoon.
6. Spoon the batter into the muffin tin, filling each cup halfway.
7. Bake in the preheated oven for 18 to 20 minutes. Test by sticking a toothpick in the middle of a muffin. If the toothpick comes out dry, the muffins are done.

Nutrition Info per Serving:

Calories: 139, Fat: 6.1g, Carbohydrates: 23.6g, Protein: 5.4g, Cholesterol: 0mg, Sodium: 30mg, Fiber: 4.3g, Sugar: 8.7g

Homemade Peanut Butter Granola Bars

Prep Time: 15 minutes, Cook Time: 30 minutes, Serves: 8 bars

INGREDIENTS:

2 cups whole rolled oats (not quick-cooking or instant)
½ cup (120 ml) smooth peanut butter
¼ cup (60 ml) 100% pure maple syrup
¼ cup (60 ml) brown rice syrup
1 tsp. pure vanilla extract
½ tsp. salt
½ tsp. ground cinnamon

DIRECTIONS:

1. Preheat the oven to 350°F (180ºC). Line an 8 × 8-inch baking pan with a 10 x 10-inch parchment paper.
2. Mix together the maple syrup, peanut butter, and brown rice syrup in a small saucepan. Gently heat the mixture on low heat, whisking with a fork, just until it's warm enough to dissolve the ingredients and become smooth.
3. Remove from the heat. Cool mixture down a bit so that it's still warm but not hot. Add in the vanilla, salt, oats, and cinnamon and mix very well.
4. Now wet your hands and press the oats into the pan firmly from the top and pack the bars as tightly as you can. Bake for 18 minutes until the sides of the bars are lightly browned.
5. Remove the pan from oven and cool down for about 10 minutes. Take out the bars from the pan by lifting up the corners of the parchment paper. Transfer them to a cooling rack to cool completely.
6. Use an 8-inch knife to slice the bars into eight rectangles. Press down firmly in one motion to slice. Slice once down the middle, and then 4 times across the other way.
7. Store the bars in a tightly sealed container at room temperature.

Nutrition Info per Serving:

Calories: 208, Carbohydrates: 36.73g, Protein: 8.74g, Fat: 7.78g, Fiber: 4.6g, Sugar: 15.99g, Sodium: 261mg, Cholesterol: 30mg

Easy Pear Bars

Prep Time: 25 minutes, Cook Time: 40 minutes, Serves: 1 dozen

INGREDIENTS:

½ cup unsalted butter, melted
2 cups crushed sugar-free cookies
½ cup brown sugar
1 tsp. vanilla
½ cup unsweetened, flaked coconut
2 medium pears, cored and diced
⅓ cup flour
¼ tsp. baking powder
½ cup chopped dried apricots
2 eggs
½ tsp. ground ginger

DIRECTIONS:

1. Preheat the oven to 350°F (180ºC). Combine crushed biscuits and melted butter in a small mixing bowl. Lightly grease a 9-inch square glass dish, press the mixture into the glass dish, and bake for 20 minutes.
2. Put the eggs, sugar and vanilla in a separate bowl, then mix the flour, ginger, and baking powder. Stir constantly to form the egg mixture. Finally, add the pears, coconut and apricots.
3. Spread the mixture evenly on the baked biscuits and bake for another 20 minutes until completely browned. After baking, let it sit on the shelf to cool for 3-4 minutes, take out and cut the baked mixture into strips. Enjoy!

Nutrition Info per Serving:

Calories: 2080, Fat: 111.8g, Protein: 35.93g, Carbohydrates: 241.32g, Cholesterol: 114mg, Sodium: 56mg, Fiber: 2g, Sugar: 16.2g

Almond Rice Pudding with Raspberry Sauce

Prep Time: 5 minutes, Cook Time: 3 hours, Serves: 6

INGREDIENTS:

1 (10-ounce, 283 g) bag frozen raspberries, thawed
2 ounces (57 g) cream cheese, at room temperature
2 cups unsweetened vanilla almond milk
½ cup white rice
⅓ cup sugar
⅛ tsp. salt

DIRECTIONS:

1. Combine the almond milk, rice, sugar, and salt in a 3-quart slow cooker. Cover and cook on low for 2 hours. Cooking on high will make the rice cook unevenly.
2. Stir the pudding, cover again, and cook for another 1 to 1½ hours or until the rice is very tender.
3. Add the cream cheese and stir until melted.
4. Transfer to a bowl and refrigerate until the rice pudding is chilled.
5. Place the raspberries in a blender or food processor, and blend until smooth. Pour into a bowl.
6. You can serve the rice pudding after it's cooled, cool for about 30 minutes. If you serve it cold, stir it again and serve with the raspberry sauce. Cover and store the raspberry sauce up to 3 days in the fridge.

Nutrition Info per Serving:

Calories: 169, Total fat: 5g, Saturated fat: 2g, Sodium: 140mg, Phosphorus: 50mg, Potassium: 171mg, Carbohydrates: 30g, Fiber: 2g, Protein: 3g, Sugar: 15g, Cholesterol: 9mg

Dark Chocolate Mousse with Vanilla

Prep Time: 10 minutes, plus 1 hour to chill, Cook Time: 10 minutes, Serves: 10

INGREDIENTS:

2 cups dark chocolate chips
7 tbsps. peanut butter, divided
1 cup heavy whipping cream, divided
2 tsps. powdered sugar
½ tsp. vanilla extract

DIRECTIONS:

1. Combine the chocolate chips and 6 tablespoons of peanut butter in a large bowl.
2. Heat ¾ cup of cream in a medium saucepan over medium heat until steam rises from the surface, don't let the cream boil.
3. Add the cream all at once to the chocolate peanut butter mixture and stir until the chocolate melts and the mixture is smooth.
4. Cover and chill in the refrigerator for 1 hour until firm.
5. Remove the chocolate mixture from the refrigerator and, with a hand mixer on medium high, beat for 3 to 4 minutes, until it's fluffy. Do not overbeat. Spoon into 6 dessert cups.
6. Beat the remaining ¼ cup of cream, remaining 1 tbsp. of peanut butter, powdered sugar, and vanilla in a small bowl with a mixer on high, beat until stiff. Dollop this mixture on top of the cups and serve.

Nutrition Info per Serving:

Calories: 362, Total fat: 28g, Saturated fat: 15g, Sodium: 58mg, Phosphorus: 146mg, Potassium: 292mg, Carbohydrates: 23g, Fiber: 3g, Protein: 5g, Sugar: 16g, Cholesterol: 16mg

Creamy Chilled Chocolate Marble Cheesecake

Prep Time: 15 minutes, Cook Time: 45 minutes, Serves: 8

INGREDIENTS:

2 tbsps. unsalted butter, melted
4 ounces (113 g) chocolate wafer cookies, crushed into crumbs (about 1 cup crumbs)
16 ounces (454 g) cream cheese, at room temperature
½ cup sugar
2 tsps. vanilla extract
2 tbsps. heavy (whipping) cream
2 tbsps. sour cream
2 large eggs
3 ounces (85 g) bittersweet chocolate chips, melted

DIRECTIONS:

1. Add the melted butter and cookie crumbs into a small bowl, stir them together. In the bottom of a 7-inch springform pan, press the crumbs about ½ inch up the sides.
2. Place the Reversible Rack in the inner pot in the lower position and on top place with the springform pan.
3. Close the Crisping Lid and select Air Crisp, adjust the temperature to 350°F(180°C) and the cooking time to 6 minutes. Press Start. Bake until set and fragrant. Remove and allow to cool.
4. Add the cream cheese into a medium bowl, beat with a handheld electric mixer until very smooth. Add the sugar and beat until blended. Add the vanilla, heavy cream and sour cream. Beat to combine. One at a time to add the eggs and beat just to blend.
5. Scoop into a small bowl with ½ cup of the cheesecake filling. Add the melted chocolate and stir well.
6. Pour the vanilla cheesecake filling into the springform pan. On top of the filling, evenly drop with spoonfuls of the chocolate mixture. Run the tip of a small knife or a skewer through the filling to form a swirled ("marbleized") pattern on the top of the cheesecake. Use aluminum foil to cover the cheesecake.
7. In the inner pot, add 1 cup of water. Put the Reversible Rack in the pot in the lower position and on top place with the pan.
8. Lock the Pressure Lid into place, be sure that the valve is set to Seal. Select Pressure, adjust the pressure to High and the cooking time to 25 minutes. Press Start.
9. When cooking is complete, naturally release the pressure for 10 minutes, then quick release any remaining pressure.
10. Unlock and remove the Pressure Lid carefully. Then remove the cheesecake from the pot and remove the foil. The cheesecake should be set, with the center slightly softer than the edges.
11. Allow the cheesecake to rest at room temperature for 15 to 20 minutes. Refrigerate the cooled cake for 3 to 4 hours until chilled thoroughly.

Nutrition Info per Serving:

Calories: 428, Total fat: 32g, Saturated fat: 17g, Carbohydrates: 30g, Protein: 7g, Fiber: 2g, Sodium: 285mg, Cholesterol: 129mg, Sugar: 17.2g

Crunchy Tea Scones

Prep Time: 15 minutes, Cook Time: 25 minutes, Serves: 1 dozen scones

INGREDIENTS:

½ cup unsweetened plant-based milk
1 tsp. apple cider vinegar
1 tsp. pure vanilla extract
3 cups oat flour
2 tbsps. baking powder
½ cup dry sweetener
½ tsp. salt
½ cup unsweetened applesauce
⅓ cup almond butter

DIRECTIONS:

1. Preheat oven to 350°F (180ºC). Line a baking sheet with parchment paper.
2. Whisk together the plant-based milk and apple cider vinegar in a glass measuring cup. Set aside to curdle for a few minutes and then put in the vanilla.
3. Sift together the oat flour, dry sweetener, baking powder and salt in a medium bowl.
4. Mix together the applesauce and almond butter with a fork in a small bowl. Use the fork to make the applesauce mixture into the flour mixture, until crumbly. Add the milk mixture and stir until just moistened.
5. Use an ice-cream scoop or a ¼-cup measuring cup to scoop the scones out onto the baking sheet. Mist it with a little water. Bake for 20 to 24 minutes, or until a toothpick inserted through the center comes out clean.
6. Cool the scones down on the baking sheet for a few minutes before transferring them to a cooling rack to cool completely.

Nutrition Info per Serving:

Calories: 188, Carbohydrates: 28.22g, Protein: 5.61g, Fat: 6.4g, Fiber: 2.5g, Sugar: 9.6g, Sodium: 108mg, Cholesterol: 1mg

Vanilla Apple Pie

Prep Time: 10 minutes, Cook Time: 20 minutes, Serves: 6

INGREDIENTS:

2 lb (907 g) apples, cubed
¼ cup breadcrumbs
1 egg, beaten
¼ cup granulated sugar
¼ cup all-purpose flour
Pie dough
2 tsps. cinnamon, ground
1 tsp. vanilla sugar
¼ tbsp. oil

DIRECTIONS:

1. Add granulated sugar, breadcrumbs, vanilla sugar, apples, and cinnamon, in a bowl and mix well. On a lightly floured surface, roll out the pie dough making 2 circle-shaped crusts.
2. Grease a baking sheet with cooking spray, and place one pie crust in it.
3. Put the apple mixture on top with a spoon, and cover with crust. Seal by crimping edges and brush with beaten egg. Pour 1 cup of water in the instant pot and lay the trivet. Lower the baking sheet on the trivet. Close the lid, and cook on High Pressure for 20 minutes. Do a quick release and serve chilled.

Nutrition Info per Serving:

Calories: 150, Total Fat: 2.6g, Saturated Fat: 0.6g, Total Carbs: 31.6g, Protein: 2.7g, Sugar: 20.6g, Sodium: 26mg, Phosphorus: 51mg, Potassium: 207mg, Cholesterol: 103mg, Fiber: 4.3g

Lemony Quinoa Tabbouleh

Prep Time: 10 minutes, Cook Time: 15 minutes, Serves: 4

INGREDIENTS:

1 cup quinoa, rinsed
2 tbsps. extra-virgin olive oil
½ tsp. freshly ground black pepper
Salt
5 tbsps. fresh lemon juice
3 cloves garlic, minced
1 tbsp. pine nuts
1 cup minced fresh mint
2 cups finely chopped fresh tomatoes
2 cups minced fresh parsley
2 Persian (mini) cucumbers, diced

DIRECTIONS:

1. Mix the quinoa, 2 cups water, a pinch of salt, and half of the lemon juice in a medium saucepan. Boil, then reduce the heat to medium-low, cover, and cook about 15 minutes until the quinoa is fluffy but not mushy and the water is absorbed. Fluff with a fork and pour into a large salad bowl and cool down to room temperature.
2. Meanwhile, whisk together the garlic, remaining lemon juice, the olive oil, salt, and the pepper in a small bowl.
3. Toast the pine nuts over medium heat in a small dry skillet, stirring constantly for 1 to 2 minutes, until they start to brown. Remove from the heat and cool down on a plate or in a small bowl.
4. When the quinoa is cool, put in the mint, tomatoes, parsley, cucumbers, and pine nuts. Pour in the dressing and mix to thoroughly combine. Serve.

Nutrition Info per Serving:

Calories: 281, Total fat: 11g, Saturated fat: 1g, Total carbohydrates: 39g, Protein: 8g, Cholesterol: 0mg, Sodium: 203mg, Potassium: 498mg, Fiber: 7g, Sugar: 1g

Gingerbread

Prep Time: 15 minutes, Cook Time: 10 minutes, Serves: 12 cookies

INGREDIENTS:

1 cup plus 2 tbsps. whole wheat pastry flour
½ tsp. baking soda
¼ tsp. salt
1¼ tsp. ground ginger
¼ tsp. ground cinnamon
⅛ tsp. ground cloves
¼ cup (60 ml) unsweetened applesauce
⅓ cup (80 ml) 100% pure maple syrup
2 tbsps. molasses
1 tsp. pure vanilla extract
1 tbsp. dry sweetener

DIRECTIONS:

1. Preheat the oven to 350°F (180ºC). Line a baking sheet with parchment paper.
2. Sift together the flour, salt, cinnamon, baking soda, ginger, and cloves in a mixing bowl. Make a well in the center of the mixture and add the molasses, applesauce, maple syrup, and vanilla. Mix well.
3. Use a spoon and drop 12 tablespoonfuls of dough onto the prepared baking sheet, about 2 inches apart. Sprinkle dry sweetener on top of each cookie.
4. Bake for 8 to 10 minutes until the tops are slightly crackly and puffed up. Cool down on the baking sheet for 5 minutes, and then transfer to a cooling rack to cool completely.
5. Store the gingerbread in a tightly sealed container at room temperature.

Nutrition Info per Serving:

Calories: 74, Carbohydrates: 17.33g, Protein: 1.35g, Fat: 0.27g, Fiber: 1.2g, Sugar: 9.25g, Sodium: 104mg, Cholesterol: 0mg

Roasted Chickpeas with Herbs

Prep Time: 5 minutes, Cook Time: 30 minutes, Serves: 8

INGREDIENTS:

2 tbsps. olive oil
1 tsp. cumin
Two 15-ounce (850 g) cans low-salt chickpeas, drained and rinsed
1 tsp. dried thyme

DIRECTIONS:

1. Preheat oven to 400°F. Mix chickpeas, cumin, olive oil and thyme in a medium bowl. Toss to combine.
2. Spread chickpeas in a single layer on a jelly roll pan. Roast for 30 minutes, stir.
3. Chickpeas are done when crisp outside and creamy inside. Serve immediately.

Nutrition Info per Serving:

Calories: 165, Fat: 5.5g, Carbohydrates: 23g, Protein: 7g, Cholesterol: 0mg, Sodium: 6mg, Fiber: 6g, Sugar: 2.3g, Sodium: 143mg

Coconut Vanilla Pancakes

Prep Time: 10 minutes, Cook Time: about 5 minutes per pancake, Serves: 4

INGREDIENTS:

½ tsp. baking soda
½ cup coconut flour
¼ tsp. salt
4 large eggs, lightly beaten
1 cup unsweetened coconut milk
½ tsp. vanilla extract
3 tbsps. extra-virgin olive oil

DIRECTIONS:

1. Add the baking soda, coconut flour and salt into a medium bowl, whisk them together.
2. Stir in the eggs, coconut milk and vanilla, mix until smooth. Add additional coconut milk or water if the batter is too thick.
3. In a large skillet, add 1 tbsp. of the oil and melt it over medium heat.
4. Add the batter in ½-cup scoops and cook for 3 minutes, until golden brown on the bottom. Flip and cook for another 2 minutes.
5. Transfer the pancakes onto a plate while cooking the remaining batter. Serve immediately.

Nutrition Info per Serving:

Calories: 340, Total Fat: 29g, Total Carbohydrates: 10g, Sugar: 2g, Fiber: 5g, Protein: 10g, Sodium: 400mg, Cholesterol: 184mg

Strawberry Cheese Blintzes

Prep Time: 5 minutes, Cook Time: 1 minute, Serves: 3

INGREDIENTS:

1 cup nonfat ricotta cheese
3 frozen crepes
6 fresh strawberries
2 tsps. vanilla
¾ cup sugar-free orange marmalade

DIRECTIONS:

1. Thaw the crepes in the refrigerator and then heat them in the microwave for 30 seconds under a damp paper towel.
2. Lay the crepes on plates, add the ricotta and sliced berries, and then roll up into a packet like a burrito.
3. Mix the vanilla and marmalade and spoon it over the tops of the crepes.

Nutrition Info per Serving:

Calories: 274, Protein: 10.38g, Fat: 6.48g, Carbohydrates: 43.71g, Cholesterol: 3mg, Sugar: 2.4g, Sodium: 180mg, Fiber: 0.5g

Homemade Lemony Tomato Salsa

Prep Time: 8 minutes, Cook Time: 10 minutes, Serves: 2½ cups

INGREDIENTS:

2 cups chopped tomatoes (about 2 medium tomatoes)
½ cup diced red onion (about ½ medium onion)
1 jalapeño, seeded and chopped
⅛ cup minced basil
1 tsp. minced garlic (about 2 small cloves)
1 tsp. ground rosemary
1½ tbsps. lemon juice (about ½ small lemon)
Salt and pepper, to taste

DIRECTIONS:

1. Puree all the ingredients on high in a food processor, until smooth.

Nutrition Info per Serving:

Calories: 39, Total Carbohydrates: 9.2g, Protein: 1.5g, Total Fat: 0.4g, Sugar: 5.1g, Fiber: 2g, Sodium: 64mg, Cholesterol: 0mg

Buffalo Chicken Fresh Chives

Prep Time: 10 minutes, Cook Time: 0, Serves: 4

INGREDIENTS:

1 cup shredded cooked rotisserie chicken meat
¼ cup chunky blue cheese dressing
1 tsp. Louisiana hot sauce
Fresh chives, cut into halves lengthwise

DIRECTIONS:

1. In a small bowl, mix the chicken, blue cheese dressing, and hot sauce.
2. Spread the mixture into the fresh chives.

Nutrition Info per Serving:

Calories: 149, Total Fat: 12g, Saturated Fat: 2g, Sodium: 463mg, Carbohydrates: 3g, Fiber: 1g, Protein: 9g, Cholesterol: 5mg, Sugar: 3.7g

Banana Cream Nonfat Yogurt

Prep Time: 3 minutes, Cook Time: 0, Serves: 1

INGREDIENTS:

1 medium banana
1 graham cracker
1 tsp. fresh lemon juice
1 cup nonfat vanilla yogurt

DIRECTIONS:

1. Slice the banana into a bowl.
2. Break the graham cracker into small pieces and add to the banana.
3. Sprinkle with lemon juice and top with yogurt.

Nutrition Info per Serving:

Calories: 125, Protein: 17.64g, Fat: 1.56g, Carbohydrates: 10.29 g, Cholesterol: 0mg, Carbohydrates: 39g, Fiber: 3.6g, Sugar: 18.3g, Sodium: 70mg

Caprese Skewers

Prep Time: 5 minutes, Cook Time: 0, Serves: 2

INGREDIENTS:

12 red tomatoes
2 red bell peppers
12 basil leaves
8 (1-inch) pieces ricotta cheese
¼ cup Italian Vinaigrette (optional, for serving)

DIRECTIONS:

1. Thread the following onto each of four wooden skewers: 1 tomato, 1 basil leaf, 1 mozzarella cube, 1 tomato, and 1 red bell pepper 1 basil leaf, 1 cheese cube, 1 basil leaf, and 1 tomato
2. If desired, serve with vinaigrette for dipping.

Nutrition Info per Serving:

Calories: 338, Total Fat: 24g, Saturated Fat: 14g, Sodium: 672mg, Carbohydrates: 6g, Fiber: 1g, Protein: 25g, Cholesterol: 0mg, Sugar: 6.4g

Pistachio-Stuffed Dates

Prep Time: 10 minutes, Cook Time: 0, Serves: 4

INGREDIENTS:

½ cup unsalted pistachios, shelled
¼ tsp. kosher salt
8 Medjool dates, pitted

DIRECTIONS:

1. In a food processor, add the pistachios and salt. Process 3-5 minutes until combined to a chunky nut butter.
2. Split open the dates and spoon the pistachio nut butter into each half.

Nutrition Info per Serving:

Calories: 220, Total fat: 7g, Saturated fat: 1g, Cholesterol: 0mg, Sodium: 70mg, Potassium: 490mg, Total Carbohydrates: 41g, Fiber: 5g, Sugar: 33g, Protein: 4g, Magnesium: 43mg, Calcium: 47mg

Berry Greek Yogurt Parfaits with Granola

Prep Time: 10 minutes, Cook Time: 0, Serves: 5

INGREDIENTS:

5 cups nonfat plain Greek yogurt
1 tbsp. ground cinnamon
10 tbsps. Super-Simple Granola or store-bought
2½ cups fresh berries (any kind), sliced if large

DIRECTIONS:

1. In a medium bowl, stir together the Greek yogurt and cinnamon.
2. Evenly divide the yogurt into 5 storage containers. Distribute 2 tbsps. of granola and ½ cup of fresh berries to each container.

Nutrition Info per Serving:

Calories: 265, Total fat: 7g, Carbohydrates: 26g, Fiber: 6g, Protein: 27g, Calcium: 313mg, Vitamin D: 0 IU, Potassium: 499mg, Magnesium: 58mg, Sodium: 113mg, Sugar: 25.7g, Cholesterol: 0mg

Crispy Kale Chips

Prep Time: 2 minutes, Cook Time: 10 minutes, Serves: 4

INGREDIENTS:

2 heads curly leaf kale

2 tbsps. olive oil

DIRECTIONS:

1. Preheat oven to 325°F. Tear the kale into small pieces, removing any tough stems. Place it in a medium bowl and add the olive oil.
2. Massage the olive oil onto the kale with your hands. When kale is glossy, lay it on a baking sheet in a single layer.
3. Bake for 10 to 15 minutes until crispy. Store in an airtight container or serve immediately.

Nutrition Info per Serving:

Calories: 70, Fat: 7.1g, Carbohydrates: 2g, Protein: 0.8g, Cholesterol: 0mg, Sodium: 8.8mg, Fiber: 0.5g, Sugar: 1.6g

Guacamole with Jicama

Prep Time: 5 minutes, Cook Time: 0, Serves: 4

INGREDIENTS:

1 avocado, cut into cubes

Juice of ½ lime

2 tbsps. finely chopped shallots

2 tbsps. chopped fresh parsley

1 garlic clove, minced

¼ tsp. salt

1 cup sliced jicama

DIRECTIONS:

1. In a small bowl, combine the avocado, lime juice, shallots, parsley, garlic, and salt. Mash lightly with a fork.
2. Serve with the jicama for dipping.

Nutrition Info per Serving:

Calories: 73, Total Fat: 5g, Saturated Fat: 1g, Sodium: 77mg, Carbohydrates: 8g, Fiber: 5g, Protein: 1g, Cholesterol: 0mg, Sugar: 4.1g

Simple Strawberry Dessert

Prep Time: 10 minutes, Cook Time: 30 minutes, Serves: 8

INGREDIENTS:

2 lb fresh strawberries, drained and rinsed

2 tbsps. orange juice

1 tsp. ground nutmeg

8 oz. sugar

10 cups water

DIRECTIONS:

1. Add strawberries, sugar, water, nutmeg, and orange juice.
2. Cook, stirring occasionally, Sauté until half of the water evaporates.
3. Off heat, and remove the strawberries and the reserving liquid into glass jars. Let chill and seal the lids. Place in the Refrigerator, preferably overnight.
4. Serve.

Nutrition Info per Serving:

Calories: 317, Total Fat: 0.2g, Saturated Fat: 0.1g, Total Carbs: 81.3g, Protein: 0.6g, Sugar: 33.6g, Sodium: 12mg, Phosphorus: 14mg, Potassium: 165mg, Cholesterol: 0mg, Fiber: 1.9g

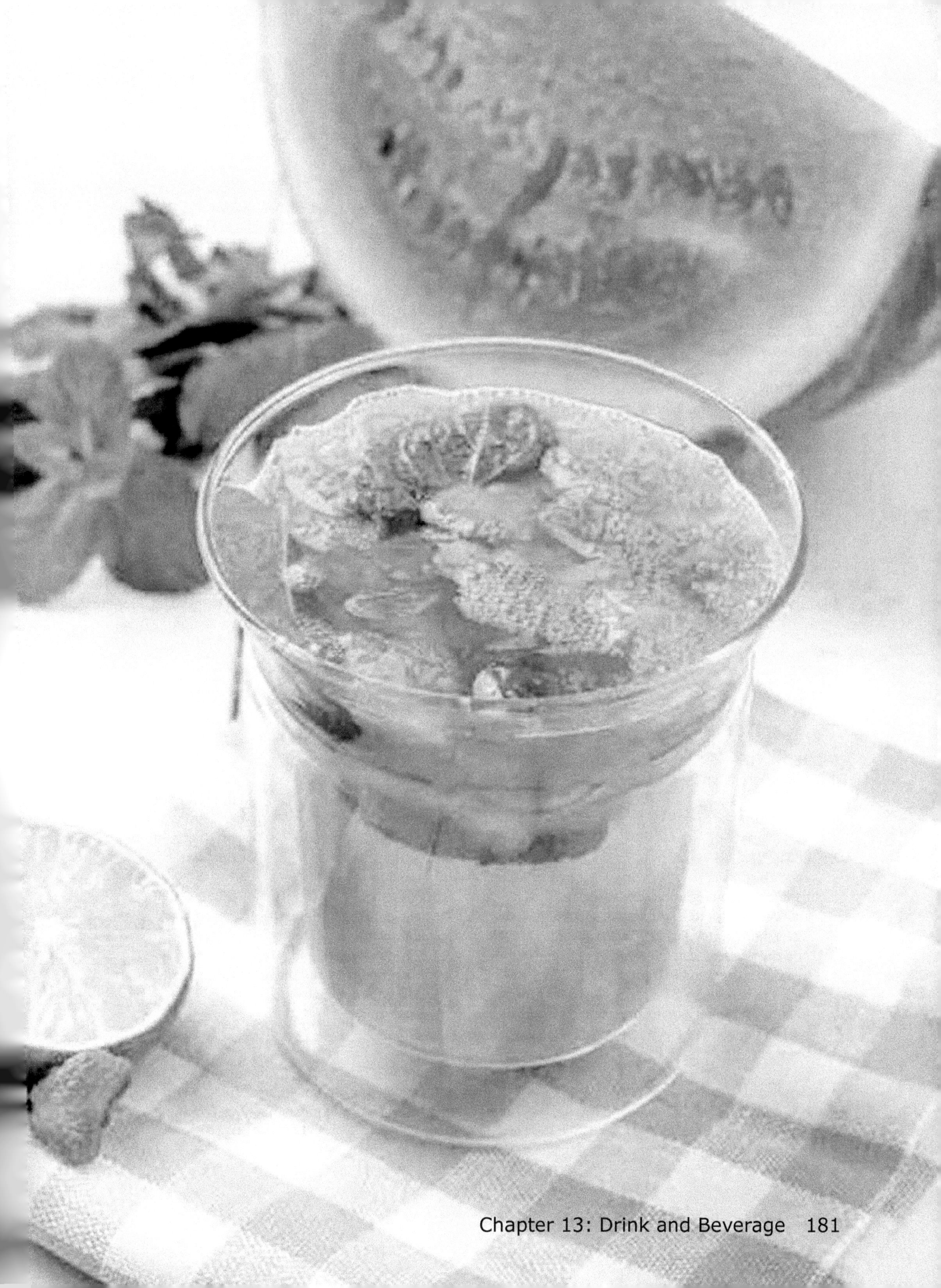

Chapter 13: Drink and Beverage

Fresh Berry Mint Infused Water

Prep Time: 5 minutes, plus 1 hour to chill, Cook Time: 1 minute, Serves: 8

INGREDIENTS:

½ cup strawberries
½ cup blackberries
3 mint sprigs
8 cups water

DIRECTIONS:

1. Mix the water, strawberries, blackberries, and mint in a large pitcher.
2. Before drinking, cover the infused water and chill for at least 1 hour.
3. Store in the refrigerator for up to 2 days.

Nutrition Info per Serving:

Calories: 7, Total Fat: 0g, Saturated Fat: 0g, Cholesterol: 0mg, Carbohydrates: 2g, Fiber: 1g, Protein: 0g, Phosphorus: 4mg, Potassium: 28mg, Sodium: 0mg, Sugar: 14.1g

Rice Milk

Prep Time: 5 minutes, plus 8 to 12 hours to soak, Cook Time: 1 minute, Serves: 4

INGREDIENTS:

1 cup long-grain white rice
4 cups water
½ tsp. vanilla extract (optional)

DIRECTIONS:

1. Toast the rice in a medium dry skillet over medium heat for 5 minutes, until lightly browned.
2. Transfer the rice to a jar or bowl, and add the water. Cover, refrigerate, and soak overnight.
3. Add the rice and water and vanilla (if using) in a blender, process until smooth.
4. Pour the milk into a glass jar or bowl over with a fine-mesh strainer. Serve immediately, or cover, refrigerate, and serve within three days. Shake before using.

Nutrition Info per Serving:

Calories: 112, Total Fat: 0g, Saturated Fat: 0g, Cholesterol: 0mg, Carbohydrates: 24g, Fiber: 0g, Protein: 0g, Phosphorus: 0mg, Potassium: 55mg, Sodium: 80mg, Sugar: 0.1g

Low-Carb Arnold Palmer

Prep Time: 10 minutes, Cook Time: 0, Serves: two 17-ounce 500-ml

INGREDIENTS:

4 cups (950 ml) brewed black tea (decaf or regular), chilled
¼ cup (60 ml) lemon juice
2 tsps. erythritol, or 6 drops liquid stevia
½ tsp. finely ground Himalayan salt

DIRECTIONS:

1. In a large jug or pitcher that holds at least 34 ounces (1 L), add all the ingredients.
2. Use a large spoon to mix well.
3. Cover and store in the refrigerator for up to 5 days.

Nutrition Info per Serving:

Calories: 6, Calories from fat: 1.8, Total fat: 0.2g, Saturated fat: 0.2g, Carbs: 0.7g, Net carbs: 0.6g, Protein: 0.2g, Sugar: 0.6g, Dietary fiber: 0.1g, Sodium: 376mg, Cholesterol: 0mg

Peach Carrot Ginger Water

Prep Time: 10 minutes, Cook Time: 0, Serves: 10

INGREDIENTS:

2 peaches, peeled, pitted, and chopped
1 large carrot, peeled and grated
1-inch piece peeled fresh ginger, lightly crushed
3 fresh thyme sprigs
10 cups water

DIRECTIONS:

1. In a large pitcher, add the peaches, carrot, ginger, and thyme.
2. Stir in the water, and mix to combine.
3. Place the pitcher in the refrigerator and leave to infuse for overnight.
4. Serve cold.

Nutrition Info per Serving:

Calories: 40, Total fat: 0g, Saturated fat: 0g, Cholesterol: 0g, Sodium: 13g, Carbohydrates: 10.7g, Fiber: 1g, Phosphorus: 8mg, Potassium: 69mg, Protein: 0.3g, Sugar: 9.7g

Turmeric Ginger Lemonade

Prep Time: 5 minutes, plus time to cool and chill, Cook Time: 5 minutes, Serves: two 12-ounce (350-ml)

INGREDIENTS:

2½ cups (590 ml) water
1 tsp. ginger powder
1 tsp. turmeric powder
¼ cup (60 ml) lemon juice
2 tsps. aloe vera (optional)
2 tsps. erythritol, or 2 drops liquid stevia (optional)
¼ tsp. finely ground Himalayan salt
Pinch of ground black pepper
6 fresh mint leaves
1 small lemon, cut into wedges

DIRECTIONS:

1. In a medium-sized saucepan, add the water, ginger, and turmeric, bring to a boil. After boiling, remove from the heat, then stir in the lemon juice, aloe vera (if using), sweetener (if using), salt, and pepper. Use a spoon to stir and let it to cool for 1 hour, until completely cooled.
2. In a 24-ounce (710-ml) or larger airtight container, place the mixture. Add the mint leaves, then squeeze in the lemon juice and drop the wedges into the lemonade. Chill in the refrigerator until cold.
3. When ready to enjoy, pour into two 12-ounce (350-ml) or larger glasses.

Nutrition Info per Serving:

Calories: 13, Total fat: 0.4g, Saturated fat: 0.3g, Carbs: 2g, Net carbs: 1.5g, Protein: 0.4g, Sugar: 0.7g, Dietary fiber: 0.5g, Sodium: 204mg, Cholesterol: 0mg

Watermelon Mint Cooler with Vodka

Prep Time: 5 minutes, Cook Time: 0, Serves: four 4-ounce, 120-ml

INGREDIENTS:

4½ ounces (128 g) fresh watermelon cubes, divided
12 mint leaves, divided
8 ice cubes, divided
4 ounces (120 ml, 113 g) vodka, divided
4 tsps. lime juice, divided
1⅛ cups (265 ml) sparkling or still water, divided

DIRECTIONS:

1. Prepare four 4-ounce (120-ml) or larger glasses. On a cutting board, place a quarter of the watermelon cubes and cut them into ¼-inch (6-mm) dice. Transfer the diced watermelon into the glasses. Then add 3 mint leaves, 2 ice cubes, 1 ounce (30 ml) of vodka, and 1 tsp. of lime juice to each glass.
2. In a bowl, add the remaining watermelon pieces and use a fork to mash until you've removed as much of the juice as possible. Pour the juice into the glasses, about 2 teaspoons per glass. Fill sparkling water into each glass and enjoy!

Nutrition Info per Serving:

Calories: 70, Calories from fat: 0, Total fat: 0g, Saturated fat: 0g, Carbs: 1.3g, Net Carbs: 1.3g, Protein: 0.1g, Sugar: 0.6g, Dietary fiber: 0g, Sodium: 2mg, Cholesterol: 0mg

Homemade Coconut Milk

Prep Time: 5 minutes, Cook Time: 0, Serves: 1 quart (950 ml)

INGREDIENTS:

10 ounces (285 g) fresh coconut flesh (from 1 whole coconut, about 1¾ pounds, 800 g)
4 cups (950 ml) water
¼ cup (25 g) unflavored MCT oil powder (optional)
1½ tsps. vanilla extract (optional)

DIRECTIONS:

1. In a blender or food processor, add the coconut and water. Blend or pulse on high for 1 to 2 minutes, until the coconut pieces are completely pulverized.
2. Set a fine-mesh strainer in or drape a piece of cheesecloth over a bowl, add the milk and drain at least 48 ounces (1.4 L). Pour the coconut mixture through the strainer or cheesecloth slowly, allowing the milk to drip into the bowl. If you're using a strainer, use a spoon to press on the pulverized coconut flesh to release the excess liquid. If you're using cheesecloth, pick up the sides of the cloth and wring out the excess liquid.
3. If you do not wish to include the optional add-ins, skip to Step 4. If using the optional add-ins, return the strained coconut milk into the blender or food processor, then add the MCT oil powder and/or vanilla and blend or pulse on low for 10 seconds, just until incorporated.
4. In a 1-quart (950-ml) airtight container, place the milk.
5. Keep in the refrigerator for up to 4 days or in the freezer for up to 1 month.

Nutrition Info per Serving:

Calories: 46, Calories from fat: 40, Total fat: 4.5g, Saturated fat: 4g, Carbs: 1.2g, Net carbs: 1.2g, Protein: 0.2g, Sugar: 0.4g, Dietary fiber: 0g, Sodium: 23mg, Cholesterol: 0mg

Cucumber-Watermelon Juice

Prep Time: 5 minutes, Cook Time: 2 minutes, Serves: 4 (makes 5 cups)

INGREDIENTS:

5 cups chopped seedless watermelon
1 cup chopped unpeeled cucumber
10 fresh mint leaves
Juice of ½ lime

DIRECTIONS:

1. Blend the watermelon and cucumber in the blender(batches if necessary) and blend in high until smooth.
2. Add the mint and lime juice in the last blend.
3. Serve chilled as a beverage or summer soup, or freeze in Popsicle molds for a light treat.

Nutrition Info per Serving:

Calories: 66, Protein: 2g, Fat: 0.9g, Carbohydrates: 15g, Fiber: 1g, Sugar: 13g, Sodium: 5mg, Cholesterol: 0mg

Mint and Cumin Salted Lassi

Prep Time: 5 minutes, Cook Time: 1 minute, Serves: 2

INGREDIENTS:

1 tsp. cumin seeds
½ cup mint leaves
1 cup plain, unsweetened yogurt
½ cup water

DIRECTIONS:

1. Toast the cumin seeds in a dry skillet over medium heat for 1 to 2 minutes, until fragrant.
2. Transfer the seeds to a blender, then add the mint, yogurt, and water, process until smooth.
3. Serve immediately.

Nutrition Info per Serving:

Calories: 114, Total Fat: 6g, Saturated Fat: 3g, Cholesterol: 15mg, Carbohydrates: 5g, Fiber: 0g, Protein: 10g, Phosphorus: 158mg, Potassium: 179mg, Sodium: 43mg, Sugar: 5.7g

Hot Chocolate

Prep Time: 5 minutes, Cook Time: 5 minutes, Serves: 4

INGREDIENTS:

4½ (1080 ml) cups unsweetened low-fat almond milk
5 ounces (142 g) dark or bittersweet chocolate (70 percent cocoa), chopped
¼ tsp. cinnamon, ground

DIRECTIONS:

1. Add milk to a saucepan over medium heat just below the simmering point, reduce the heat to low, and add the chocolate. Stir gently to mix the chocolate into the milk.
2. Put in the cinnamon when the chocolate is melted. Whisk vigorously and serve immediately.

Nutrition Info per Serving:

Calories: 65, Fat: 4.3g, Carbohydrates: 4.4g, Protein: 1.4g, Cholesterol: 0mg, Sodium: 202mg, Fiber: 0.3g, Sugar: 28.7g

Papaya Mint Infused Water

Prep Time: 5 minutes, Cook Time: 0, Serves: 10

INGREDIENTS:

1 cup fresh papaya, peeled, seeded, and diced
2 tbsps. chopped fresh mint leaves
10 cups distilled or filtered water

DIRECTIONS:

1. In a large pitcher, add the papaya and mint. Then pour in the water.
2. Stir well, and refrigerate the pitcher to infuse, overnight if possible.
3. Serve cold.

Nutrition Info per Serving:

Calories: 2, Total fat: 0g, Saturated fat: 0g, Cholesterol: 0g, Sodium: 0g, Carbohydrates: 0g, Fiber: 0g, Phosphorus: 0mg, Potassium: 4mg, Protein: 0g, Sugar: 1.8g

Appendix 1: Measurement Conversion Chart

Volume Equivalents (Dry)	
US STANDARD	METRIC (APPROXIMATE)
1/8 teaspoon	0.5 mL
1/4 teaspoon	1 mL
1/2 teaspoon	2 mL
3/4 teaspoon	4 mL
1 teaspoon	5 mL
1 tablespoon	15 mL
1/4 cup	59 mL
1/2 cup	118 mL
3/4 cup	177 mL
1 cup	235 mL
2 cups	475 mL
3 cups	700 mL
4 cups	1 L

Temperatures Equivalents	
FAHRENHEIT (F)	CELSIUS(C) (APPROXIMATE)
225 °F	107 °C
250 °F	120 °C
275 °F	135 °C
300 °F	150 °C
325 °F	160 °C
350 °F	180 °C
375 °F	190 °C
400 °F	205 °C
425 °F	220 °C
450 °F	235 °C
475 °F	245 °C
500 °F	260 °C

Volume Equivalents (Liquid)		
US STANDARD	US STANDARD (OUNCES)	METRIC (APPROXIMATE)
2 tablespoons	1 fl.oz.	30 mL
1/4 cup	2 fl.oz.	60 mL
1/2 cup	4 fl.oz.	120 mL
1 cup	8 fl.oz.	240 mL
1 1/2 cup	12 fl.oz.	355 mL
2 cups or 1 pint	16 fl.oz.	475 mL
4 cups or 1 quart	32 fl.oz.	1 L
1 gallon	128 fl.oz.	4 L

Weight Equivalents	
US STANDARD	METRIC (APPROXIMATE)
1 ounce	28 g
2 ounces	57 g
5 ounces	142 g
10 ounces	284 g
15 ounces	425 g
16 ounces (1 pound)	455 g
1.5 pounds	680 g
2 pounds	907 g

Appendix 2: Dirty Dozen and Clean Fifteen

The Environmental Working Group (EWG) is a widely known organization that has an eminent guide to pesticides and produce. More specifically, the group takes in data from tests conducted by the US Department of Agriculture (USDA) and then categorizes produce into a list titled "Dirty Dozen," which ranks the twelve top produce items that contain the most pesticide residues, or alternatively the "Clean Fifteen," which ranks fifteen produce items that are contaminated with the least amount of pesticide residues.

The EWG has recently released their 2021 Dirty Dozen list, and this year strawberries, spinach and kale – with a few other produces which will be revealed shortly – are listed at the top of the list. This year's ranking is similar to the 2020 Dirty Dozen list, with the few differences being that collards and mustard greens have joined kale at number three on the list. Other changes include peaches and cherries, which having been listed subsequently as seventh and eighth on the 2020 list, have now been flipped; the introduction – which the EWG has said is the first time ever – of bell and hot peppers into the 2021 list; and the departure of potatoes from the twelfth spot.

DIRTY DOZEN LIST	
Strawberries	Cherries
Spinach	Peaches
Kale, collards and mustard greens	Pears
Nectarines	Bell and hot peppers
Apples	Celery
Grapes	Tomatoes

CLEAN FIFTEEN LIST	
Avocados	Broccoli
Sweet corn	Cabbage
Pineapple	Kiwi
Onions	Cauliflower
Papaya	Mushrooms
Sweet peas (frozen)	Honeydew melon
Eggplant	Cantaloupe
Asparagus	

These lists are created to help keep the public informed on their potential exposures to pesticides, which then allows for better and healthier food choices to be made.

This is the advice that ASEQ-EHAQ also recommends. Stay clear of the dirty dozen by opting for their organic versions, and always be mindful of what you are eating and how it was grown. Try to eat organic as much as possible – whether it is on the list, or not.

Appendix 3: Recipes Index

Lightning Source UK Ltd.
Milton Keynes UK
UKHW032015180123
415590UK00009B/241

9 781801 215411